Medical Nutrition & Disease

A CASE-BASED APPROACH

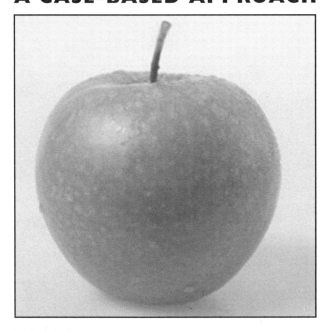

Third Edition

JOHN A. PERROTTO, M.S., D.C.
PRE-CHIROPRACTIC ADVISOR
BIOLOGY DEPARTMENT
NASSAU COMMUNITY COLLEGE

Medical Nutrition & Disease

A CASE-BASED APPROACH

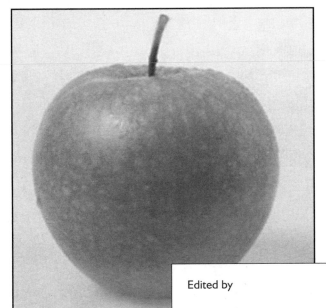

Third Edition

Edited by

Lisa Hark, PhD, RD
Director, Nutrition Education and Prevention Program
University of Pennsylvania School of Medicine
Philadelphia, Pennsylvania

Gail Morrison, MD
Vice Dean for Education
Professor of Medicine
University of Pennsylvania School of Medicine
Philadelphia, Pennsylvania

Blackwell
Publishing

Blackwell Publishing, Inc., 350 Main Street, Malden, Massachusetts 02148-5018, USA
Blackwell Publishing Ltd, 9600 Garsington Road, Oxford OX4 2DQ, UK
Blackwell Science Asia Pty Ltd, 550 Swanston Street, Carlton, Victoria 3053,
   Australia

03 04 05 06 5 4 3 2 1

ISBN: 0-632-04658-9

Library of Congress Cataloging-in-Publication Data
Medical nutrition and disease : a case-based approach / edited by Lisa
   Hark, Gail Morrison.—3rd ed.
      p. ; cm.
   Includes bibliographical references and index.
   ISBN 0-632-04658-9
   1. Dietetics.   2. Diet therapy.   3. Nutrition.
   [DNLM: 1. Nutrition—Case Report.   2. Diet Therapy—Case Report.
   3. Nutritional Support—Case Report. WB 400 M4896 2003]
   I. Hark, Lisa.   II. Morrison, Gail.

   RM216.M456   2003
   613.2—dc21   2003001496

A catalogue record for this title is available from the British Library

Acquisitions: Nancy Anastasi Duffy
Development: Selene Steneck
Production: Debra Lally
Cover design: Mary McKeon
Typesetter: TechBooks in New Delhi, India
Printed and bound by Capital City Press in Berlin, VT

For further information on Blackwell Publishing, visit our website:
www.blackwellpublishing.com

Notice: The indications and dosages of all drugs in this book have been recommended in
the medical literature and conform to the practices of the general community. The
medications described and treatment prescriptions suggested do not necessarily have
specific approval by the Food and Drug Administration for use in the diseases and
dosages for which they are recommended. The package insert for each drug should be
consulted for use and dosage as approved by the FDA. Because standards for usage
change, it is advisable to keep abreast of revised recommendations, particularly those
concerning new drugs.

Contents

Editors-In-Chief

Lisa A. Hark, PhD, RD
Director, Nutrition Education and
   Prevention Program
University of Pennsylvania School of Medicine
Philadelphia, Pennsylvania

Gail Morrison, MD
Vice Dean for Education
Professor of Medicine
University of Pennsylvania School of Medicine
Philadelphia, Pennsylvania

Associate Editors

Frances M. Burke, MS, RD
Coordinator, Nutrition Education Program
University of Pennsylvania School of Medicine
Senior Nutritionist, Cardiac Risk
   Intervention Program
University of Penn Health System
Philadelphia, Pennsylvania

Darwin D. Deen, MD, MS
Clinical Associate Professor
Director, Medical Student Education
Department of Family Medicine and
   Community Health
Albert Einstein College of Medicine
Bronx, New York

Gabriella A. Maldonado, MS
Editorial Research Associate
University of Pennsylvania School of Medicine
Philadelphia, Pennsylvania

Lisa D. Unger, MD, FACP
Attending Physician
Clinical Nutrition Support Services
Hospital of the University of Pennsylvania
Philadelphia, Pennsylvania

Contributors

Maryanne Petrella Aloupis, RD, CNSD
Clinical Nutrition Specialist
Clinical Nutrition Support Services
Hospital of the University of Pennsylvania
Philadelphia, Pennsylvania

Diane Barsky, MD, FAAP, FACN
Assistant Professor of Pediatrics

The Children's Hospital of Philadelphia
Philadelphia, Pennsylvania

Lisa Bellini, MD
Assistant Professor of Medicine
Vice Chair for Education and
   Inpatient Services
Department of Medicine
University of Pennsylvania Health System
Philadelphia, Pennsylvania

Marjorie Bowman, MD, MPA
Professor and Chair
Department of Family Practice and
   Community Medicine
University of Pennsylvania Health System
Philadelphia, Pennsylvania

Frances Burke, MS, RD
Coordinator, Nutrition Education Program
University of Pennsylvania School of Medicine
Senior Nutritionist, Cardiac Risk
   Intervention Program
University of Pennsylvania Health System
Philadelphia, Pennsylvania

Jo Ann S. Carson, PhD, RD, LD
Associate Professor
Department of Clinical Nutrition
University of Texas Southwestern
   Medical Center
Dallas, Texas

Peter Cherouny, MD
Associate Professor, Obstetrics
   and Gynecology
University of Vermont
Chair, Medical Staff and Women's
   Health Care
Service Quality Improvement
Committees, Fletcher Allen Health Care
Burlington, Vermont

Michael D. Cirigliano, MD, FACP
Associate Professor of Medicine
University of Pennsylvania School of Medicine
Philadelphia, Pennsylvania

Charlene Compher, PhD, RD, FADA, CNSD
Assistant Professor in Nutrition Science

University of Pennsylvania School of Nursing
Philadelphia, Pennsylvania

Ara DerMarderosian, PhD
Professor of Pharmacognosy
Research Professor of Medicinal Chemistry
University of the Sciences in Philadelphia
Philadelphia, Pennsylvania

Darwin D. Deen, MD, MS
Clinical Associate Professor
Director, Medical Student Education
Department of Family Medicine and
    Community Health
Albert Einstein College of Medicine
Bronx, New York

Cade Fields-Gardner, MS, RD, LD, CD
Director of Services
The Cutting Edge
Cary, Illinois

Larry N. Finkelstein, DO
Assistant Professor of Family Medicine
Philadelphia College of Osteopathic Medicine
Philadelphia, Pennsylvania

Marian L. Fitzgibbon, PhD
Professor of Psychiatry and
    Preventive Medicine
Northwestern University Medical School
Chicago, Illinois

Judith Fish, MMSc, RD, LD, CNSD
Nutrition Consultant
Private Practice
Asheville, North Carolina

Gary D. Foster, PhD
Clinical Director, Weight and Eating
    Disorders Program
University of Pennsylvania School of Medicine
Philadelphia, Pennsylvania

Allison Sarubin Fragakis, MS, RD
Nutrition Consultant
Private Practice
Greenbrae, California

David C. Frankenfield, MS, RD
Surgical Nutrition Support Dietitian

Milton S. Hershey Medical Center
Department of Clinical Nutrition
Hershey, Pennsylvania

Marion J. Franz, MS, RD, CDE
Nutrition Concepts by Franz, Inc.
Minneapolis, Minnesota

**M. Patricia Fuhrman, MS, RD, LD, FADA,
    CNSD**
Chair of Dietetics
Jewish Hospital College of Nursing and
    Allied Health
St. Louis, Missouri

Katherine Galluzzi, DO
Professor and Chair
Department of Geriatrics
Philadelphia College of Osteopathic Medicine
Philadelphia, Pennsylvania

Henry Ginsberg, MD
Irving Professor of Medicine
Columbia-Presbyterian Medical Center
New York, New York

Samuel N. Grief, MD
Assistant Professor in Clinical Family
    Medicine
University of Illinois at Chicago
Chicago, Illinois

Scott M. Grundy, MD, PhD
Director, Center for Human Nutrition
Professor, Department of Internal Medicine
University of Texas Southwestern Medical
    Center
Dallas, Texas

Richard J. Ham, MD
Director, Center on Aging
Professor of Geriatric Medicine and
    Psychiatry
Robert C. Byrd Health Sciences Center
West Virginia University
Morgantown, West Virginia

Lisa A. Hark, PhD, RD
Director, Nutrition Education and Prevention
    Program

University of Pennsylvania School of Medicine
Philadelphia, Pennsylvania

Jo Ann Tatum Hattner, MPH, RD, CSP
Hattner/Coulston Nutrition
Palo Alto, California

Stephen Havas, MD, MPH, MS
Professor
Department of Epidemiology and
    Preventive Medicine & Department
    of Medicine
University of Maryland School of Medicine
Baltimore, Maryland

Janet Hines, MD
Assistant Professor of Medicine
University of Pennsylvania School
    of Medicine
Philadelphia, Pennsylvania

Ann Honebrink, MD
Medical Director
Women and Children's Health Services
Pennsylvania Hospital
University of Pennsylvania Health System
Philadelphia, Pennsylvania

Barbara Hopkins, MMSc, RD, LD
Director, Dietetic Internship Program
Department of Nutrition
Georgia State University
Atlanta, Georgia

Balint Kacsoh, MD, PhD
Associate Professor of Anatomy, Physiology
    and Pediatrics
Division of Basic Medical Sciences and
    Department of Pediatrics
Mercer University School of Medicine
Macon, Georgia

Wahida Karmally, MS, RD, CDE
Associate Research Scientist
Irving Center for Clinical Research
Columbia University College of Physicians
    and Surgeons
New York, New York

John Kerner, MD
Professor of Pediatrics
Lucile Packard Children's Hospital at
    Stanford
Stanford, California

Ruth A. Lawrence, MD
Professor of Pediatrics and
    Obstetrics/Gynecology
Director, Breastfeeding and Human Lactation
    Study Center
University of Rochester School of Medicine
    and Dentistry
Rochester, New York

Carine M. Lenders, MD, MS
Instructor, Harvard Medical School
Co-Director, Obesity Program
Combined Program of Gastroenterology
    and Nutrition
Children's Hospital-HUNG
Boston, Massachusetts

Gary R. Lichtenstein, MD
Associate Professor of Medicine
University of Pennsylvania School
    of Medicine
Director, Inflammatory Bowel Disease
    Program
Hospital of the University of Pennsylvania
Philadelphia, Pennsylvania

Gregg Y. Lipschik, MD
Assistant Professor of Medicine
Pulmonary and Critical Care Division
University of Pennsylvania School
    of Medicine
Philadelphia, Pennsylvania

**Laura E. Matarese, MS, RD, LD, FADA,
    CNSD**
Director, Nutrition Intestinal Rehabilitation
The Cleveland Clinic Foundation
Cleveland, Ohio

Maria R. Mascarenhas, MBBS
Assistant Professor of Pediatrics
University of Pennsylvania School of Medicine

Director, Nutrition Support Service
Children's Hospital of Philadelphia
Division of Gastroenterology and
    Nutrition
Philadelphia, Pennsylvania

Gail Morrison, MD
Vice Dean for Education
Professor of Medicine
University of Pennsylvania School
    of Medicine
Philadelphia, Pennsylvania

Cathy Nonas, MS, RD, CDE
Nutrition Consultant
Obesity Research Center
St. Lukes-Roosevelt Hospital
New York, New York

Judith Roepke, PhD, RD
Dean, School of Continuing Education and
    Public Service
Emeritus Professor of Family and
    Consumer Sciences
Ball State University
Muncie, Indiana

Elizabeth Ross, MD, LDN
Physician/Nutritionist
Tufts University School of Nutrition Science
    and Policy
Boston, Massachusetts

José Antonio Ruy-Díaz Reynoso, MD, FICS
Chief, Division of Metabolic and
    Nutrition Support
Hospital General "Dr. Manuel Gea Gonzalez"
Chairman, Department of Clinical Nutrition
School of Medicine, Anahuac University
    Mexico City
Huixquilucan, Estado de México

Doug Seidner, MD
Clinical Associate Professor
Ohio State School of Medicine
Staff Physician, Department of
    Gastroenterology

The Cleveland Clinic Foundation
Cleveland, Ohio

F. Xavier Pi-Sunyer, MD, MPH
Professor of Medicine, Columbia University
Chief, Division of Endocrinology, Metabolism
    and Nutrition
Director, Obesity Research Center
St. Luke's Roosevelt Hospital
New York, New York

Linda G. Snetselaar, PhD, RD
Associate Professor
College of Public Health and College of
    Medicine
University of Iowa
Iowa City, Iowa

Ezra Steiger, MD
Consultant in General Surgery
Department of General Surgery
Co-Director, Nutrition Support
Director, Intestinal Rehabilitation Program
The Cleveland Clinic Foundation
Cleveland, Ohio

Jean Stover, RD
Renal Dietitian
Gambro Healthcare
Philadelphia, Pennsylvania

Philippe Szapary, MD
Assistant Professor of Medicine
Division of General Internal Medicine
University of Pennsylvania School of Medicine
Philadelphia, Pennsylvania

Andrew M. Tershakovec, MD
Director
Regulatory Affairs Domestic
Merck Research Laboratories
Blue Bell, Pennsylvania

Cynthia A. Thomson, PhD, RD
Assistant Professor, Nutritional Sciences
University of Arizona School of Medicine
Tucson, Arizona

Brian W. Tobin, PhD, FACN, CNS
Associate Professor of Nutrition,
     Biochemistry and Pediatrics
Division of Basic Medical Sciences
Mercer University School of Medicine
Macon, Georgia

Lisa D. Unger, MD, FACP
Attending Physician
Clinical Nutrition Support Services
Hospital of the University of Pennsylvania
Philadelphia, Pennsylvania

Linda Van Horn, PhD, RD
Professor
Department of Preventive Medicine
Northwestern University Medical School
Chicago, Illinois

Judith Wylie-Rosett, EdD, RD
Professor and Head
Division of Health, Behavior and Nutrition
Epidemiology and Social Medicine
Albert Einstein College of Medicine
Bronx, New York

Jane White, PhD, RD, FADA
Professor
Department of Family Medicine
Graduate School of Medicine
University of Tennessee-Knoxville
Knoxville, Tennessee

Jennifer M. Williams, MS, RD, CNSD
Clinical Nutrition Specialist
University of Pennsylvania Health System
Philadelphia, Pennsylvania

Part Editors/Reviewers

Part 1: Fundamentals of Nutrition Assessment

Marilyn S. Edwards, PhD, RD
Associate Professor, Department of Internal
  Medicine
Division of Gastroenterology, Hepatology,
  and Nutrition
The University of Texas Medical School
Houston, Texas

Patrick E. McBride, MD, MPH
Professor of Medicine
Director, Preventive Cardiology
Department of Medicine-Cardiology and
  Family Medicine
University of Wisconsin Medical School
Madison, Wisconsin

Sachiko T. St. Jeor, PhD, RD
Professor and Director
Nutrition Education and Research Program
University of Nevada School of Medicine
Reno, Nevada

Part 2: Nutrition Throughout the Lifecycle

Richard Neill, MD
Residency Director, Family Practice
  Residency
University of Pennsylvania
Department of Family Practice and
  Community Medicine
Philadelphia, Pennsylvania

Kathryn M. Kolasa, PhD, RD, LDN
Professor and Section Head
Nutrition Education and Services
Department of Family Medicine

The Brody School of Medicine at East
  Carolina University
Greenville, North Carolina

Part 3: Nutrition and Pathophysiology

Peter Jones, PhD
Professor
University of Tennessee Medical School
  in Memphis
Department of Molecular Sciences
Memphis, Tennessee

Linda G. Snetselaar, PhD, MS
Associate Professor
College of Public Health and
College of Medicine
University of Iowa
Iowa City, Iowa

Charles B. Eaton, MD, MS
Associate Professor
Center for Primary Care and Prevention
Department of Family Medicine
Brown University
Pawtucket, Rhode Island

Part 4: Fundamentals of Nutrition Support

Gordon L. Jensen, MD, PhD
Director, Vanderbilt Center for
  Human Nutrition
Nashville, Tennessee

Marion Winkler, MS, RD, LDN, CNSD
Surgical Nutrition Specialist
Rhode Island Hospital
Senior Teaching Associate of Surgery
Brown University School
  of Surgery
Cranston, Rhode Island

Preface: *Medical Nutrition & Disease: A Case-Based Approach*

We are extremely proud to introduce the third edition of *Medical Nutrition & Disease*. This edition has been significantly revised and updated in a number of important ways. First, we have included several new contributors and editors, many of whom represent Nutrition Academic Award (NAA) Program participants. The NAA Program, sponsored by the National Heart, Lung, and Blood Institute (NHLBI) and the National Institute of Diabetes, Digestive and Kidney Diseases (NIDDK), has funded 21 U.S. medical schools to design, implement, and evaluate model nutrition education programs for undergraduate and graduate medical education that would be disseminated to other medical schools and postgraduate programs. The third edition has also been significantly updated to illustrate key nutrition issues and concerns in the 21st century both in the U.S. and abroad.

The scientific evidence supporting medical nutrition therapy continues to be elucidated and the importance of nutrition in health promotion and disease prevention is becoming more apparent. With this growth in knowledge, skills and attitudes, major changes have occurred in curriculum development and national nutrition guidelines have been amended. Numerous groups have identified nutrition as a major component of their recommendations including the National Cholesterol Education Program, American Cancer Society, American Heart Association, American Diabetes Association, *Healthy People 2010*, and the Joint National Committee on the Prevention, Detection, Evaluation, and Treatment of High Blood Pressure. These recommendations have been incorporated where appropriate into this edition.

All of the chapters have been revised and updated and include the most current evidenced-based medical nutrition therapy. A new chapter on Herbal Medicine has been added to reflect the interest in complementary and alternative medicine and several new cases have been written. The new cases cover Obesity and Metabolic Syndrome; Iron Deficiency Anemia; Drug-Herb Interaction; Overweight Children and Insulin Resistance; HIV and Opportunistic Infection; Diabetic Ketoacidosis in Type 1 Diabetes; Management of Type 2 Diabetes; and Parenteral Nutrition in Colon Cancer with Post-Operative Sepsis.

All chapters and cases continue to be co-authored by teams of physicians and registered dietitians. Learning objectives covered in the 3rd edition of *Medical Nutrition & Disease* have been adapted from the NAA *Nutrition Curriculum Guide for Training Physicians*, which has been a major project of the NAA Program and can be accessed via the Web at *http://www.nhlbi.nih.gov/funding/training/naa/products.htm.*

United States Medical Licensing Examinations (USMLE)

In 2000, the Michigan Medical Nutrition Education Consortium submitted a proposal to the National Board of Medical Examiners requesting a nutrition sub-score for the USMLE Step 1 exam. They suggested that because nutrition is integral to human health and well-being, it is critical for physicians in training to understand the role of nutrition in medical care. Their proposal led to the creation of a nutrition sub-score on the USMLE Step 1 exams which will allow medical schools to evaluate the effectiveness of their teaching efforts. This sub-score will provide important feedback to students and institutions regarding the adequacy of their nutrition curriculum and will serve as a critical evaluation and research tool for assessing the impact of present and future nutrition education programs in U.S. medical schools. Schools that are not teaching nutrition adequately will be apprised of this fact through the nutrition sub-score and may be encouraged to address this deficiency. Updating exams to reflect what physicians need to know will help students recognize the importance of their nutrition curriculum. This initiative could ultimately contribute to the health of the general public by assuring that physicians in practice have some degree of knowledge in nutrition.

Conclusion

Health professionals need to be prepared to address lifestyle interventions. At a time when the Surgeon General has called upon the nation to respond to an impending health crisis and a Senate panel is considering the Improved Nutrition and Physical Activity Act to increase the public school education regarding the importance of diet and exercise to our health, most medical schools are still challenged to integrate nutrition across their undergraduate and graduate medical curriculum. Nutritional interventions are considered first line therapy for obesity, diabetes, hypertension, hyperlipidemia, and atherosclerosis. The metabolic syndrome represents an identifiable (and modifiable) risk factor for these diseases that can and should be addressed. The effectiveness of dietary interventions in these conditions has been well documented. Unfortunately, health professionals may not feel prepared to effectively counsel their patients about diet and lifestyle changes. This will only change as medical educators rise to the challenge to improve nutrition education.

For more information on how to successfully incorporate nutrition education into your undergraduate and post-graduate residency training programs, contact:

Lisa Hark, PhD, RD
Director, Nutrition Education and Prevention Program
University of Pennsylvania School of Medicine
3450 Hamilton Walk
Suite 100, Stemmler Hall
Philadelphia, PA 19104-6087
215-349-5795, fax: 215-573-7075, lhark@mail.med.upenn.edu

Contact our home page for resources for nutrition education, including PowerPoint slides that can be downloaded for educational purposes, as well as for References called out within the text: *http://www.med.upenn.edu/nutrimed*

Lisa Hark, PhD, RD, and Gail Morrison, MD

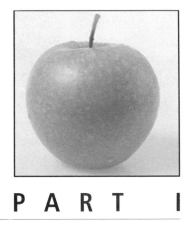

P A R T   I

Fundamentals of Nutrition Assessment

1

Overview of Nutrition in Clinical Care

Lisa Hark, Marjorie Bowman, and Lisa Bellini

Objectives*

- Recognize the value of nutrition assessment in the comprehensive care of ambulatory and hospitalized patients.
- Describe the diagnosis, prevalence, health consequences, and etiology of obesity and undernutrition.
- Recognize overweight and obesity as a worldwide public health problem in both children and adults.
- Take an appropriate patient history, including medical, family, social, nutrition/dietary, physical activity, and weight histories; use of prescription medicines, over-the-counter medicines, and dietary and herbal supplements; and consumption of alcohol and other recreational drugs.
- Demonstrate how to conduct an appropriate physical examination, body mass index, and waist circumference and evaluate growth and development and signs of nutritional deficiency or excess.
- Identify the most common physical findings associated with obesity, undernutrition, and vitamin/mineral deficiencies or excesses.
- List the laboratory measurements commonly used to assess the nutritional status of patients.

* SOURCE: Objectives for chapter and case adapted from the *NIH Nutrition Curriculum Guide for Training Physicians* (*http://www.nhlbi.nih.gov/funding/training/naa*).

Purpose of Nutrition Assessment in Clinical Care

Nutrition assessment is the evaluation of an individual's nutritional status based on the interpretation of clinical information obtained from the medical history, diet history, review of systems, physical examination, and laboratory data. The purposes of the nutrition assessment are to evaluate an individual's dietary intake and nutritional status accurately; to determine if medical nutrition therapy or counseling, or both, is needed; and to monitor changes in nutritional status and evaluate the effects of nutritional interventions. Nutrition assessment is an important tool in clinical medicine because malnutrition (both obesity and undernutrition) are common clinical findings and many patients can benefit from medical nutrition therapy (MNT) using established evidenced-based protocols.

Overweight and Obesity

Health Consequences

Obesity is a complex, multifactorial disease that is becoming increasingly common among adults and children in developed countries. According to the US Surgeon General's *Call to Action to Prevent and Treat Overweight and Obesity,* approximately 300,000 deaths per year in the United States are currently associated with overweight and obesity. In addition, obese individuals have 50% to 100% increased risk of premature death from all causes compared to individuals of normal weight. The National Heart, Lung, and Blood Institute (NHLBI) *Clinical Guidelines on the Identification, Evaluation, and Treatment of Overweight and Obesity in Adults* states that "next to smoking, obesity is the second leading cause of preventable death in the US today." Overweight and obese individuals have an increased risk of diabetes, coronary heart disease, hyperlipidemia, hypertension, stroke, gallbladder disease, sleep apnea, osteoarthritis, respiratory problems, and certain types of cancers (endometrium, breast, prostate, and colon), all of which increase their risk of mortality (Figure 1-1). In 2000, the total costs associated with obesity in the United States were estimated at $117 billion, mostly due to the costs of type 2 diabetes, coronary heart disease, and hypertension.

Strong evidence has shown that a modest weight loss of 10% of body weight results in a reduction of blood pressure, fasting glucose, and lipid levels. Treatment for obese individuals with three or more of the following risk factors should be aggressive: cigarette smoking, hypertension, high low-density lipoprotein cholesterol (LDL-C) levels, low high-density lipoprotein cholesterol (HDL-C) levels, elevated fasting glucose levels, family history of coronary heart disease, and age over 45 and 55 years in men and women, respectively (see Chapter 7).

Healthy People 2010, initiated by the US Department of Health and Human Services, is a plan to improve the health of the Nation during the first decade of the twenty-first century. *Healthy People 2010* is composed of goals, objectives, determinants of health, and health status. A total of 28 areas are covered;

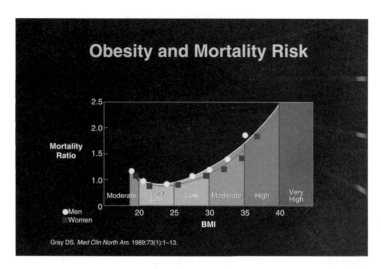

Figure 1-1   Obesity and mortality risk. BMI, body mass index.

SOURCE: Reproduced by permission from Gray DS. Diagnosis and prevalence of obesity. Med Clin North Am 1989; 73(1):1–13.

focus areas include Diabetes, Nutrition and Overweight, Physical Activity and Fitness, Food Safety, and Heart, Kidney, and Pulmonary Diseases. One goal of *Healthy People 2010* is to promote health and reduce chronic diseases associated with diet and overweight. The objectives to reach these goals are related to weight status and growth, food and nutrient consumption, iron deficiency and anemia, school work site and nutrition counseling, and food security (*http://www.healthgov/healthypeople/document*).

Etiology

The etiology of obesity can be explained by biologic and environmental factors. Biologic factors that have been identified include an individual's genetic predisposition, resting energy expenditure (REE), and the size and number of adipose cells.

Genetics

More than 300 genes have been identified that influence obesity in humans. Genetic studies over the past several decades investigating adopted twins and their biologic and adoptive parents show that adoptees' weight correlates most strongly with that of their biologic parents' weight. Additional research has shown that children of one overweight parent have a 40% chance of becoming an overweight adult; this risk increases to 80% if both parents are overweight. Regardless of the strong evidence for genetic influences on human obesity, genetics accounts for no more than one third of the variance in body weight. Because there has been no change in the gene pool over the past decade, the dramatic increase in the prevalence of obesity, both in children and adults in the United States, likely reflects environmental influences.

Adipose Cell Size and Number

The size and number of fat cells have been researched for many years and vary between normal, overweight, and obese individuals. During infancy, adolescence, and pregnancy, fat cells normally increase in number. With modest weight gain, they increase in size, and with significant weight gain, they increase in size and number. With weight loss, fat cells decrease in size but not in number. The lack of reduction in fat cells may explain why it is difficult for obese individuals to lose a significant amount of weight and maintain this weight loss for an extended period of time.

Resting Energy Expenditure (REE)

The amount of energy required to maintain vital organ function in a resting state is referred to as *REE* and is approximately 10% above the basal metabolic rate (BMR). The BMR is taken when an individual awakens in the morning and is generally impractical to measure. Thus, the REE is used. REE accounts for approximately 65% of total daily energy expenditure and varies considerably among individuals with different height, weight, age, body composition, and sex. REE is significantly correlated with lean body mass; thus, regular physical activity, especially weight-bearing exercises that can increase lean muscle mass, can increase REE. Since REE decreases as people age because of the loss of lean body mass over time, regular exercise can play a significant role in maintaining REE, especially in older adults. Behavioral (and therefore modifiable) factors that have been identified with obesity as contributory to overweight and obesity include excessive caloric intake and inadequate physical activity.

Excess Caloric or Energy Intake

Humans require energy (calories) to support normal metabolic functions, physical activity, and growth and repair of tissues (Tables 1-1 to 1-3). According to the National Health and Nutrition Examination Survey (NHANES) III (conducted from 1988 to 1994), Americans are eating 220 more calories per day than they were 20 years ago. This increase in calories can be partially attributed to a combination of increased portion sizes or "super-size" servings, the increased frequency of eating outside the home, especially at fast food restaurants, and the increased consumption of fat-free foods, which may be high in carbohydrates and calories but perceived as low calorie or calorie free.

Decreased Physical Activity

The dramatic increase in sedentary activities and labor-saving devices (sitting at the computer; watching television; using the remote control; taking escalators, elevators, or moving sidewalks; using drive-through windows to pick up food; and using garage door openers) has reduced the amount of energy we expend as a society. Currently, 70% of the population does not get enough exercise. According to the Centers for Disease Control and Prevention's (CDC) National

Table 1-1 Definition of energy/calorie.

Energy is expressed in kilocalories (kcal) and is produced by the oxidation of dietary protein, fat, carbohydrate, and alcohol.

• 1 g **protein** yields approximately 4 kcal.
• 1 g **carbohydrate** yields approximately 4 kcal.
• 1 g **fat** yields approximately 9 kcal.
• 1 g **alcohol** yields approximately 7 kcal.

A calorie is the amount of heat required to raise the temperature of 1 g water by 1°C. A kilocalorie is thus the amount of heat required to raise the temperature of 1 kcal water by 1°C.

Table 1-2 Harris-Benedict equation to estimate calorie requirements.

The Harris-Benedict equations estimate the basal (resting) energy expenditure in adults, which varies with body size and gender.

Resting energy expenditure (REE) equation for men:

$$66 + [13.7 \times \text{weight (kg)}] + [5.0 \times \text{height (cm)}] - [6.8 \times \text{(age)}] = \text{kcal/d}$$

REE equation for women:

$$655 + [9.7 \times \text{weight (kg)}] + [1.85 \times \text{height (cm)}] - [4.7 \times \text{(age)}] = \text{kcal/d}$$

The Harris-Benedict equation should be modified by using an adjusted body weight for patients who are obese because adipose tissue is not as metabolically active as lean body mass. The REE would be overestimated if this factor were not taken into account. The equation for calculating an adjusted body weight is:

$$[(\text{Current body weight} - \text{goal weight}) \times 25\%] + \text{goal weight}$$

Total energy expenditure (TEE):
Multiply the REE by an activity factor to estimate the TEE: Use 1.2 for those confined to bed, 1.3 for those with a sedentary lifestyle and low physical activity. Healthy, active individuals can use a factor of 1.5 to estimate caloric needs for weight maintenance.

Table 1-3 Estimating total energy expenditure based on physical activity (use adjusted body weight for obese individuals).

ACTIVITY LEVEL	MEN	WOMEN
Light	30 kcal/kg	30 kcal/kg
Moderate	40 kcal/kg	37 kcal/kg
Heavy	50 kcal/kg	44 kcal/kg

SOURCE: National Research Council, 1989.

Health Interview Survey, 40% of US adults say they never engage in any exercise, sports, or physically active hobbies during their leisure time. Women are more likely to be sedentary than are men, and African-American and Hispanic populations have higher rates of sedentary behavior when compared to whites. In addition, the Behavioral Risk Factor Surveillance System indicates that participation in physical activity declines as people age. The combination of increased caloric intake and decreased physical activity over the past several decades is the most likely environmental factor associated with the significant increase in overweight and obesity seen in the United States and developed countries.

Because regular physical activity modestly contributes to weight loss as well as reduces abdominal fat and increases cardiorespiratory fitness, it should be strongly encouraged, along with a reduced-calorie diet, to improve the health of overweight and obese individuals. Recent studies from the National Weight Control Registry have indicated that regular physical activity is the single best predictor of long-term weight control in overweight and obese individuals. *Healthy People 2010* goals are to increase the percentage of adults who engage in regular physical activity, preferably daily, for at least 30 minutes per day, and the Center for Disease Control and Prevention (CDC) and Institute of Medicine (IOM) recommends that children and adults respectively participate in at least 1 hour of physical activity every day (see Case 1).

Diagnosis and Assessment

Body Mass Index (BMI)

Overweight and obesity are now defined using BMI, which can be derived from Figure 1-2, determined from the web site *http://www.nhlbisupport.com/bmi*, or calculated using the following equation:

$$BMI = \frac{weight\ (kg)}{height\ (m^2)}$$

According to the NHLBI's Clinical Guidelines, BMI provides a more accurate measure of total body fat than body weight alone. The BMI value is also more accurate than the ideal height-weight tables that were based on a homogeneous population, primarily white, with higher than average socioeconomic status. These values did not accurately reflect body fat content in the general population. In addition, these values were gender specific, whereas the BMI uses a direct calculation comparing weight relative to height, regardless of gender. BMI has also been shown to more accurately estimate obesity even compared to bioelectrical impedance tests. BMI should therefore be used, along with waist circumference and other risk factors, to assess an individual's risk. However, it has some limitations: BMI may overestimate body fat in very muscular people and underestimate body fat in some underweight people who have lost lean tissue, such as the elderly.

The NHLBI Clinical Guidelines classify BMI as shown in Table 1-4. Since many people with a BMI of 25 or greater begin to experience health problems associated with obesity, such as elevated LDL-C and total cholesterol levels, high blood pressure, and glucose intolerance, as shown in Figure 1-1, the guidelines define overweight individuals as those with a BMI of 25 to 29.9 kg/m^2 and obese individuals as those with a BMI of 30 kg/m^2 and above.

Prevalence

The percentage of the population between age 20 and 70 with a BMI of 25 to 29.9 kg/m^2 (overweight) and BMI greater than 30 kg/m^2 (obese) has increased

Body Mass Index Chart

in/cm	lbs/kg 100/45	105/48	110/50	115/52	120/55	125/56	130/59	135/61	140/64	145/66	150/68	155/70	160/73	165/75	170/77	175/79	180/82	185/84	190/86	195/89	200/91	205/93	210/95	215/98	220/100	225/102	230/104	235/107	240/109	245/111	250/114
5'0"/153	20	21	21	22	23	24	25	26	27	28	29	30	31	32	33	34	35	36	37	38	39	40	41	42	43	44	45	46	47	48	49
5'1"/155	19	20	21	22	23	24	25	26	26	27	28	29	30	31	32	33	34	35	36	37	38	39	40	41	42	43	43	44	45	46	47
5'2"/158	18	19	20	21	22	23	24	25	26	27	27	28	29	30	31	32	33	34	35	36	37	37	38	39	40	41	42	43	44	45	46
5'3"/160	18	19	19	20	21	22	23	24	25	26	27	27	28	29	30	31	32	33	34	35	35	36	37	38	39	40	41	42	43	43	44
5'4"/163	17	18	19	20	21	21	22	23	24	25	26	27	27	28	29	30	31	32	33	33	34	35	36	37	38	39	39	40	41	42	43
5'5"/165	17	17	18	19	20	21	22	22	23	24	25	26	27	27	28	29	30	31	32	32	33	34	35	36	37	37	38	39	40	41	42
5'6"/168	16	17	18	19	19	20	21	22	23	23	24	25	26	27	27	28	29	30	31	31	32	33	34	35	36	36	37	38	39	40	40
5'7"/171	16	16	17	18	19	20	20	21	22	23	23	24	25	26	27	27	28	29	30	31	31	32	33	34	34	35	36	37	38	38	39
5'8"/173	15	16	17	17	18	19	20	21	21	22	23	24	24	25	26	27	27	28	29	30	30	31	32	33	33	34	35	36	36	37	38
5'9"/176	15	16	16	17	18	18	19	20	21	21	22	23	24	24	25	26	27	27	28	29	30	30	31	32	32	33	34	35	35	36	37
5'10"/178	14	15	16	17	17	18	19	19	20	21	22	22	23	24	24	25	26	27	27	28	29	29	30	31	32	32	33	34	34	35	36
5'11"/181	14	15	15	16	17	17	18	19	20	20	21	22	22	23	24	24	25	26	27	27	28	29	29	30	31	31	32	33	33	34	35
6'0"/183	14	14	15	16	16	17	18	18	19	20	20	21	22	22	23	24	24	25	26	26	27	28	28	29	30	31	31	32	33	33	34
6'1"/186	13	14	15	15	16	16	17	18	18	19	20	20	21	22	22	23	24	24	25	26	26	27	28	28	29	30	30	31	32	32	33
6'2"/188	13	13	14	15	15	16	17	17	18	19	19	20	21	21	22	22	23	24	24	25	26	26	27	28	28	29	30	30	31	31	32
6'3"/191	13	13	14	14	15	16	16	17	18	18	19	19	20	21	21	22	23	23	24	24	25	26	26	27	28	28	29	29	30	31	31
6'4"/193	12	13	13	14	15	15	16	16	17	18	18	19	19	20	21	21	22	23	23	24	24	25	26	26	27	27	28	29	29	30	30

Underweight	Normal	Overweight	Obese
<18.5	19 - 24.9	25 - 29.9	>30

Figure 1-2   Classification of obesity according to body mass index.

SOURCE: National Heart, Lung and Blood Institute, Bethesda, MD.

Table 1-4   Classification of body mass index.

Underweight	$<18.5 \text{ kg/m}^2$
Normal weight	$18.5–24.9 \text{ kg/m}^2$
Overweight	$25.0–29.9 \text{ kg/m}^2$
Obesity (class 1)	$30.0–34.9 \text{ kg/m}^2$
Obesity (class 2)	$35.0–39.9 \text{ kg/m}^2$
Extreme obesity (class 3)	$\geq 40 \text{ kg/m}^2$

SOURCE: National Heart, Lung, and Blood Institute, National Institutes of Health, 1998.

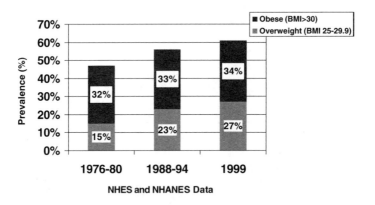

Figure 1-3   Age-adjusted prevalence of overweight and obesity among US adults aged 20 to 70 years. BMI, body mass index; NHES, National Health and Nutrition Examination Survey; NHANES, National Health and Nutrition Examination Surveys.

SOURCE: Centers for Disease Control and Prevention.

significantly since 1976 according to the Nutrition Health Examination Survey (NHES) I (1971–1974) and National Health and Nutrition Examination Survey (NHANES) II (1976–1980) and III (1988–1994), as shown in Figure 1-3 (*http://www.cdc.gov/nchs/nhanes.htm*).

Minority groups, such as African-Americans and Mexican-Americans, as well as those with lower incomes and less education, are especially prone. In addition, 13% of children aged 6 to 11 years and 14% of adolescents aged 12 to 19 are considered overweight, rates that have more than doubled since 1970 (Figure 1-4).

Health professionals should routinely assess height, weight, and BMI and evaluate growth and development in infants, children, and adolescents. Patients who are of normal weight or those with no other risk factors should be encouraged to maintain their weight as they age. Overweight patients with comorbidities, such as diabetes, hypertension, or heart disease, should be advised to lose weight by increasing their physical activity level and reducing their total calorie and saturated fat intake.

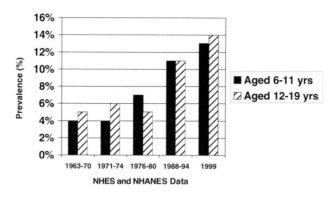

Figure 1-4   Prevalence of overweight among US children and adolescents. NHES, National Health and Nutrition Examination Survey; NHANES, National Health and Nutrition Examination Surveys.

SOURCE: Centers for Disease Control and Prevention.

Growth Charts

Between 1962 and 1974, the US Public Health Service performed a series of measurements on a large population of formula-fed infants from diverse racial, socioeconomic, and geographic backgrounds. Growth charts developed from this cross section have been used for many years as reference standards to plot infant, child, and adolescent height (length), weight, and head circumference according to age and gender.

Recently, new growth charts, based on NHANES data collected from 1971 to 1994, have been developed by the CDC (*http://www.cdc.gov/growthcharts*). These charts more appropriately represent the combined growth patterns of breast-fed and formula-fed infants, including all racial and ethnic groups, and include BMI-for-age and gender values. As children grow, their body composition changes, and therefore, all growth parameters should be plotted and interpreted over time. BMI provides a guideline based on weight and height to assess the degree of undernutrition, overweight, and obesity. Since the development of body fat varies according to age and gender, BMI should be plotted on age and gender-specific charts.

If BMI-for-age and gender-specific values are below the fifth percentile, children may be underweight. From the fifth up to the eighty-fifth percentile, they have an acceptable weight. Greater than the eighty-fifth percentile they are at risk of being overweight, since excess adipose tissue is not easily assessed in overweight children. Greater than the ninety-fifth percentile and above is used to diagnose overweight in children and adolescents. According to the Bogalusa Heart Study, 60% of children and teenagers with a BMI-for-age above the ninety-fifth percentile have at least one risk factor for cardiovascular disease. Once a diagnosis is made, intervention is necessary to help overweight children reduce their rate of weight gain rather than lose weight, as losing weight may interfere with their height growth velocity (see Chapter 5).

Waist Circumference

Waist circumference is an independent measure of risk in normal-weight as well as overweight and obese individuals. Excess fat located in the abdominal area (termed *visceral adipose tissue*), is reflected in the waist circumference measurement. Waist circumference is an independent predictor of morbidity and is considered an independent risk factor for diabetes, dyslipidemia, hypertension, and cardiovascular disease, even when BMI is not markedly increased, although this may differ among ethnic groups. In patients with a BMI greater than 35, there is little additional risk from elevated waist circumference, as severe risk is already present. Therefore, measuring waist circumference is recommended in patients with a BMI of less than 35 kg/m^2. The waist circumference measurement may be particularly important for patients who have a family history of diabetes and are borderline overweight.

In order to obtain an accurate waist circumference measurement, patients should be standing in only their underwear. A horizontal mark should be drawn just above the uppermost lateral border of the right iliac crest, which should then be crossed with a vertical mark in the midaxillary line. The measuring tape is placed in a horizontal plane around the abdomen at the level of this marked point on the right side of the trunk. The plane of the tape should be parallel to the floor, and the tape should be snug but not tight. The patient should be advised to breathe normally when the measurement is taken. Waist circumference values greater than 102 cm (40 in.) in men and greater than 88 cm (35 in.) in women are considered indicators of increased risk. These values also represent one of the diagnostic criteria of metabolic syndrome (see Case 1). Tracking waist circumference over time in individuals who are attempting to lose weight is recommended.

Undernutrition

Health Consequences

According to the World Health Organization (WHO; *http://www.who.org*), undernutrition affects all age groups across the entire lifespan, from conception to older adults. Health consequences of underweight range from intrauterine brain damage and growth failure to reduced physical and mental capacity in childhood to an increased risk of developing diet-related chronic diseases later in life.

Reduced food intake results in loss of fat, muscle, and ultimately viscera bone. This reduction in tissue mass results in weight loss. The smaller tissue mass has reduced nutritional requirements likely reflecting more efficient utilization of ingested food and a reduction in work capacity at the cellular level. The combination of decreased tissue mass and reduction in work capacity impedes homeostatic responses, including responses to critical illness or surgery. The stress of critical illness inhibits the body's natural conservation response to undernutrition. In addition, undernourished individuals experience nutrient deficiencies and imbalances that exacerbate the natural reduction in cellular work that occurs with undernutrition and suffer a decrease in the inflammatory response and immune function as well. These alterations result in increased morbidity and mortality among malnourished patients. Adequate nutrition is essential for reversing the physiologic derangements and to recover from illness. Aggressive nutritional support, instituted early in critical illness, may reduce the adverse effects of the critically ill patient's response to injury.

Prevalence

Children, older adults, and hospitalized and nursing home patients are particularly prone to undernutrition. According to the *Healthy People 2010* objectives, 8% of low-income children under the age of 5 years were growth retarded due to undernutrition in 1997. According to WHO, 49% of the 10.7 million deaths in children under 5 years of age in developing countries are associated with undernutrition. Some degree of undernutrition occurs during most hospitalizations regardless of the type of injury or illness. The prevalence of undernutrition in the outpatient population is poorly documented. Risk factors for undernutrition include chronic diseases, multiple prescription medications, poverty, inadequate nutritional knowledge, homebound or nonambulatory status or both, poor social support structure, major psychiatric diagnosis, and alcoholism. Undernutrition in nursing home patients has been reported to range from 10% to 50%.

Food insecurity is defined by the US Department of Agriculture (USDA) as lack of access to enough food to meet basic needs fully at all times due to lack of financial resources. Households that are insecure, even when hunger is not present, are so limited in resources that they may run out of food and cannot afford balanced meals. *Hungry households* have been defined as those that lack adequate financial resources to the point at which family members, especially children, are hungry on a regular basis and adults' food intake is severely reduced.

According to the USDA report from the Census Bureau, 31 million Americans (12 million children and 19 million adults) suffer from hunger or live on the edge of hunger. In addition, the number of US children in insecure and hungry households was 10.6 million and 2.64 million, respectively, in 1999. Children are almost twice as likely as adults to be living in hungry/food insecure households (16.9% of all children compared to 9.5% of all adults). Unfortunately, with the shift from welfare to work, many low-income working families who are eligible for Food Stamps do not participate in the program, leaving children more vulnerable to food insecurity than ever before. Bills have been introduced in Congress to improve the Food Stamp Program to better target low-income working families and those making the transition from public assistance. Other federally funded programs, such as the Women, Infants, and Children (WIC) Program, provide nutrition resources for low-income pregnant women and children.

Etiology/Causes

Decreased Oral Intake

Poverty, poor dentition, gastrointestinal obstruction, abdominal pain, anorexia, dysphagia, depression, social isolation, and pain from eating are some of the many possible causes of decreased oral intake.

Increased Nutrient Loss

Glycosuria, bleeding in the digestive tract, diarrhea, malabsorption, nephrosis, a draining fistula, and protein-losing enteropathy can all result in nutrient loss.

Increased Nutrient Requirements

Any hypermetabolic state or excessive catabolic process can result in increased nutrient requirements. Common examples of situations that can dramatically affect nutrient requirements include surgery, trauma, fever, burns, hyperthyroidism, severe infection, malabsorption syndromes, critical illness, and human immunodeficiency virus/acquired immunodeficiency syndrome (HIV/AIDS). Pregnant women and children are at increased risk due to increased nutritional requirements for growth.

Diagnosis: Marasmus and Kwashiorkor

Undernutrition is a suboptimal or deficient supply of nutrients that interferes with an individual's growth, development, general health, or recovery from illness. A BMI of less than 18.5 kg/m^2 defines adults who are consistently underweight and at risk for undernutrition. Infants and children who consistently fall below the fifth percentile for weight-for-age or BMI-for-age on the pediatric growth charts should be evaluated further. In acute undernutrition, a child's weight-for-age percentile on the growth chart falls first, followed by an arrest in height growth. In extreme cases of undernutrition or starvation, a child's head circumference growth may also plateau, since the body naturally conserves its nutrient supply to preserve brain function. The importance of plotting pediatric growth parameters over time is paramount, as poor weight gain, weight loss, and crossing percentiles for height or head circumference are key to diagnosing undernutrition, failure to thrive, and other medical conditions, such as cystic fibrosis. Many of these conditions are associated with poor weight gain in the pediatric population.

Marasmus

Marasmus results when the body's requirements for calories and protein are not met by dietary intake. Marasmus is characterized by severe tissue wasting, excessive loss of lean body mass and subcutaneous fat stores, dehydration, and weight loss. Decreased protein intake is usually associated with decreased calorie intake but can occur independently.

Kwashiorkor

Kwashiorkor describes a predominant protein deficiency. It is characterized by lethargy, apathy, irritability, retarded growth, changes in skin (dermatitis) and hair pigmentation, edema, and low serum albumin.

Both marasmus and kwashiorkor are associated with weakness, weight loss, decline in functional status (increased difficulties associated with activities of daily living), impaired immune function with increased susceptibility to infection, and increased risk of morbidity and mortality.

Percent Weight Change

Weight loss is very common in hospitalized and nursing home patients. It is also frequently seen in older adults or those with significant appetite changes due to chronic illnesses, such as cancer or gastrointestinal problems, or secondary to surgery, chemotherapy, or radiation therapy. If weight loss was identified in the medical history or review of systems, it is essential to take a diet history and determine the percent weight change over that period of time using the patient's current body weight and usual weight. Severity of weight loss is defined by percent change in a defined period of time (Table 1-5).

$$\text{Percent weight change} = \frac{\text{usual weight} - \text{current weight} \times 100}{\text{usual weight}}$$

Table 1-5   Interpretation of percent weight change.

TIME	SIGNIFICANT WEIGHT LOSS	SEVERE WEIGHT LOSS
1 wk	1.0–2.0%	>2.0%
1 mo	5.0%	>5.0%
3 mo	7.5%	>7.5%
6 mo	10.0%	>10.0%
1 yr	20.0%	>20.0%

Energy and Protein Needs in Hospitalized or Critically Ill Patients

Activity factors are added to the REE as necessary to calculate total daily caloric needs, which vary for hospitalized and nonhospitalized patients (see Table 1-2). Total energy expenditure (TEE) is equal to the REE times the appropriate physical activity factor. The physical activity factor for hospitalized patients or those confined to bed is 1.2, and for nonhospitalized, sedentary patients, it is 1.3.

Protein requirements in the critically ill patient depend on the degree of catabolic stress that the patient is experiencing. Protein calories should be calculated separately. Some guidelines are as follows:

- In unstressed well-nourished individuals, protein needs range from 0.6 to 1.0 g/kg body weight per day.

- In postsurgical patients, protein needs range from 1.5 to 2.0 g/kg body weight per day.

- In highly catabolic patients (burns, infection, fever), protein needs can be greater than 2 g/kg body weight per day.

Integrating Nutrition into the Medical History and Physical Examination

The following illustrates how to integrate nutrition into all components of the clinical evaluation and nursing assessment, including the medical history, diet history, review of systems, physical examination, laboratory assessment, and treatment plan.

Importance of Taking a Diet History

The purpose of obtaining dietary information from patients is to assess their nutritional status and, if necessary, formulate a treatment plan. Infants, children, adolescents, pregnant women, older adults, and those with a family history of or who have diabetes, hypertension, heart disease, hyperlipidemia, obesity, eating disorders, alcoholism, osteoporosis, gastrointestinal (GI) or renal disease, cancer, weight loss, or weight gain should always be asked about their eating habits and need careful dietary assessment even during a routine visit. Dietary information can be collected using any of the methods described in this section. In addition, the patient's past or current patterns of food intake, or both, such as vegetarian or kosher diet practices; their cultural background; and their social situation should be considered during the interview process. Family members who purchase and prepare the food should be involved in the interview process as much as possible. Diet-related questions can take only a few minutes if properly directed.

24-Hour Recall

Purpose This informal, qualitative, questioning method elicits all the foods and beverages the patient has consumed in the preceding 24 hours. This method is recommended for patients with diabetes because of the ability to assess the timing of meals, snacks, and insulin injections.

Questions "Please describe everything that you ate and drank within the past 24 hours (meals and snacks), including quantities and how you prepared these foods." Begin with the last meal eaten and work backwards or ask for a description of everything that the patient ate the day before. Family members are usually consulted if the patient is a child or unable to convey information. Patients can be asked to write down what they ate the day before while they are waiting to be seen. Hospitalized patients can be monitored through calorie counts reported by the nursing or dietary staff, who record the daily amounts of food and drink the patient consumes. Keep in mind that the 24-hour recall method, when used alone, may underestimate or overestimate a person's usual caloric intake since the patient's recollection may not reflect long-term dietary habits.

Usual Intake/Diet History

Purpose Similar to the 24-hour recall, a usual intake/diet history is a retrospective means of obtaining dietary information by asking the patient to recall his or her normal daily intake pattern, including amounts of foods consumed. This method is suggested for older adults who frequently skip meals and for those interviewing pediatric patients whose diets may not be varied. This approach provides more information about usual intake patterns than others and tends to reflect long-term dietary habits with greater accuracy.

Questions "What do you usually eat and drink during the day for meals and snacks?" As a busy clinician, this question may be all that you will have time to ask, but it can serve as a screening mechanism to identify patients who need further counseling with a registered dietitian. When using this approach it is important to be flexible. Begin by asking patients to describe their usual intake, and if they do not recall their usual diet, ask what they ate and drank the day before (a switch to the 24-hour recall method). You can then ask if this 24 hours is typical. Also bear in mind that some patients tend to report having eaten only those foods that they know are healthy.

Food Frequency Questionnaire

Purpose The food frequency questionnaire is another retrospective approach used to determine trends in the patient's usual frequency of consumption of specific foods.

Questions The patient is usually asked several questions regarding the frequency of intake of particular foods. Frequencies can be listed to identify daily, weekly, or monthly consumption patterns. Patients can be asked several questions during the history, or these items can be added to the written form for new patients while they are in the waiting room or mailed before their visit. For the clinician, these questions can be geared toward the patient's existing medical conditions, which is why this method is best for patients with diabetes, heart disease, hypertension, or osteoporosis and for evaluating current intake of fruits, vegetables, dairy products, or meats, for example (Table 1-6).

Medical History

Past Medical History

Standard past medical history, such as immunizations, hospitalizations, surgeries, major injuries, chronic illnesses, and significant acute illnesses, can have nutritional implications. Detailed information should be obtained about current or recent prescription medications and use of vitamins, minerals, laxatives, topical medications, over-the-counter medications, and products such as nutritional or herbal supplements that patients frequently do not recognize as medications. Nutritional supplements include any products that patients use to increase their caloric, vitamin, or protein intake. Whether the patient has any known food allergies or suffers from milk (lactose) intolerance is also important.

Family History

Patients are asked to identify their parents, siblings, children, and partner; give their respective ages and health status; and indicate the cause of death of any

Table 1-6   Key diet history questions for brief intervention.

Questions for all patients
- How many meals and snacks do you eat every day?
- How often do you eat out? What kinds of restaurants?
- What do you like to drink during the day, including alcohol? How many glasses?
- How often do you eat fruits and vegetables?
- How often do you eat dairy products? Low fat or regular type?
- Do you usually finish what is on your plate or leave food?
- How often do you exercise, including walking?

In addition to the questions above

Questions for patients with hyperlipidemia (see Chapter 7)
- How often do you eat fatty meats? (hot dogs, bacon, sausage, salami, pastrami, corned beef)?
- How often do you eat fish? How is it prepared?
- What do you spread on your bread?
- What types of fats do you use in cooking?
- What type of snacks and desserts do you eat?

Questions for patients with hypertension (see Chapter 7)
- Do you use a salt shaker at the table or in cooking?
- Do you read food labels for sodium content? (<400 mg/serving permitted)
- How often do you eat canned, smoked, frozen, and processed foods?

Questions for patients with diabetes (see Chapter 9)
- What time do you take your diabetes medication (including insulin)?
- What time do you eat your meals and snacks?
- Do you ever skip meals during the day?
- How many servings of starchy foods, such as breads, cereals, pastas, corn, peas, or beans do you eat during a typical day?

SOURCE: Lisa Hark, PhD, RD, University of Pennsylvania School of Medicine. Used with permission.

deceased family members. Familial occurrences of disease also are recorded here. Nutrition assessment questions should probe for any family history of diabetes, heart disease, obesity, hypertension, osteoporosis, eating disorders, or alcoholism.

Social History

Pertinent nonmedical information recorded here includes the patient's occupation, daily exercise pattern, and marital and family status. Information is also solicited regarding the patient's education, economic status, residence, emotional response and adjustment to illness, and any other information that might influence the patient's understanding of his or her illness and adherence to a nutritional program. Details concerning the duration and frequency of the patient's use of substances such as alcohol, tobacco, illicit drugs, and caffeine are also recorded here. These data can be extremely useful when formulating the treatment plan. Economic limitations that influence access to an adequate diet, difficulties shopping for or preparing food, or participation in feeding programs (WIC, Meals on Wheels) are relevant to nutritional assessment.

Review of Systems

This subjective re-examination of the patient's history is organized by body systems. It differs from the past medical history by concentrating on symptoms, not diagnoses, and by emphasizing current more than past information. All positive and negative findings are listed. Nutrition questions vary according to the patient's age. One goal of this part of the history is to determine whether any dietary changes have occurred in the patient's life, either voluntarily or as a consequence of illness, medication use, or psychological problems. Examples within the review of systems that may have nutritional implications (and their significance) include weakness and fatigue (anemia), clothes tighter or looser (weight gain or loss), vomiting, nausea, diarrhea (poor nutrition intake, lactose intolerance), dehydration, constipation (low fiber or fluid intake), and amenorrhea (anorexia nervosa).

Physical Examination

The physical examination begins with the patient's vital signs (blood pressure, heart rate, respiration rate, temperature), height, weight, BMI, and general appearance. For example, "On examination, she is a well-developed, thin woman." When terms such as *obese, overweight, undernourished, thin, well nourished, well developed,* or *cachectic* (profound, marked state of ill health and undernutrition) are used, they should be supported by findings in the physical examination and noted in the problem list. Nutrition-oriented aspects of the physical examination focus on the skin, head, hair, eyes, mouth, nails, extremities, abdomen, skeletal muscle, and fat stores. Areas to examine closely for muscle wasting include the temporal muscles and the interosseous muscles on the hands. The skeletal muscles of the extremities also serve as an indicator of undernutrition. Subcutaneous fat stores should be examined for losses due to a sudden decrease in weight or for excess accumulation that commonly occurs in obesity. Specific signs that are attributable to a vitamin or mineral deficiency are listed in Table 1-7 and defined in the Glossary. Isolated vitamin deficiencies such as scurvy and pellagra are rarely seen in modern clinical practice. At the present time, the most commonly encountered nutritional problem seen in clinical practices in the United States and many developed countries is obesity. Additional clinical signs with their nutritional implications appear in Table 1-7.

Laboratory Data to Diagnose Nutritional and Medical Problems

No single blood test or group of tests accurately measures nutritional status. Therefore, clinical judgment is important in deciding what tests to order based on the individual's history and physical findings. The following tests are grouped according to the medical condition.

Table 1-7   **Clinical signs with nutritional implications and significance on physical examination.**

Vital signs:	temperature, blood pressure, pulse, respiratory rate, height, weight, body mass index, waist circumference, percent weight change
General:	Wasted, cachectic, overweight, obese
Skin:	Acanthosis nigricans (obesity, diabetes)
	Ecchymosis (vitamin K and C deficiency)
	Dermatitis (marasmus, niacin, riboflavin, zinc, biotin, essential fatty acid deficiency)
	Follicular hyperkeratosis (vitamin A deficiency)
	Petechiae (vitamin A, C, or K deficiency)
	Pigmentation changes (niacin, marasmus)
	Pressure ulcers/delayed healing (kwashiorkor, diabetes)
	Psoriasiform rash, eczematous scaling (zinc deficiency)
	Purpura (vitamin C or K deficiency)
	Scrotal dermatosis (riboflavin)
	Pallor (iron, folic acid, vitamin B_{12}, copper, vitamin E deficiency)
	Thickening and dryness of skin (linoleic acid deficiency)
Hair:	Dyspigmentation, easy pluckability (protein), alopecia (zinc, biotin deficiency)
Head:	Temporal muscle wasting (marasmus and cachexia)
	Delayed closure of fontanelle (pediatric undernutrition or growth retardation)
Eyes:	Night blindness, xerosis, Bitôt's spots, keratomalacia (vitamin A deficiency)
	Photophobia, blurring, conjunctival inflammation, corneal vascularization (riboflavin deficiency)
Mouth:	Angular stomatitis (riboflavin, iron deficiency)
	Bleeding gums (vitamin C, K, riboflavin deficiency)
	Cheilosis (riboflavin, niacin, vitamin B_6 deficiency)
	Dental caries (fluoride deficiency)
	Hypogeusia (zinc, vitamin A deficiency)
	Glossitis (riboflavin, niacin, folic acid, vitamin B_{12}, vitamin B_6 deficiency)
	Nasolabial seborrhea (vitamin B_6 deficiency)
	Papillary atrophy or smooth tongue (riboflavin, niacin, iron deficiency)
	Fissuring, scarlet or raw tongue (niacin, folate, B_{12}, B_6 deficiency)
Neck:	Goiter (iodine deficiency)
	Parotid enlargement (marasmus)
Thorax:	Thoracic rosary (vitamin D deficiency)
Abdomen:	Abdominal obesity
	Diarrhea (niacin, folate, vitamin B_{12} deficiency; marasmus)
	Hepatomegaly/ascites (kwashiorkor, alcoholism)
Cardiac:	Heart failure (thiamine, selenium deficiency, anemia)
Genital/urinary:	Delayed puberty (marasmus)
	Hypogonadism (zinc deficiency)
Extremities:	Ataxia (vitamin B_{12} deficiency, vitamin B_6 toxicity)
	Bone ache, joint pain (vitamin C deficiency)
	Bone tenderness, kyphosis, thickening of costochondral junction (vitamin D deficiency)

Table 1-7 (continued)

	Edema (thiamine and protein deficiency)
	Growth retardation, failure to thrive (energy deficiency)
	Hyporeflexia (thiamine deficiency)
	Kyphosis (calcium, vitamin D deficiency)
	Muscle wasting and weakness (vitamin D, protein-energy undernutrition)
	Softening of bone (vitamin D, calcium, phosphorus deficiency)
	Squaring of shoulders–loss of deltoid muscles (kwashiorkor)
Nails:	Spooning (koilonychias) (iron deficiency)
	Transverse lines (kwashiorkor)
Neurologic:	Dementia, delirium, disorientation (niacin, thiamine, vitamin E deficiency)
	Loss of reflexes, wrist drop, foot drop (thiamine deficiency)
	Ophthalmoplegia (vitamin E, thiamine deficiency)
	Decreased sensation (thiamine, vitamin B_{12} deficiency)
	Tetany (vitamin D, calcium, magnesium deficiency)

SOURCE: Lisa Hark, PhD, RD, University of Pennsylvania School of Medicine. Used with permission.

Undernutrition

Protein Status Clinically, visceral protein status may be depleted by increased protein losses in the stool and urine, as a result of wounds involving severe blood loss, or by poor dietary protein intake. The following serum protein levels may prove useful in conjunction with other nutrition assessment parameters. Once again, however, each of these tests has limitations because serum protein levels are affected not only by nutritional and hydration status but by disease states, surgery, and liver function.

The half-life ($t_{1/2}$) of each protein is given because knowing its duration allows the clinician to use these tests to diagnose acute and chronic protein-energy undernutrition.

- **Serum albumin.** Serum albumin has a $t_{1/2}$ of 18 to 20 days and reflects nutritional status over the previous 3 months. Levels may decrease with acute stress, overhydration, trauma, surgery, liver disease, and renal disease. False increases often occur with dehydration. This test is not a good indicator of recent dietary status or acute changes (less than 3 weeks) in nutritional status given its long $t_{1/2}$. Significantly reduced levels of serum albumin are associated with increased morbidity and mortality.

- **Serum transferrin.** Serum transferrin has a half-life of 8 to 9 days. Changes in serum transferrin levels are influenced by iron status, as well as by protein and calorie intake. Results of this test reflect intake over the preceding several weeks.

- **Serum prealbumin.** With a half-life of 2 to 3 days, serum prealbumin reflects nutritional status as well as protein and calorie intake over the previous week. Prealbumin levels may be falsely elevated with renal disease. However, as with albumin, the level is reduced with severe liver disease.

Alcoholism Aspartate aminotransferase (AST), alanine aminotransferase (ALT), thiamine, folate, vitamin B_{12}

Anemia Complete blood count (CBC), serum iron and ferritin, total iron-binding capacity (TIBC), transferrin saturation, mean corpuscular volume (MCV), reticulocyte count, red blood cell folate, serum vitamin B_{12}

Diabetes Serum glucose, hemoglobin (Hgb) A1c, insulin levels, C-reactive protein, serum and urinary ketone bodies

Eating Disorders Potassium, albumin

Fluid, Electrolyte and Renal Function Sodium, potassium, chloride, calcium, phosphorus, magnesium, blood urea nitrogen (BUN), creatinine, urine urea nitrogen, urinary and serum oxalic acid, and uric acid

Hyperlipidemia Cholesterol, triglyceride, LDL-C, HDL-C, homocysteine, thyroid-stimulating hormone (TSH; secondary cause)

Malabsorption Vitamins A, D, E, and K

Refeeding Syndrome Albumin, calcium, phosphorous, magnesium, potassium

Assessment and Problem List: Medical Nutrition Therapy

The health care professional clinically assesses the individual patient based on the medical history, diet history, physical examination, and laboratory data. Active problems are listed in order of their importance. Inactive problems are also recorded. Evidence of a nutrition disorder should be considered primary if it occurs in an individual with no other etiology that explains signs and symptoms of undernutrition. A primary nutrition problem is usually the result of imbalances, inadequacies, or excesses in the patient's nutrient intake. Manifestations may include obesity, weight loss, undernutrition, or poor intake of vitamins or minerals, such as iron, calcium, folate, or vitamin B_{12}.

Secondary nutrition problems occur when a primary pathologic process results in inadequate food intake, impaired absorption and utilization of nutrients, increased loss or excretion of nutrients, or increased nutrient requirements. Common causes of secondary nutrition disorders include anorexia nervosa, malabsorption, diabetes, trauma, acute medical illness, and surgery. Often undernutrition occurs as a result of a chronic condition or a critical illness complicating the underlying disease. After assessing each problem, medical nutrition therapy should be recommended that includes both a diagnostic component and a treatment plan. Patient education is an essential part of medical nutrition therapy (Table 1-8).

Effective Counseling for Lifestyle and Behavior Change

Behavior change for major lifestyle changes often requires many attempts, large and small, over many years. The first principle of behavior change is to understand the long-term nature of lifestyle changes, both to encourage a person who

Table 1-8   Key dietary issues by age and disease.

Infants	Fluoride, iron, calories for growth and development
Children	Fluoride, iron, calcium, calories for growth and development
Teenagers	Iron, calcium, calories for pubertal development (screen for eating disorders)
Pregnancy	Folate, iron, calcium, appropriate weight gain
Alcoholism	Folate, thiamine, vitamin B_{12}, calories
Anemia	Iron, vitamin B_{12}, folate
Ascites	Sodium, protein
Beriberi	Thiamine
Cancer	Adequate calories and fiber
Congestive heart failure	Sodium
COPD, asthma	Vitamin D, calcium, weight loss, calories
Diabetes	Carbohydrates, saturated fat, cholesterol, calories, fiber
Heart disease	Saturated fat, monounsaturated fat
Hyperlipidemia	Cholesterol, folate, fiber
Hypertension	Sodium, calcium, potassium, alcohol, total calories
Kidney stones	Calcium, oxalate, uric acid, protein, sodium, fluid
Liver disease	Protein, sodium, fluid
Malabsorption	Vitamins A, D, E, and K
Obesity	Total calories, saturated fat
Osteoporosis	Vitamin D and calcium
Pellagra	Niacin
Renal failure	Protein, sodium, potassium, phosphorus, fluid
Rickets	Vitamin D and calcium
Scurvy	Vitamin C
Vegetarian	Protein, vitamin B_{12}, iron, calcium

COPD, chronic obstructive pulmonary disease.
SOURCE: Lisa Hark, PhD, RD, University of Pennsylvania School of Medicine. Used with permission.

has not met goals or has relapsed and for health care providers, who also can become discouraged with apparent lack of immediate success.

In making a change, people move through a series of steps: precontemplation, contemplation, preparation, action, maintenance, and relapse (Prochaska Stage of Change Model). This model is often used to clarify for people and their providers their readiness for change. Health care providers can provide information and motivational counseling to help patients move from one stage to another. Providers can help the patient by considering behavioral beliefs, such as personal perceived risk of negative outcome from the behavior, normative beliefs (similar behavior by family members and individuals important to them), and efficacy beliefs (they believe they can make the change). People often need skills (label reading and menu planning) to help turn their intention to action. Providers who model or perform a specific behavior are more likely to help patients perform this behavior. Reviewing barriers to a change, the circumstances of previous behavior change and relapse, and motivations to change can also provide useful insights to patients. Important questions that could be asked of all individuals seen for follow-up to assess their level of change include:

- How have you changed your diet or exercise since the last visit?
- What problems did you encounter in making these changes?
- Do you feel confident that you can maintain the changes you have made?
- What changes would you still like to make in your diet or exercise pattern to improve your health?
- How can I help you with these changes?
- What one behavior could you change that would result in the most significant change in your health?
- What one or two behaviors would you be unlikely to change now?

For a list of references for this chapter, please visit the University of Pennsylvania School of Medicine's Nutrition Education and Prevention Program web site: *http://www.med.upenn.edu/nutrimed/articles.html*

Case 1

Obese Woman with Metabolic Syndrome

Cathy Nonas, Xavier Pi-Sunyer, and Gary Foster

Objectives

- Identify methods to appropriately diagnose obesity and the metabolic syndrome in adults.
- Describe the metabolic and health consequences associated with being overweight or obese.
- Given the anthropometric and laboratory data, and usual diet of a patient, assess the patient's risk for metabolic complications associated with excess weight gain.
- Describe the components of a successful weight management program, including specific nutrition and physical activity recommendations.
- Identify the biochemical and metabolic effects of diets varying in macronutrient content.
- Describe the efficacy of pharmacologic and surgical approaches for the treatment of obesity.

RS is a 44-year-old woman who works as a management consultant. She presents to her family physician with elevated blood pressure (BP) and obesity. She has a history of dieting but has been unable to maintain a healthy weight. This is approximately the twelfth time in the past 15 years that she has tried a weight-loss diet. RS states that her weight problems began when she had her first child 18 years ago. Although she understands the medical consequences associated with being overweight, she is primarily motivated to lose weight for cosmetic reasons.

Past Medical History

RS has no history of cardiovascular or gallbladder disease. [She has not had an electrocardiogram (ECG) for the past 5 years.] She takes no medications, vitamins, or herbal supplements, although she states that she should be taking calcium. When asked about sleep disturbances, she admits to snoring at night but denies waking up in the middle of the night or falling asleep during daytime activities.

Family History

The family history is positive for overweight and obesity. RS's one brother and a sister are overweight. Her father and another sister are of normal weight. Her mother is obese and hypertensive and had a myocardial infarction at the age of 67. RS states that her mother does not have diabetes, although her blood glucose was elevated in a recent blood test.

Social History

RS does not smoke. She averages two to three glasses of wine per week. She eats three meals per day and admits to nibbling whenever food is available at work or when she is bored. She states she has no time to exercise because of her work and family schedule. RS is currently at her highest adult weight.

Review of Systems

Skin: No history of rashes or unusual skin pigmentation

Head, ears, eyes, nose, throat (HEENT): No visual complaints

Neurologic: No headaches, tremors, seizures, or depression

Endocrine: Normal menstrual cycle; denies abnormal heat or cold intolerances

Cardiovascular: Normal rate and rhythm; no orthopnea or dyspnea

Joints: No swelling, heat, or redness

Physical Examination

Vital Signs

Temperature: 98.4°F (36.9°C)

Heart rate: 88 beats per minute (BPM)

BP: 135/88 mm Hg

Height: 5′3″ (160 cm)

Current weight: 208 lb (94.5 kg)

BMI: 36.8 kg/m^2

Waist circumference: 38 in. (96.5 cm)

Weight history: Her highest adult weight is her current weight; her lowest weight of 150 lb (68 kg) was before she had children at age 25. Her average weight has been 175 lb (79.4 kg).

Obstetric history: RS delivered three healthy, full-term children, who are now 18, 13, and 10 years old. She gained 35 to 40 lb (16 to 18 kg) with each pregnancy and lost approximately 20 lb (9 kg) after each birth but did not return to her prepregnancy weight. RS has never been able to reach her prepregnancy weight.

General: Obese woman in no acute distress; no cushingoid features

Examination: Nonpalpable thyroid; negative hirsutism or striae; no dorsal, cervical, or supraclavicular fat; no acanthosis nigricans. Her limbs are not edematous. She has no stretch marks.

Laboratory Data

Patient's Fasting Values	Normal Values
Glucose: 116 mg/dL	70–110 mg/dL
Potassium: 3.8 mEq/L	3.5–5.0 mEq/L
Cholesterol: 216 mg/dL	Desirable <200 mg/dL
Triglycerides: 175 mg/dL	Desirable <150 mg/dL
HDL: 42 mg/dL	Desirable for female ≥50 mg/dL
Calculated LDL: 139 mg/dL	Desirable <130 mg/dL

RS provides vague information on serving sizes, particularly when she feels guilty about them. The following is what was extrapolated from her usual diet:

Breakfast (home)	Coffee	8 oz (240 mL)
	Half-and-half cream	1 oz (30 mL)
	Bagel	1 large
	Cream cheese	2 Tbsp.
	Orange juice	8 oz (240 mL)
Lunch (home)	Chef salad (turkey, ham, cheese, boiled egg)	2 cups
	French dressing	3 Tbsp.
	Bread sticks	2 small
	Ice tea (presweetened)	12 oz (360 mL)
Snack (home)	Pretzels	1.5-oz bag
	Diet soda	12 oz (360 mL)
Dinner (home)	Spaghetti	2 cups
	Tomato sauce	1/2 cup
	Beef meatballs	3 oz (85 g)
	Garlic bread	1 piece
	Red wine	5 oz (150 mL)
Snack (home)	Vanilla wafers	10 small
	Lemonade	12 oz (360 mL)

Total calories: 2691 kcal
Protein: 94 g (14% of calories)
Fat: 90 g (30% of calories)
Saturated fat: 33 g (11% of calories)
Monounsaturated fat: 21 g (7% of calories)
Cholesterol: 334 mg
Carbohydrate: 355 g (53% of calories)
Dietary fiber: 13 g
Sodium: 4800 mg
Calcium: 601 mg

Case Questions

1. How are overweight and obesity clinically assessed in this patient?
2. What are the medical risks associated with obesity in this patient?
3. Does RS meet the criteria to diagnose metabolic syndrome?
4. What are the appropriate treatment goals for RS?
5. RS is interested in trying a high-protein, low-carbohydrate diet. Describe the biochemical and metabolic effects of high-protein, low-carbohydrate diets.
6. Is this popular diet appropriate for RS based on her medical history?
7. What dietary and exercise guidelines would you recommend for RS considering her diagnosis of metabolic syndrome and her current diet?
8. On a subsequent visit, RS is interested in medication for weight loss. Discuss the current criteria and options for pharmacologic therapy.
9. Is RS a candidate for surgical treatment of obesity?

Case Answers

1. **How are overweight and obesity clinically assessed in this patient?**

    BMI is a useful clinical calculation for documenting obesity because it assesses the relative risk of excess weight (see Figure 1-2). BMI is defined as weight (kg)/height (m^2). An alternative method of calculating BMI is to take the weight (in pounds) multiplied by a factor of 703. Divide this number by the height (in inches) squared.

    The amount of intra-abdominal adipose tissue, independent of BMI, correlates strongly with increased risk of cardiovascular disease, stroke, dyslipidemia, hypertension, and type 2 diabetes in both men and women. Abdominal obesity can be assessed by measuring the patient's waist circumference, in the horizontal plane around the abdomen at the level of the iliac crest.

    RS is clinically assessed as having class II obesity (see Table 1-4) because she has a BMI of 36.8 kg/m^2. In addition, she has excess adipose tissue located in her abdomen, as indicated by her waist circumference of 38 in. (96.5 cm), increasing her risk for heart disease and diabetes.

2. **What are the medical risks associated with obesity in this patient?**

    Obesity increases a person's risk of developing cardiovascular disease, dyslipidemia, hypertension, type 2 diabetes, osteoarthritis, gallstones, respiratory disease, cholecystitis, and certain types of cancer. Obesity also increases a patient's risk during surgical procedures because increased subcutaneous fat can make surgery technically more difficult and prolongs the procedure. Postoperation complications are more common in obese patients.

Evidence exists to indicate that RS is experiencing some signs of physical stress related to obesity that include the following:

1. RS complains of snoring, which, combined with obesity, places her at risk for sleep apnea in the future.
2. Borderline high LDL according to the Adult Treatment Panel (ATP III; 2001) Guidelines from the National Cholesterol Education Program (NCEP) (see Chapter 7).
3. Elevated fasting glucose level, suggesting impaired glucose tolerance and insulin resistance, although not frank diabetes. It is unclear whether RS's mother has diabetes, but RS is at risk for type 2 diabetes due to the constellation of risk factors: obesity, abdominal fat distribution, sedentary lifestyle, and impaired glucose tolerance.
4. Elevated BP adding to her risk of disease according to the Sixth Report of the Joint National Committee on Prevention, Detection, Evaluation, and Treatment of High BP (JNC VI).
5. Elevated triglyceride level and a low HDL level for a woman.

3. **Does RS meet the criteria to diagnose metabolic syndrome?**

   Recent attention regarding risk for coronary heart disease has focused on a cluster of metabolic abnormalities that arise primarily out of obesity. According to the NCEP ATP III guidelines, a patient can be diagnosed with metabolic syndrome if he or she exhibits three of the five conditions listed in Table 1-9. (Note the differences in low normal ranges for HDL cholesterol for identifying men and women with metabolic syndrome.) RS has all five of the criteria for metabolic syndrome.

4. **What are the appropriate treatment goals for RS?**

   The first line of treatment for patients with obesity and the metabolic syndrome are weight reduction and increased physical activity. However, one does not need to lose a lot of weight to be successful.

Weight Reduction

Clinical research has demonstrated that obese individuals who achieve and maintain a 10% reduction in body weight, regardless of initial BMI, are likely to lower their BP, serum glucose, and LDL-cholesterol and triglyceride levels, thereby reducing their risk of developing diabetes and

Table 1-9   Identification of metabolic syndrome.

1. Abdominal obesity: waist circumference greater than 40 in. (102 cm) in men and 35 in. (89 cm) in women

2. Elevated fasting triglycerides (>150 mg/dL)

3. Low high-density lipoprotein cholesterol (<40 mg/dL in men and <50 mg/dL in women)

4. Hypertension (>130/85 mm Hg) or taking antihypertensive medications

5. Insulin resistance or diabetes (fasting glucose >110 mg/dL)

SOURCE: National Cholesterol Education Program. NHLBI, 2002.

cardiovascular disease. The Diabetes Prevention Program (DPP), a national study comparing lifestyle changes to medication, found that type 2 diabetes can be prevented or delayed with just a 5% to 7% weight loss due to lifestyle changes. For a more complete review of the Diabetes Prevention Program (DPP), see Chapter 9, Case 2.

Lifestyle modifications may also prevent the onset of hypertension as well as reduce elevated BP. RS has a BP of 135/88 mm Hg. According to JNC VI, patients with a BP in the high normal range of 130/85 to 139/89 mm Hg should begin an aggressive lifestyle modification program to lower BP to less than 130/85 mm Hg to reduce the risk of cardiovascular disease.

A linear association has been demonstrated between excess body weight (BMI greater than 27) and severity of hypertension. A mean weight loss of 20 lb (9.2 kg) is associated with a 6.3 mm Hg reduction in systolic BP and a 3.1 mm Hg reduction in diastolic BP. In addition, weight loss enhances the BP-lowering effect of antihypertension medications.

The incidence of other health problems associated with obesity, such as sleep apnea and osteoarthritis, also decreases with moderate weight loss. Thus, if RS were to lose 20 lb (9.2 kg) or approximately 10% of her weight, it is likely that the clinical abnormalities associated with the metabolic syndrome would improve.

Increased Physical Activity

Exercise has been shown to be the single best predictor of long-term weight maintenance and therefore should always be encouraged for weight loss. Patients who participate in regular exercise have lower BP levels as well as a reduced risk of cardiovascular disease and osteoporosis compared to those who do not exercise. The Centers for Disease Control (CDC) and Prevention recommends a minimum of 30 minutes a day of physical activity 5 days a week for adults. The current Institute of Medicine (IOM) recommendations are to reach 1 hour a day of exercise, which is consistent with the CDC'S recommendations for physical activity for children and teenagers. Current research indicates that this level of physical activity can be accumulated over the day. Both observational and interventional studies suggest that even brisk walking 3 hours per week can reduce the risk of cardiovascular disease and type 2 diabetes by at least 30%.

An active lifestyle has also been shown to prevent or delay the development of type 2 diabetes, since both moderate and vigorous exercise decrease the risk of impaired glucose tolerance and type 2 diabetes. It is likely that the beneficial effects of exercise on the prevention of cardiovascular disease are associated with improvements in the metabolic syndrome. In hypertensive patients with hyperinsulinemia, regular exercise has consistently demonstrated a reduction in BP levels. Regular exercise has also been shown to reduce levels of triglyceride-rich very-low-density lipoprotein (VLDL) particles.

5. RS is interested in trying a high-protein, low-carbohydrate diet. Describe the biochemical and metabolic effects of high-protein, low-carbohydrate diets.

High-protein, low-carbohydrate diets remain popular today, with the most controversial being those that exclude almost all carbohydrate (less than 5% of total calories). These extremely low-carbohydrate diets, such as the Atkins diet, may consist of greater than 150 g protein, 100 g total fat (much of which is saturated fat), 500 mg cholesterol, and less than 28 g carbohydrate per day during the induction phase of the diet.

These diets are ketogenic, meaning they cause the body to go into ketosis. *Ketosis* can be defined as the production of ketone bodies, namely acetoacetic acid and beta–hydroxybutyric acid, from the breakdown of free fatty acids. Ketosis also occurs during starvation, but due to lack of calories and protein, significant lean body mass is lost. In the weight-loss diets that try to promote ketosis, the dietary protein is excessive, and therefore, lean body mass seems to be preserved (although research is sparse).

When ketone bodies build up in excess amounts (ketonemia), they spill into the urine (ketonuria) and are excreted as sodium or potassium salts, resulting in a net loss of sodium and potassium. Excess dietary animal protein may also lead to hyperuricemia (increased uric acid in the blood) and hyperuricosuria (increased excretion of uric acid in urine), which increase the patient's risk of developing gout, uric acid kidney stones, and possibly bone loss. It is therefore critical to drink at least 64 oz (1920 ml) water per day on this high-protein diet and to maintain an adequate electrolyte intake.

The question then is why do people lose weight on high-protein, low-carbohydrate diets? Most experts agree that when patients adhere to any weight-loss program, plan their meals, and focus on what and how much they are eating, they lose weight. In addition, when entire food groups, such as carbohydrates, are avoided, caloric intake is significantly reduced.

Until recently, little scientific data existed regarding the safety and efficacy of very low-carbohydrate diets. Researchers at the University of Pennsylvania, the University of Colorado, and Washington University investigated the effects of the Atkins diet compared to those of conventional low-fat (less than 30 percent), low-saturated-fat, high-carbohydrate (greater than 55%) diets. Preliminary 12-week data indicated that people on the Atkins diet lose an average of 10% of their original body weight compared to 5% on the conventional diet. Those on the Atkins diet also had an increase in HDL and a decrease in triglyceride levels compared to those following the conventional high-carbohydrate diet. The conventional high-carbohydrate diet was associated with more favorable effects on total and LDL cholesterol levels, as one would expect from a low-saturated-fat, low-cholesterol diet. The short- and long-term effects of extremely low-carbohydrate, high-protein diets are currently under investigation.

The rationale for this low-carbohydrate, high-protein diet is the theory that high-carbohydrate diets promote insulin resistance and cause obesity. Insulin resistance occurs as a result of increased body weight, lack of exercise, or medical conditions such as type 2 diabetes. Protein also stimulates insulin secretion. Consuming more calories than your body requires from any food source potentially leads to weight gain if not balanced with increased exercise.

6. **Is this popular diet appropriate for RS based on her medical history?**

Given the cardiovascular concerns and the lack of controlled data, a ketogenic weight-loss diet may not be appropriate for RS. If she feels that she is eating too many carbohydrates from starches and simple sugars, we can suggest that she become more aware of serving sizes and eat more vegetables and fruits and predominantly whole grains.

On a ketogenic diet, when carbohydrates are reduced to 28 g per day, fat and protein intake are significantly increased. Depending on the choice of protein-containing foods, a high saturated fat diet may result. It is well established from epidemiologic data and clinical trials that a high saturated fat intake increases serum LDL levels and therefore the risk of cardiovascular disease. The current ATP III Therapeutic Lifestyle Changes diet advocates less than 7% of the total calories coming from saturated fat, fewer than 200 mg cholesterol and up to 20% of calories from monounsaturated fat per day (see Chapter 7).

In addition, in order to keep carbohydrates low enough so that ketosis occurs, fruits, fruit juices, grains, and dairy products are severely limited or avoided. Therefore, these diets are lacking in vitamins (A, B, C, D) and minerals (calcium). Patients are advised in these self-help books to take many vitamin and mineral supplements.

Additional data from the Dietary Approaches to Stop Hypertension (DASH) diet, a multicenter randomized, controlled trial that assessed the effects of dietary patterns on BP, support eating plenty of fruits, vegetables, and dairy foods for patients with high BP. This trial enrolled 459 adults with mean baseline BP levels of 131.3/84.7 mm Hg. Subjects were randomized to the control diet rich in fruits and vegetables with an average fat content or a combination diet with low-fat dairy and reduced total and saturated fat. Results showed a 5.5 mm Hg greater decrease in systolic pressure and 3.0 mm Hg greater decrease in diastolic pressure with the intervention diet as compared to the control diet. The average sodium intake was 3000 mg per day. Reduction in BP began within 2 weeks and was maintained for the duration of the study. Further BP reductions were achieved with sodium restriction.

7. **What dietary and exercise guidelines would you recommend for RS considering her diagnosis of metabolic syndrome and her current diet?**

Considering the fact that RS has tried unsuccessfully to diet 12 times over the past 15 years, it is important to assess what she feels is her biggest vulnerability and also what lifestyle changes she is willing to incorporate.

Clearly, RS needs to focus on decreasing her total caloric intake and increasing her level of physical activity to lose weight and improve her metabolic syndrome.

Dietary Goals

Specifically, RS would benefit from decreasing her consumption of saturated fat, low fiber, simple carbohydrates, and sodium intake. The current IOM report recommends 45% to 65% of total calories coming from carbohydrates and 20% to 35% from fat. Because of the beneficial effects of increasing monounsaturated fat (MUFA) on triglyceride and HDL levels, RS could replace saturated fat with MUFA by using olive oil on her salad instead of French dressing and substituting low-fat cream cheese for the full-fat varieties. Snacking on hummus and raw carrots rather than pretzels, crackers, or cookies should also be suggested. She could also choose carbohydrate-containing, high-fiber foods such as fresh fruits, vegetables, and whole grain breads instead of bagels and pasta. RS needs to be counseled on reducing her serving size of pasta. She can add cooked frozen vegetables to her spaghetti to fill her up at dinner. Water and other noncaloric drinks should be substituted for sugar-sweetened drinks or fruit juice, as these drinks are contributing a significant number of empty-calorie carbohydrates to her diet.

As shown in the revised menu, we recommended that RS substitute a small amount of peanut butter, a good source of MUFA and protein, for butter or cream cheese at breakfast. We also suggested that she skip the cheese and egg yolk on the chef salad at lunch. Turkey, boiled ham, and egg whites are good sources of lean, low-fat protein. If RS skips the garlic bread with dinner and limits her pasta to one cup cooked, she will be successful in decreasing calories, carbohydrate, saturated fat, and cholesterol. By adding vegetables RS will improve the nutritional value of her diet while keeping total calories low. Finally, RS should be advised to take a calcium supplement (500 mg per day) since her calcium intake is far below her daily requirement of 1200 mg per day.

Physical Activity Goals

RS states that she does not have time to exercise because of her work and children's schedule. She currently works as a management consultant and travels several times a month. Therefore, in order to realistically encourage RS to increase her activity, it would be helpful to address these time barriers and to help her identify strategies to achieve increased physical activity. When she is traveling, she could bring her exercise clothes and sneakers. When she is at home, she could take a walk at night after dinner, or she could walk during her lunch break at work. In RS's case, she may benefit from using a pedometer that measures the number of steps taken each day. Metabolic fitness goals could be set at 5000 steps (or

30 minutes) per day, which can be gradually achieved over time. Keeping a record of her exercise may help RS stick with her commitment.

Realistic Weight Goals

The health care provider should discuss the appropriate rate of weight loss. A safe rate of weight loss is 1 to 2 lb or 1% of body weight per week. RS's current weight is 208 lb (94.3 kg), and she is 63 in. (160 cm) tall. If RS is able to adhere to these dietary recommendations and increase her physical activity, she should be able to reduce her weight by 10 to 20 lb (4.5 to 9.0 kg) over a period of 6 months. Studies have shown that weight loss slows or stops after approximately the twenty-fourth week of most diets. This "plateau" occurs because the calories consumed and energy expended are now sufficient to maintain, rather than to allow for additional weight loss.

After this goal is attained, a new weight goal can be negotiated. Since RS would like to lose more, it is helpful to reiterate how much healthier she will be when she meets her first goal and the fact that she is very successful if she maintains that weight loss. A potential next goal of 175 lb (79.4 kg) can be set.

Recommended Revised Diet for Obesity

Breakfast (home)	Coffee	8 oz (240 mL)
	Whole grain bread	1 slice
	Peanut butter	1 Tbsp.
	Low-fat milk (1%)	4 oz (120 mL)
	Banana	1 small
Lunch (home)	Chef salad (no cheese) (turkey, ham, egg whites, tomato, raw broccoli)	2 cups
	Olive oil	2 Tbsp.
	Balsamic vinegar	2 Tbsp.
	Diet soda or water	12 oz (360 mL)
Snack (home)	Hummus	4 Tbsp.
	Raw carrots	2 oz (57 g)
	Water	8 oz (240 mL)
Dinner (home)	Spaghetti	1 cup
	Mixed vegetables	10 oz (283 g)
	Lean beef meatballs	3 oz (85 g)
	Water	8 oz (240 mL)
Snack (home)	Fat-free yogurt	8 oz (240 mL)

Total calories: 1506 kcal
Protein: 78 g (20% of calories)

Fat: 59 g (34% of calories)
Saturated fat: 11 g (7% of calories)
Monounsaturated fat: 29 g (17% of calories)
Carbohydrate: 178 g (46% of calories)
Dietary fiber: 34 g
Sodium: 1934 mg
Calcium: 785 mg

8. **On a subsequent visit, RS is interested in medication for weight loss. Discuss the current criteria and options for pharmacologic therapy.**

Pharmacologic interventions to facilitate weight loss include enhancing satiety, decreasing fat absorption, and decreasing appetite. Two medications for weight loss are currently approved by the Food and Drug Administration (FDA) for long-term use: sibutramine (Meridia) and orlistat (Xenical). It is important to note that although most people consider stopping the drug after weight loss has resulted, this may precipitate weight regain. Similarly, it would be inappropriate to stop a cholesterol-lowering medication after blood cholesterol has been reduced or to discontinue a hypertension medication because BP has normalized.

It is also important to note that sibutramine and orlistat have very low abuse potential and both have good safety records. However, weight reduction with either of these medications is modest (7 to 11 lb or 3 to 5 kg) over a 1-year period. Many over-the-counter weight-loss products are available, but their safety and efficacy are not assured by clinical trials.

Sibutramine (Meridia)

Sibutramine is a serotonin and norepinephrine reuptake inhibitor (SNRI). Research shows that this drug reduces body weight by decreasing food intake. Research findings in humans indicate that patients receiving 10 to 15 mg per day of sibutramine had a 6% to 8% weight loss, compared to a 2% weight loss with placebo. This drug is indicated for patients with a BMI greater than 30 or greater than 27 in the presence of risk factors. Sibutramine is prescribed in the following dosages: 5, 10, or 15 mg once per day. It can be taken in the morning to reduce any effect of insomnia; however, the medication is best prescribed based on the patient's high risk eating time, as the medication seems to peak at about 7 hours in the fed state.

Since sibutramine is a serotonergic medication, it should be monitored in patients who are also taking selective serotonin reuptake inhibitors [SSRIs; e.g., paroxetine (Paxil), sertraline (Zoloft), fluoxetine]. Sibutramine is contraindicated in patients who take monoamine oxidase (MAO) inhibitors or those with poorly controlled hypertension, a history of coronary artery disease, congestive heart failure, arrhythmia, or stroke. Regular BP and heart rate monitoring is required since norepinephrine effects can increase heart rate (4 BPM in clinical studies) and cause small increases in systolic and diastolic pressure (2 to 4 mm Hg). The long-term effects of these changes are unknown. Other common side effects include dry mouth and constipation. In one double-blind, 2-year study, weight loss was better maintained at 1 year and HDL-C was raised significantly in those subjects prescribed sibutramine compared with those taking placebo.

Orlistat (Xenical)

Orlistat's activity occurs in the stomach and small intestine and promotes weight loss by inhibiting gastric and pancreatic lipases, thus partially blocking the hydrolysis of triglycerides. Thirty percent of ingested fat is unabsorbed and excreted in the stool. Patients are required to follow a low-fat diet ($\leq 30\%$) in order to minimize side effects, specifically steatorrhea, associated with fat malabsorption. Orlistat is prescribed at a dose of 120 mg three times a day with meals containing fat. Because fat-soluble vitamins may also be malabsorbed, a multivitamin should be prescribed once per day to be taken at least 2 hours before or after the medication. Orlistat is contraindicated for pregnant and lactating women and those with chronic malabsorption syndromes and cholestasis. In a 2-year study, patients given orlistat lost more weight, maintained more weight loss, and reduced serum cholesterol, LDL-C, and BPs compared with subjects who took a placebo.

It is incumbent on the physician to bring the patient back for a follow-up visit within a month to assess the effectiveness of the medication as well as any side effects. One criterion of success for either medication is a 4 lb (1.8 kg) weight loss in the first month. If this has not occurred, it is important for the physician and patient to re-evaluate the effectiveness of this medication for improvement in behavior, adherence, and so forth.

9. **Is RS a candidate for surgical treatment of obesity?**

Patient selection criteria for surgical treatment:

- BMI of 40 or greater or 35 or greater for those with weight-related comorbidities
- History of failed conservative weight loss approaches
- No substance abuse and/or psychiatric disorders

Several surgical options are available for severe obesity; however, the most common are the vertical banded gastroplasty (VBG) and the gastric bypass (GBP; Figures 1-5 and 1-6). The procedures result in a weight loss of 25% to 50% of initial weight, and the weight loss is generally well maintained. The GBP results in a greater weight loss than does the VBG. Follow-up data up to 14 years reveal very good success after gastric bypass. Significant improvements in comorbidities also occur. Nutritional side effects include, but are not limited to, undernutrition, nutrient malabsorption, and dumping syndrome. It is important, therefore, to make

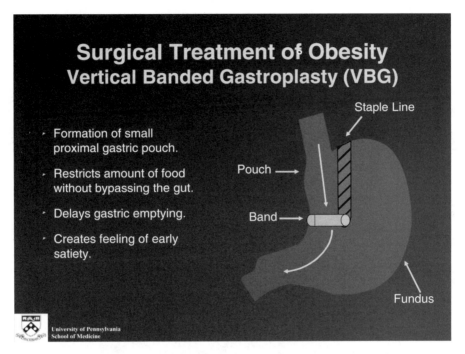

Figure 1-5 Surgical treatment of obesity: vertical banded gastroplasty (VBG).

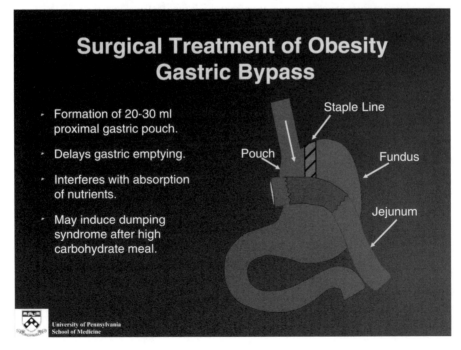

Figure 1-6 Surgical treatment of obesity: gastric bypass.

sure that the patient will be able to follow the structure of the postsurgical diet, which includes eating minuscule amounts of food, mostly protein, for the first 6 weeks or so and taking vitamins and minerals daily.

See Chapter Review Questions, pages A-7 to A-9.

2

Vitamins, Minerals, and Phytochemicals

Cynthia Thomson and Allison Sarubin-Fragakis

Objectives

- Identify the functions and sources of vitamins and minerals and their role in the promotion and maintenance of health.
- Identify populations at risk for vitamin and mineral deficiencies.
- Define the role of oxidative injury and dietary antioxidants in the pathogenesis of disease.
- Evaluate the role of antioxidant therapy in the prevention and treatment of disease.
- Become familiar with the use of dietary reference intakes (DRIs) and upper intake levels (ULs) for vitamins and minerals in order to avoid the risk of adverse effects.

Vitamins and minerals are classified as micronutrients, chemical substances required for normal growth and metabolism. Vitamins are organic compounds essential for a multitude of metabolic reactions in vivo that result in the release of energy from carbohydrates, fats, and proteins. Minerals are inorganic elements that do not furnish energy but play vital roles in a multitude of physiologic functions. For the most part, humans rely on exogenous sources to supply their vitamin and mineral needs. Known exceptions are the production of vitamin K and biotin by certain intestinal micro-organisms; the synthesis of vitamin D from its precursor, cholesterol; and the synthesis of niacin from its precursor, tryptophan.

* SOURCE: Objectives for chapter and cases adapted from the *NIH Nutrition Curriculum Guide for Training Physicians* (*http://www.nhlbi.nih.gov/funding/training/naa*).

Although the major functions of vitamins and minerals were elucidated in the early 1950s, they were historically studied in relation to classic diseases associated with profound deficiency states. More recently scientists have focused research beyond overt deficiency in an effort to understand the more complex role of micronutrients in disease prevention and treatment. Annual expenditure for over-the-counter dietary supplements in the United States is estimated to be in excess of 16 billion dollars. It is important that clinicians responsible for educating their patients with respect to appropriate use of vitamin and mineral supplementation understand the role of vitamins and minerals in health and disease.

In the United States, the Food and Drug Administration (FDA) is the agency mandated to regulate dietary supplements. Under the Dietary Supplement and Education Act, supplements are regulated independent of foods and as such have a separate set of standards for labeling. In addition, the US government established the Office of Dietary Supplements at the National Institutes of Health to further evaluate scientific evidence for the use of dietary supplements as well as to monitor safety. Given the complexity of issues surrounding the use of dietary supplements, it is imperative that health care professionals identify and utilize reliable information resources in developing care plans for patients and clients.

Recommended Intake Levels

Deficiency states are relatively common throughout parts of the world where the food supply remains inadequate. Developed countries, however, are now more concerned with the importance of a varied diet in the prevention and treatment of disease. People are asking new questions: Will folic acid prevent heart disease? Will phytochemicals and antioxidants protect against cancer? Will a contemporary public health initiative to fortify breads and cereals with folic acid reduce the incidence of neural tube defects?

Vitamins and minerals are crucial throughout life for proper growth, development, and metabolism. The required quantities of each vitamin, however, change throughout the life cycle. For example, the cellular requirements for vitamins increase during infancy, adolescence, pregnancy, and lactation.

The Food and Nutrition Board of the National Research Council established a recommended daily allowance (RDA) for most nutrients based on a review of published scientific data. A considerable body of knowledge exists for certain vitamins and minerals, and designated RDAs for various gender and age categories have been established. These levels are set at two standard deviations above the mean requirement to cover the needs of practically all healthy persons.

Two caveats concerning these recommendations exist: The suggested levels were established for groups of healthy people, and the requirements of individuals with special nutritional needs or medical conditions are not addressed by the Food and Nutrition Board. In addition, the RDAs were developed to prevent classic nutrient deficiencies, not to enhance overall health and well-being.

In an effort to better meet the changing nutritional needs of the American population, the Institute of Medicine (IOM) of the National Academy of Sciences established the first dietary reference intakes (DRIs) in 1997. The new DRIs move beyond the traditional RDAs to focus on the prevention of chronic disease. The DRIs provide a range of safe and appropriate intakes as well as tolerable upper limits (when the data are available). To date, DRIs have been established for vitamin A, the B vitamins, vitamin C, vitamin D, vitamin E, vitamin K, choline, calcium, chromium, copper, fluoride, iodine, iron, magnesium, manganese, molybdenum, phosphorus, selenium, and zinc. Recommendations regarding the intake of other nutrients will be available over the next decade as the scientific evidence is evaluated. Tables 2-1 and 2-2 outline the current DRIs for vitamins and minerals, and Table 2-3 lists current tolerable ULs. The UL is the maximum level of daily intake that is likely to pose no risk of adverse effects.

Functions and Sources of Vitamins

Vitamins occur in minute quantities in foods and are classified as fat soluble or water soluble. Vitamins A (retinol, carotenoids), D (cholecalciferol), E (tocopherols), and K (phylloquinone, menaquinone, and menadione) are fat soluble (Table 2-4). Vitamin C (ascorbic acid) and the B complex—thiamine (vitamin B_1), riboflavin (vitamin B_2), niacin (vitamin B_3), pantothenic acid (vitamin B_5), pyridoxine (vitamin B_6), cobalamin (vitamin B_{12}), folate (folic acid), and biotin—are water soluble (Table 2-5). Individual vitamins differ in their chemical structure and function and produce characteristic symptoms of deficiency or toxicity. Fat-soluble vitamins are readily stored in adipose tissue, whereas water-soluble vitamins, when consumed in excess, are excreted in urine. Acute and chronic toxicities have been reported with vitamins from both classes, particularly vitamins A and D, niacin, pyridoxine, and fluoride.

Recommended Vitamin Intakes

Vitamin Deficiency

To determine the adequacy of an individual's vitamin intake, the clinician should take a dietary history to determine the variety of foods that are commonly consumed and whether food groups such as fruits, vegetables, or dairy are being avoided. In addition, laboratory tests will reveal whether a biochemical basis for deficiency or inadequacy exists. When suspected the clinician should perform a physical examination to diagnose any overt lesions commonly associated with classic nutrient deficiencies (see Tables 2-4 and 2-5). Outlined below are several factors that may contribute to micronutrient inadequacy.

Inadequate Intake

A major factor contributing to inadequate vitamin intake is a poor or energy-deficient diet. This may be related to poverty, limited knowledge of nutrition,

Table 2-1 Dietary reference intakes: recommended intakes for individuals, vitamins.

LIFE STAGE GROUP	VITAMIN A (μg/d)[a]	VITAMIN C (mg/d)	VITAMIN D (μg/d)[b,c]	VITAMIN E (mg/d)[d]	VITAMIN K (μg/d)	THIAMINE (mg/d)	RIBOFLAVIN (mg/d)	NIACIN (mg/d)[e]	VITAMIN B_6 (mg/d)	FOLATE (μg/d)[f]	VITAMIN B_{12} (μg/d)	PANTOTHENIC ACID (mg/d)	BIOTIN (μg/d)	CHOLINE[g] (mg/d)
Infants														
0–6 mo	400*	40*	5*	4*	2.0*	0.2*	0.3*	2*	0.1*	65*	0.4*	1.7*	5*	125*
7–12 mo	500*	50*	5*	5*	2.5*	0.3*	0.4*	4*	0.3*	80*	0.5*	1.8*	6*	150*
Children														
1–3 yr	300	15	5*	6	30*	0.5	0.5	6	0.5	150	0.9	2*	8*	200*
4–8 yr	400	25	5*	7	55*	0.6	0.6	8	0.6	200	1.2	3*	12*	250*
Males														
9–13 yr	600	45	5*	11	60*	0.9	0.9	12	1.0	300	1.8	4*	20*	375*
14–18 yr	900	75	5*	15	75*	1.2	1.3	16	1.3	400	2.4	5*	25*	550*
19–30 yr	900	90	5*	15	120*	1.2	1.3	16	1.3	400	2.4	5*	30*	550*
31–50 yr	900	90	5*	15	120*	1.2	1.3	16	1.3	400	2.4	5*	30*	550*
51–70 yr	900	90	10*	15	120*	1.2	1.3	16	1.7	400	2.4[h]	5*	30*	550*
>70 yr	900	90	15*	15	120*	1.2	1.3	16	1.7	400	2.4[h]	5*	30*	550*
Females														
9–13 yr	600	45	5*	11	60*	0.9	0.9	12	1.0	300	1.8	4*	20*	375*
14–18 yr	700	65	5*	15	75*	1.0	1.0	14	1.2	400[i]	2.4	5*	25*	400*
19–30 yr	700	75	5*	15	90*	1.1	1.1	14	1.3	400[i]	2.4	5*	30*	425*
31–50 yr	700	75	5*	15	90*	1.1	1.1	14	1.3	400[i]	2.4	5*	30*	425*
51–70 yr	700	75	10*	15	90*	1.1	1.1	14	1.5	400	2.4[h]	5*	30*	425*
>70 yr	700	75	15*	15	90*	1.1	1.1	14	1.5	400	2.4[h]	5*	30*	425*

Pregnancy													
≤18 yr	750	80	5*	15	1.4	1.4	18	1.9	600ʲ	2.6	6*	30*	450*
19-30 yr	770	85	5*	15	1.4	1.4	18	1.9	600ʲ	2.6	6*	30*	450*
31-50 yr	770	85	5*	15	1.4	1.4	18	1.9	600ʲ	2.6	6*	30*	450*
Lactation													
≤18 yr	1200	115	5*	19	1.6	1.6	17	2.0	500	2.8	7*	35*	550*
19-30 yr	1300	120	5*	19	1.6	1.6	17	2.0	500	2.8	7*	35*	550*
31-50 yr	1300	120	5*	19	1.6	1.6	17	2.0	500	2.8	7*	35*	550*

NOTE: This table [taken from the dietary reference intake (DRI) reports; see http://www.nap.edu) presents recommended dietary allowances (RDAs) in **bold type** and adequate intakes (AIs) in ordinary type followed by an asterisk (*). RDAs and AIs may both be used as goals for individual intake. RDAs are set to meet the needs of almost all (97% to 98%) individuals in a group. For healthy breastfed infants, the AI is the mean intake. The AI for other life stage and gender groups is believed to cover needs of all individuals in the group, but lack of data or uncertainty in the data prevent being able to specify with confidence the percentage of individuals covered by this intake.

ᵃ As retinol activity equivalents (RAEs). 1 RAE = 1 μg retinol, 12 μg beta-carotene, 24 μg alpha-carotene, or 24 μg β-cryptoxanthin. The RAE for dietary provitamin A carotenoids is twofold greater than retinol equivalents (RE), whereas the RAE for preformed vitamin A is the same as RE.

ᵇ Cholecalciferol. 1 μg cholecalciferol = 40 IU vitamin D.

ᶜ In the absence of adequate exposure to sunlight.

ᵈ As α-tocopherol. α-Tocopherol includes RRR-α-tocopherol, the only form of α-tocopherol that occurs naturally in foods, and the $2R$-stereoisomeric forms of α-tocopherol (RRR-, RSR-, RRS-, and RSS-α-tocopherol) that occur in fortified foods and supplements. It does not include the $2S$-stereoisomeric forms of α-tocopherol (SRR-, SSR-, SRS-, and SSS-α-tocopherol), also found in fortified foods and supplements.

ᵉ As niacin equivalents (NE). 1 mg niacin = 60 mg tryptophan; 0–6 mo = preformed niacin (not NE).

ᶠ As dietary folate equivalents (DFE). 1 DFE = 1 μg food folate = 0.6 μg folic acid from fortified food or as a supplement consumed with food = 0.5 μg of a supplement taken on an empty stomach.

ᵍ Although AIs have been set for choline, there are few data to assess whether a dietary supply of choline is needed at all stages of the life cycle, and it may be that the choline requirement can be met by endogenous synthesis at some of these stages.

ʰ Because 10% to 30% of older people may malabsorb food-bound B_{12}, it is advisable for those older than 50 yr to meet their RDA mainly by consuming foods fortified with B_{12} or a supplement containing B_{12}.

ⁱ In view of evidence linking folate intake with neural tube defects in the fetus, it is recommended that all women capable of becoming pregnant consume 400 μg from supplements or fortified foods in addition to intake of food folate from a varied diet.

ʲ It is assumed that women will continue consuming 400 μg from supplements or fortified food until their pregnancy is confirmed and they enter prenatal care, which ordinarily occurs after the end of the periconceptional period—the critical time for formation of the neural tube.

SOURCE: Food and Nutrition Board, Institute of Medicine, National Academies. Copyright 2001 by the National Academy of Sciences. All rights reserved.

Table 2-2 Dietary reference intakes: recommended intakes for individuals, elements.

LIFE STAGE GROUP	CALCIUM (mg/d)	CHROMIUM (μg/d)	COPPER (μg/d)	FLUORIDE (mg/d)	IODINE (μg/d)	IRON (mg/d)	MAGNESIUM (mg/d)	MANGANESE (mg/d)	MOLYBDENUM (μg/d)	PHOSPHORUS (mg/d)	SELENIUM (μg/d)	ZINC (mg/d)
Infants												
0–6 mo	210*	0.2*	200*	0.01*	110*	0.27*	30*	0.003*	2*	100*	15*	2*
7–12 mo	270*	5.5*	220*	0.5*	130*	11*	75*	0.6*	3*	275*	20*	3
Children												
1–3 yr	500*	11*	340	0.7*	90	7	80	1.2*	17	460	20	3
4–8 yr	800*	15*	440	1*	90	10	130	1.5*	22	500	30	5
Males												
9–13 yr	1300*	25*	700	2*	120	8	240	1.9*	34	1250	40	8
14–18 yr	1300*	35*	890	3*	150	11	410	2.2*	43	1250	55	11
19–30 yr	1000*	35*	900	4*	150	8	400	2.3*	45	700	55	11
31–50 yr	1000*	35*	900	4*	150	8	420	2.3*	45	700	55	11
51–70 yr	1200*	30*	900	4*	150	8	420	2.3*	45	700	55	11
>70 yr	1200*	30*	900	4*	150	8	420	2.3*	45	700	55	11
Females												
9–13 yr	1300*	21*	700	2*	120	8	240	1.6*	34	1250	40	8
14–18 yr	1300*	24*	890	3*	150	15	360	1.6*	43	1250	55	9
19–30 yr	1000*	25*	900	3*	150	18	310	1.8*	45	700	55	8
31–50 yr	1000*	25*	900	3*	150	18	320	1.8*	45	700	55	8
51–70 yr	1200*	20*	900	3*	150	8	320	1.8*	45	700	55	8
>70 yr	1200*	20*	900	3*	150	8	320	1.8*	45	700	55	8

Pregnancy												
≤18 yr	1300*	29*	1000	3*	220	27	400	2.0*	50	1250	60	13
19–30 yr	1000*	30*	1000	3*	220	27	350	2.0*	50	700	60	11
31–50 yr	1000*	30*	1000	3*	220	27	360	2.0*	50	700	60	11
Lactation												
≤18 yr	1300*	44*	1300	3*	290	10	360	2.6*	50	1250	70	14
19–30 yr	1000*	45*	1300	3*	290	9	310	2.6*	50	700	70	12
31–50 yr	1000*	45*	1300	3*	290	9	320	2.6*	50	700	70	12

NOTE: This table presents recommended dietary allowances (RDAs) in **bold type** and adequate intakes (AIs) in ordinary type followed by an asterisk (*). RDAs and AIs may both be used as goals for individual intake. RDAs are set to meet the needs of almost all (97% to 98%) individuals in a group. For healthy breastfed infants, the AI is the mean intake. The AI for other life stage and gender groups is believed to cover needs of all individuals in the group, but lack of data or uncertainty in the data prevent being able to specify with confidence the percentage of individuals covered by this intake.

SOURCE: *Dietary Reference Intakes for Calcium, Phosphorous, Magnesium, Vitamin D, and Fluoride* (1997); *Dietary Reference Intakes for Thiamin, Riboflavin, Niacin, Vitamin B$_6$, Folate, Vitamin B$_{12}$, Pantothenic Acid, Biotin, and Choline* (1998); *Dietary Reference Intakes for Vitamin C, Vitamin E, Selenium, and Carotenoids* (2000); and *Dietary Reference Intakes for Vitamin A, Vitamin K, Arsenic, Boron, Chromium, Copper, Iodine, Iron, Manganese, Molybdenum, Nickel, Silicon, Vanadium, and Zinc* (2001). These reports may be accessed via *http://www.nap.edu.* Food and Nutrition Board, Institute of Medicine, National Academies.

Table 2-3 Vitamins

Dietary reference intakes: tolerable upper intake levels[a]

LIFE STAGE GROUP	VITAMIN A (μg/d)[b]	VITAMIN C (mg/d)	VITAMIN D (μg/d)	VITAMIN E (mg/d)[c,d]	VITAMIN K	THIAMINE	RIBOFLAVIN	NIACIN (mg/d)[d]	VITAMIN B6 (mg/d)	FOLATE (μg/d)[d]	VITAMIN B12	PANTOTHENIC ACID	BIOTIN	CHOLINE (g/d)	CAROTENOIDS[e]
Infants															
0–6 mo	600	ND[f]	25	ND	ND	ND	ND	ND	ND	ND	ND	ND	ND	ND	ND
7–12 mo	600	ND	25	ND	ND	ND	ND	ND	ND	ND	ND	ND	ND	ND	ND
Children															
1–3 yr	600	400	50	200	ND	ND	ND	10	30	300	ND	ND	ND	1.0	ND
4–8 yr	900	650	50	300	ND	ND	ND	15	40	400	ND	ND	ND	1.0	ND
Males, females															
9–13 yr	1700	1200	50	600	ND	ND	ND	20	60	600	ND	ND	ND	2.0	ND
14–18 yr	2800	1800	50	800	ND	ND	ND	30	80	800	ND	ND	ND	3.0	ND
19–70 yr	3000	2000	50	1000	ND	ND	ND	35	100	1000	ND	ND	ND	3.5	ND
>70 yr	3000	2000	50	1000	ND	ND	ND	35	100	1000	ND	ND	ND	3.5	ND
Pregnancy															
≤18 yr	2800	1800	50	800	ND	ND	ND	30	80	800	ND	ND	ND	3.0	ND
19–50 yr	3000	2000	50	1000	ND	ND	ND	35	100	1000	ND	ND	ND	3.5	ND
Lactation															
≤18 yr	2800	1800	50	800	ND	ND	ND	30	80	800	ND	ND	ND	3.0	ND
19–50 yr	3000	2000	50	1000	ND	ND	ND	35	100	1000	ND	ND	ND	3.5	ND

[a] Upper intake levels (UL) = The maximum level of daily nutrient intake that is likely to pose no risk of adverse effects. Unless otherwise specified, the UL represents total intake from food, water, and supplements. Due to lack of suitable data, ULs could not be established for vitamin K, thiamin, riboflavin, vitamin B12, pantothenic acid, biotin, or carotenoids. In the absence of ULs, extra caution may be warranted in consuming levels above recommended intakes.

[b] As preformed vitamin A only.

[c] As α-tocopherol; applies to any form of supplemental α-tocopherol.

[d] The ULs for vitamin E, niacin, and folate apply to synthetic forms obtained from supplements, fortified foods, or a combination of the two.

[e] Beta-carotene supplements are advised only to serve as a provitamin A source for individuals at risk of vitamin A deficiency.

[f] ND = Not determinable due to lack of data of adverse effects in this age group and concern with regard to lack of ability to handle excess amounts. Source of intake should be from food only to prevent high levels of intake.

Elements

LIFE STAGE GROUP	ARSENIC[b]	BORON (mg/d)	CALCIUM (g/d)	CHROMIUM	COPPER (μg/d)	FLUORIDE (mg/d)	IODINE (μg/d)	IRON (mg/d)	MAGNESIUM (mg/d)[c]	MANGANESE (mg/d)	MOLYBDENUM (μg/d)	NICKEL (mg/d)	PHOSPHORUS (g/d)	SELENIUM (μg/d)	SILICON[d]	VANADIUM (mg/d)[e]	ZINC (mg/d)
Infants																	
0–6 mo	ND[f]	ND	ND	ND	ND	0.7	ND	40	ND	ND	ND	ND	ND	45	ND	ND	4
7–12 mo	ND	ND	ND	ND	ND	0.9	ND	40	ND	ND	ND	ND	ND	60	ND	ND	5
Children																	
1–3 yr	ND	3	2.5	ND	1000	1.3	200	40	65	2	300	0.2	3	90	ND	ND	7
4–8 yr	ND	6	2.5	ND	3000	2.2	300	40	110	3	600	0.3	3	150	ND	ND	12
Males, females																	
9–13 yr	ND	11	2.5	ND	5000	10	600	40	350	6	1100	0.6	4	280	ND	ND	23
14–18 yr	ND	17	2.5	ND	8000	10	900	45	350	9	1700	1.0	4	400	ND	ND	34
19–70 yr	ND	20	2.5	ND	10,000	10	1100	45	350	11	2000	1.0	4	400	ND	1.8	40
>70 yr	ND	20	2.5	ND	10,000	10	1100	45	350	11	2000	1.0	3	400	ND	1.8	40

Elements (continued)

LIFE STAGE GROUP	ARSENIC[b] (mg/d)	BORON (mg/d)	CALCIUM (g/d)	CHROMIUM	COPPER (μg/d)	FLUORIDE (mg/d)	IODINE (μg/d)	IRON (mg/d)	MAGNESIUM (mg/d)[c]	MANGANESE (mg/d)	MOLYBDENUM (μg/d)	NICKEL (mg/d)	PHOSPHORUS (g/d)	SELENIUM (μg/d)	SILICON[d]	VANADIUM (mg/d)[e]	ZINC (mg/d)
Pregnancy																	
≤18 yr	ND	17	2.5	ND	8000	10	900	45	350	9	1700	1.0	3.5	400	ND	ND	34
19–50 yr	ND	20	2.5	ND	10,000	10	1100	45	350	11	2000	1.0	3.5	400	ND	ND	40
Lactation																	
≤18 yr	ND	17	2.5	ND	8000	10	900	45	350	9	1700	1.0	4	400	ND	ND	34
19–50 yr	ND	20	2.5	ND	10,000	10	1100	45	350	11	2000	1.0	4	400	ND	ND	40

[a] UL = The maximum level of daily nutrient intake that is likely to pose no risk of adverse effects. Unless otherwise specified, the UL represents total intake from food, water, and supplements. Due to lack of suitable data, ULs could not be established for arsenic, chromium, and silicon. In the absence of ULs, extra caution may be warranted in consuming levels above recommended intakes.

[b] Although the UL was not determined for arsenic, there is no justification for adding arsenic to food or supplements.

[c] The ULs for magnesium represent intake from a pharmacologic agent only and do not include intake from food and water.

[d] Although silicon has not been shown to cause adverse effects in humans, there is no justification for adding silicon to supplements.

[e] Although vanadium in food has not been shown to cause adverse effects in humans, there is no justification for adding vanadium to food, and vanadium supplements should be used with caution. The UL is based on adverse effects in laboratory animals, and these data could be used to set a UL for adults but not children and adolescents.

[f] ND = Not determinable due to lack of data of adverse effects in this age group and concern with regard to lack of ability to handle excess amounts. Source of intake should be from food only to prevent high levels of intake.

SOURCE: *Dietary Reference Intakes for Calcium, Phosphorous, Magnesium, Vitamin D, and Fluoride* (1997); *Dietary Reference Intakes for Thiamin, Riboflavin, Niacin, Vitamin B₆, Folate, Vitamin B₁₂, Pantothenic Acid, Biotin, and Choline* (1998); *Dietary Reference Intakes for Vitamin C, Vitamin E, Selenium, and Carotenoids* (2000); and *Dietary Reference Intakes for Vitamin A, Vitamin K, Arsenic, Boron, Chromium, Copper, Iodine, Iron, Manganese, Molybdenum, Nickel, Silicon, Vanadium, and Zinc* (2001). These reports can be accessed via *http://www.nap.edu*. Food and Nutrition Board, Institute of Medicine, National Academies. Copyright 2001 by the National Academy of Sciences. All rights reserved.

TABLE 2-4   Fat-soluble vitamin summary.

VITAMINS	METABOLISM/ FUNCTION	DEFICIENCY (D) OR EXCESS (E)	FOOD SOURCES
Vitamin A			
Retinol	• Bile needed for absorption	(D) Reduced bone growth (D) Night blindness (D) Keratomalacia	• Fortified dairy products
Retinal	• Mineral oil prevents absorption	(D) Depressed immunity	
Retinoic acid	• Stored in liver	(D) Severe: drying and scaling of skin; eye infections; blindness (E) Jaundice; spleen enlargement	• Liver, kidney
Provitamin A	• Bone and tooth structure	(E) Overdoses are toxic: skin, hair, and bone changes, petechiae	• Milk, cream, cheese
Carotenes	• Healthy skin and mucous membranes • Vision in dim light		• Dark-green leafy and deep-yellow vegetables • Deep-yellow fruits
Vitamin D	• Some storage in liver • Liver synthesizes calcidiol	(D) Rickets Soft bones	• Fortified milk • Concentrates:

Precursors:
  Ergosterol in plants; 7-dehydrocholesterol in skin
	• Kidney converts calcidiol to calcitriol
	• Functions as hormone in absorption of calcium and phosphorus; mobilization and mineralization of bone
		Enlarged joints
		    Enlarged skull
		    Deformed chest
		    Spinal curvature
		    Bowed leg
		(D) Osteomalacia
		(D) Renal osteodystrophy
		(E) Even small excess is toxic
			calciferol; viosterol
			• Fish-liver oils
			• Exposure to ultraviolet rays of sun

Vitamin E Tocopherols	• Prevents oxidation of vitamin A in intestine • Protects cell membranes against oxidation • Protects red blood cells • Limited stores in body • Polyunsaturated fats increase need	(D) Deficiency not common (D) Red cell hemolysis in malnourished infants (E) Low toxicity (E) Augments effects of anticoagulants	• Salad oils, shortenings, margarines • Whole grains, legumes, nuts, dark leafy vegetables
Vitamin K	• Forms prothrombin for normal blood clotting • Synthesized in intestines	(D) Prolonged clotting time (D) Hemorrhage, especially in newborn infants, and biliary tract disease (E) Large amounts toxic	• Synthesized by intestinal bacteria • Dark-green leafy vegetables

SOURCE: Adapted from: Weigley ES, Muller DH, Robinson CH. *Basic Nutrition and Diet Therapy.* 8th ed. Upper Saddle River, NJ: Prentice Hall, 1997.

TABLE 2-5   Water-soluble vitamin summary.

VITAMINS	METABOLISM/ FUNCTION	DEFICIENCY (D) OR EXCESS (E)	FOOD SOURCES

Ascorbic acid
Vitamin C
	• Form collagen
	• Teeth firm in gums
	• Hormone synthesis
	• Resistance to infection
	• Improve iron absorption
		(D) Poor wound healing
		(D) Poor bone, tooth
		   development
		(D) Scurvy
		   Bruising and
		   hemorrhage
		   Bleeding gums
		   Loose teeth
			• Citrus fruit
			• Strawberries,
			   cantaloupe
			• Tomatoes, broccoli
			• Raw green
			   vegetables
			• Potatoes, peppers

Thiamine
Vitamin B$_1$
	• Coenzyme for breakdown
	   of glucose for energy
	• Healthy nerves
	• Good digestion
	• Normal appetite
	• Good mental outlook
		(D) Beriberi
		   Fatigue
		   Poor appetite
		   Constipation
		   Depression
		   Neuropathy
		   Angular stomatitis
		   Polyneuritis
		   Edema
		   Heart failure/
		   enlarged heart
			• Pork, liver, other
			   meats, poultry
			• Dry beans and
			   peas, peanut butter
			• Enriched and
			   whole-grain bread
			• Milk, eggs

Riboflavin
Vitamin B$_2$
	• Coenzymes for protein
	   and glucose metabolism
	• Fatty acid synthesis
	• Healthy skin
	• Normal vision in bright
	   light
		(D) Cheilosis
		   Scaling skin
		(D) Burning, itching,
		   sensitive eyes
		(D) Magenta tongue
			• Dairy products
			• Meat, poultry, fish
			• Dark-green leafy
			   vegetables
			• Enriched and
			   whole-grain
			   breads, cereals

Niacin
Nicotinic acid
Niacinamide
	• Coenzymes for energy
	   metabolism
	• Normal digestion
	• Healthy nervous system
	• Healthy skin
	• Tryptophan a precursor:
	   60 mg = 1 mg niacin
		(D) Pellagra
		   Dermatitis
		   Angular stomatitis
		   Diarrhea
		   Depression
		   Disorientation
		   Delirium
		(E) Toxicity: flushing,
		   abnormal liver
		   function test
			• Meat, poultry, fish
			• Dark-green leafy
			   vegetables
			• Whole-grain or
			   enriched breads,
			   cereals

Vitamin B$_6$
Pyridoxine
Pyridoxal
Pyridoxamine
	• Coenzymes for protein
	   metabolism
	• Conversion of tryptophan
	   to niacin
	• Formation of heme
		(D) Cheilosis
		(D) GI upsets
		(D) Weak gait
		(D) Irritability
		(D) Neuropathy
		(D) Convulsions
			• Meat
			• Whole-grain
			   cereals
			• Dark-green leafy
			   vegetables
			• Potatoes

TABLE 2-5 (continued)

VITAMINS	METABOLISM/ FUNCTION	DEFICIENCY (D) OR EXCESS (E)	FOOD SOURCES
Vitamin B_{12}	• Formation of mature red blood cells • Synthesis of DNA, RNA • Requires intrinsic factor from stomach for absorption	(D) Pernicious anemia: lack of intrinsic factor, or after gastrectomy (D) Macrocytic anemia: neurologic degeneration, pallor	• Animal foods only: milk, eggs, meat, poultry, fish
Folate Folacin Folic acid	• Maturation of red blood cells • Synthesis of DNA, RNA	(D) Macrocytic anemia in pregnancy, sprue, pallor, NTD	• Dark-green leafy vegetables • Meat, fish, poultry • Eggs • Fortified flour • Whole-grain cereals • Citrus fruit
Biotin	• Components of coenzymes in metabolism • Some synthesis in intestine • Avidin, a protein in raw egg white, interferes with absorption	(D) Occurs only when large amounts of raw egg whites are eaten (D) Dermatitis, loss of hair	• Organ meats • Egg yolk • Legumes • Nuts • Yeast • Mushrooms • Synthesized in GI tract
Pantothenic acid	• Component of coenzyme A • Synthesis of sterols, fatty acids, heme	(D) Occurs rarely (D) Neuritis of arms, legs; burning sensation of feet (D) Vomiting	• Meat, poultry, fish • Legumes • Whole-grain cereals • Lesser amounts in milk, fruits, and vegetables

GI, gastrointestinal; DNA, deoxyribonucleic acid; RNA, ribonucleic acid; NTD, neural tube defect.
SOURCE: Adapted from: Weigley ES, Muller DH, Robinson CH. Basic Nutrition and Diet Therapy. 8th ed. Upper Saddle River, NJ: Prentice Hall, 1997.

and/or illness. A multivitamin and mineral supplement that furnishes 100% of the RDAs should be routinely prescribed for:

• Women of childbearing age
• People on low-calorie diets
• Older adults (>65 years old)
• Physically or mentally challenged individuals

- Those unable to eat a varied diet
- Individuals who choose to eat a restricted array of foods
- Individuals with diagnosed eating disorders or those with other conditions considered high risk, such as alcoholics

Increased Nutrient Requirements

Requirements for the majority of vitamins and minerals increase during pregnancy. Therefore, most pregnant women are now routinely prescribed a prenatal vitamin before and during pregnancy.

Increased Metabolic Demands

Vitamin supplements are also required to meet the increased cellular needs of patients under physiologic stress due to infection, fever, injury, burns, surgery, or chronic disease. Furthermore, recent data suggest that supplements of vitamins C and A and the mineral zinc may improve immune function.

Maldigestion and Malabsorption

Patients with gastrointestinal abnormalities who could benefit from vitamin and mineral supplementation include those with chronic pancreatitis, intractable diarrhea, surgical resection of a portion of the small intestine (short bowel syndrome), cystic fibrosis, sprue, inflammatory bowel disease, or bile duct obstruction.

Food-Nutrient or Nutrient-Nutrient Interactions

In certain cases, one nutrient can alter the bioavailability of another nutrient or foods can reduce absorption of a nutrient. For example, long-term beta-carotene supplementation can reduce serum vitamin E levels.

Treatment-Nutrient Interactions

Medications and medical treatments should always be evaluated for food and nutrient interactions, and all patients receiving such therapies should be considered at risk for iatrogenic vitamin deficiencies. For example, patients with elevated serum cholesterol levels taking bile acid sequestrants may malabsorb fat-soluble vitamins and require supplementation. Some anticonvulsant medications interfere with hepatic synthesis of vitamin D precursors.

Vitamin Excess or Toxicity

Toxic effects of vitamins usually result from food faddism, misuse of supplements, or dosage errors. Individuals who consume large doses of vitamins, whether self-prescribed or medically indicated, need education and close monitoring. Toxicity as a result of excessive vitamin intake is more commonly reported as a result of intake of fat-soluble vitamins. Early symptoms of vitamin A toxicity include cracked lips, headaches, dry rough skin, and alopecia of the eyebrows. Anorexia, nausea, and vomiting may be indicative of vitamin D toxicity. Large doses of B-complex vitamins can produce symptoms ranging from flushing, itching, burning, or tingling sensations (niacin) to progressive sensory ataxia and profound impairment of the lower-limb position and vibration senses (pyridoxine). Usually symptoms disappear when the offending vitamin is withdrawn. Excessive doses of vitamin C have been reported to predispose individuals to oxalate urinary calculi. Vitamin C increases intestinal absorption of iron. If this occurs chronically in an individual who possesses the gene for hemochromatosis, iron overload with resultant liver injury can result.

Finally, intake of certain vitamins can cause erroneous interpretation of therapy outcomes. For example, vitamin C can produce false-negative urine glucose test results in patients with diabetes mellitus as well as false-positive heme tests in stool. Vitamin supplements containing pyridoxine should be avoided by patients taking levodopa to treat Parkinson's disease, because together they form a vitamin-drug complex that makes the drug systemically unavailable.

The National Academy of Sciences is currently evaluating the available data related to vitamin and mineral toxicity. Based on the findings, ULs have been and will continue to be designated for the specific nutrients for which adequate research is available. Currently, ULs have been determined for vitamins A, C, D, E, niacin, vitamin B$_6$, folate, choline, boron, calcium, copper, fluoride, magnesium, molybdenum, nickel, phosphorus, selenium, and zinc. Due to a lack of data, ULs have not been established for vitamin K, thiamine, riboflavin, vitamin B$_{12}$, pantothenic acid, biotin, carotenoids, arsenic, chromium, and silicon (see Table 2-3).

Vitamin Therapy

Several vitamins, in pharmacologic doses, have been used as medical therapy. For example, niacin has been shown to effectively lower serum levels of total cholesterol, low-density lipoprotein (LDL) cholesterol, and triglycerides, while raising high-density lipoprotein (HDL) cholesterol. Patients need to be counseled about possible side effects, such as dyspepsia, peptic ulcer, esophageal reflux, facial flushing, and elevated serum glucose and uric acid levels, as well as liver enzymes. Pharmacologic doses of vitamin A derivatives are a standard component of acne treatment. Monthly injections of supraphysiologic doses of vitamin B$_{12}$ are indicated for patients with a diagnosis of pernicious anemia.

Minerals

Functions and Sources of Minerals

Mineral elements are inorganic substances that occur in simple forms such as sodium chloride (NaCl) or in combination with organic compounds such as the iron in hemoglobin and the sulfur in almost all proteins (Table 2-6). Minerals are classified as macrominerals or microminerals, based on their percentages of total body weight.

TABLE 2-6   Macromineral and micromineral summary.

ELEMENTS	FUNCTION	UTILIZATION, DEFICIENCY (D) OR EXCESS (E)	FOOD SOURCES
Calcium	• 99% in bones, teeth • Nervous stimulation • Muscle contraction • Blood clotting • Activates enzymes	• 10–40% absorbed • Aided by vitamin D and lactose; hindered by oxalic acid • Parathyroid hormone regulates blood levels (D) Fragile bones, osteoporosis (D) Hypertension	• Dairy products • Mustard and turnip greens • Cabbage, broccoli • Clams, oysters, salmon • Fortified foods: juice, rice, cereals
Phosphorus	• 80–90% in bones, teeth • Acid balance • Transport of fats • Enzymes for energy metabolism; protein synthesis	• Vitamin D favors absorption and use by bones (E) Renal disease	• Dairy products • Meat, poultry, fish • Whole-grain cereals, nuts, legumes
Magnesium	• 60% in bones, teeth • Transmits nerve impulses • Muscle contraction • Enzymes for energy metabolism	• Salts relatively insoluble • Acid favors absorption (D) Dietary deficiency unlikely; occurs in alcoholism, renal failure	• Milk • Meat • Green leafy vegetables • Legumes • Whole-grain cereals
Sodium	• Extracellular fluid • Water balance • Acid-base balance • Nervous stimulation • Muscle contraction	• Almost completely absorbed • Body levels regulated by adrenal; excess excreted in urine and by skin (D) Rare; occurs with excessive perspiration (E) Hypertension	• Table salt • Baking powder, baking soda • Milk, eggs • Meat, poultry, fish • Processed, cured, smoked foods
Potassium	• Intracellular fluid • Protein and glycogen synthesis • Water balance • Transmits nerve impulse • Muscle contraction	• Almost completely absorbed • Body levels regulated by adrenal; excess excreted in urine (D) Starvation (D) Diuretic therapy (D) Hypertension	• Ample amounts in meat, cereals, fruits, fruit juices, vegetables • Molasses • Salt substitute
Iron	• Mostly in hemoglobin • Muscle myoglobin	• 5–20% absorption • Acid and vitamin C aid absorption	• Organ meats, meat, fish, poultry

TABLE 2-6 (continued)

ELEMENTS	FUNCTION	UTILIZATION, DEFICIENCY (D) OR EXCESS (E)	FOOD SOURCES
	• Oxidizing enzymes for release of energy	• Daily losses in urine and feces • Menstrual loss (D) Anemia (D) Cheilosis (D) Pallor	• Whole-grain and enriched cereal • Green vegetables • Dried fruits
Iodine	• Forms thyroxine for energy metabolism	• Chiefly in thyroid gland (D) Endemic goiter	• Iodized salt • Shellfish, saltwater fish
Fluoride	• Prevents tooth decay	• Storage in bones and teeth (E) Leads to tooth mottling	• Fluoridated water • Fluoridated toothpaste
Copper	• Utilization of iron for hemoglobin formation • Pigment formation • Myelin sheath of nerves	• In form of ceruloplasmin in blood • Abnormal storage in Wilson's disease (D) Rare	• Liver, meats, shellfish • Nuts, legumes • Whole-grain cereals
Zinc	• Enzymes for transfer of carbon dioxide • Taste, protein synthesis	(D) Growth retardation (D) Altered taste (D) Depressed immunity	• Plant and animal proteins • Oysters
Selenium	• Protects cells from oxidation	(D) Anemia (D) Cardiomyopathy	• Meats • Fish, shellfish • Brazil nuts • Molasses • Wheat germ

SOURCE: Adapted from: Weigley ES, Muller DH, Robinson CH. Basic Nutrition and Diet Therapy. 8th ed. Upper Saddle River, NJ: Prentice Hall, 1997.

Macrominerals constitute more than 0.005% of the body's weight, or 50 parts per million (ppm). Examples include calcium, chloride, phosphorus, potassium, magnesium, sodium, and sulfur.

Microminerals fall into two categories:

• Minerals with identified roles in health maintenance, including chromium, cobalt, copper, fluoride, iodide, iron, manganese, molybdenum, selenium, and zinc

• Minerals with unestablished roles in health maintenance, such as arsenic, boron, cadmium, nickel, silicon, tin, and vanadium

In foods, minerals occur as salts, such as sodium chloride. Because minerals are water soluble, some loss occurs during cooking. The body is capable of storing minerals. Deficiencies, therefore, are less common than for the water-soluble vitamins, which are generally not stored.

Functions of Minerals

Minerals function together for tissue anabolism and catabolism and in the regulation of body metabolism. Examples of their functions include the following.

Bone Formation

Bone consists of a collagen matrix in which minerals are deposited. Most of the body's calcium, phosphorus, and magnesium is deposited in bones and teeth. Bones also store a reservoir of minerals to maintain proper cellular functioning in the event of an intake deficiency. Thus, although minerals are transported via the circulatory system, blood levels of minerals provide limited indication of the actual biochemical flux and body stores of minerals.

Tooth Formation

Tooth enamel and dentine (hydroxyapatite) contain appreciable amounts of calcium and phosphorus. When fluoride is incorporated into the structure, the resulting fluoroapatite is less soluble in an acid medium and therefore more resistant to the development of caries. Because enamel and dentine are not supplied with blood vessels, a decayed tooth cannot repair itself.

Coenzymes and Cofactors

Minerals are constituents of various regulatory compounds. Sulfur is part of the thiamine molecule. Cobalt is present in the vitamin B_{12} molecule. Zinc forms part of carbonic anhydrase. Iodine is present in the thyroxine molecule. Some minerals are cofactors; for example, calcium activates pancreatic lipase. In other instances, minerals catalyze reactions: Copper is needed to incorporate iron into the hemoglobin molecule, and zinc is necessary for the formation of insulin by the pancreas (see Table 2-6).

Cellular Regulation

Exact amounts of sodium, potassium, calcium, and magnesium are necessary to regulate the various cellular pumps and membrane ion channels. These elements control the passage in and out of cells of the materials that regulate the transmission of nerve impulses and muscle contractions (see Table 2-6).

Fluid Balance

Fluid balance between the intracellular and extracellular spaces depends in large part on the concentrations of extracellular sodium and intracellular potassium. Acid-base regulation also involves minerals, especially as buffer salts such as phosphate and sulfate.

Food Sources of Minerals

No single food is the best source for all minerals. Consuming a wide variety of foods usually ensures an adequate and balanced mineral intake. Some minerals are deleted in processing. Iron and chromium, for example, are removed from whole grains during the refining process. As a result, select minerals may be replenished during processing. Refined grains bearing the label "enriched" contain iron added to compensate for the amounts lost during processing. However, other nutrients, such as chromium and zinc, are not routinely replenished.

Sodium, mainly as sodium chloride, is added to numerous foods to enhance their taste and to serve as a preservative. Iodine is added routinely to table salt. Orange juice, cereals, and other foods may be fortified with calcium.

Water contains varying amounts of numerous minerals. Fluoride is present naturally in many water sources, and many municipal water supplies are fluoridated. However, well water may be very low in fluoride. Hard water contains calcium and magnesium. These minerals can be removed via ion exchange with sodium to produce soft water. Water is also a source of iron in some geographic regions.

Recommended Mineral Intakes

The Food and Nutrition Board of the National Research Council has established dietary reference intakes for calcium, magnesium, fluoride, phosphorus, chromium, copper, iodine, iron, manganese, molybdenum, selenium, and zinc (see Table 2-2).

Mineral Deficiency and Therapy

With proper selection from the abundant food and water supplies in the United States, healthy individuals should be able to meet their mineral requirements. Because the bioavailability of minerals varies, recognition of factors favoring or hindering absorption is important. Factors that influence individual needs and bioavailability of nutrients include the following:

Physiologic Need

The amount of a mineral that the body absorbs depends to some extent on its needs. Women and growing children absorb a higher percentage of calcium and iron than do men. Likewise, iron-deficient individuals absorb a higher percentage of ingested iron.

Bioavailability

The term *bioavailability* refers to the amount of an ingested nutrient that is digested and absorbed. Bioavailability differs depending on the chemical form of the mineral. For example, calcium citrate is more bioavailable than calcium carbonate. Supplementation with lower doses of the more bioavailable form will achieve the desired physiologic outcome. Heme iron, found in flesh foods, is more available than the nonheme iron, found in eggs and plant foods. Thus, the iron in meat is more readily absorbed than the iron in raisins.

Intestinal pH

Absorption of minerals occurs at various pH levels, depending on where it takes place in the intestine. The acid medium found in the stomach increases the solubility of calcium and iron salts in food, resulting in increased absorption. People suffering from achlorhydria (absence of acid production in the stomach) or individuals who take antacid medication may be at risk for malabsorption of calcium and iron. Inadequate bicarbonate secretion can also alter mineral absorption.

Nutrient-Nutrient Interactions

- Vitamin C enhances the absorption of calcium, iron, and zinc. Combining iron-containing foods with orange juice in the diet converts the iron in the meat from the ferric to the more absorbable ferrous form.
- Long-term zinc supplementation has been shown to reduce serum copper levels; therefore, patients taking zinc supplements are also advised to increase their copper intake or consider concurrent copper supplementation.
- Calcium supplements have been used therapeutically to reduce undesirable rises in serum phosphorus levels that occur in patients with chronic renal failure.

The most prevalent mineral deficiencies in the United States are iron (iron-deficiency anemia), calcium (osteoporosis), iodine (goiter), and fluoride (dental caries). Because the body stores and reuses minerals, deficiencies may not be detected for years. Causes of primary deficiencies include inadequate intake, malabsorption, and increased losses. Examples are:

- ***Chelating substances:*** Dietary oxalic acid (spinach, green beans, tea), phytic acid (whole grains), and tannins (tea, coffee) bind minerals in such a way that they are poorly absorbed. Certain medications bind directly with minerals. For example, aluminum hydroxide antacids combine with food phosphates, and other antacids bind with bile salts. Hypocholesterolemic agents and aminoglycosides may also cause decreased absorption of iron, calcium, and electrolytes.
- ***Intestinal motility:*** Mineral oil, laxatives, and diarrhea increase motility, thereby decreasing both transit time and the time for absorption of minerals.
- ***Increased intestinal loss:*** Diseases such as Crohn's disease, steatorrhea, or surgical resection of a portion of the small bowel can seriously interfere with the absorption of nutrients. In developing countries, intestinal parasites harbored by many children are a major cause of mineral undernutrition.
- ***Increased urinary loss:*** Excessive alcohol consumption can increase magnesium excretion. Digoxin and glucocorticoids increase urinary losses of calcium, magnesium, potassium, and zinc. Although the desired effect of furosemide and other loop diuretics is to increase sodium and water excretion, they also increase excretion of potassium, calcium, magnesium, and zinc.
- ***Increased loss via perspiration:*** High body and ambient temperatures commonly cause loss of sodium, chloride, potassium, and magnesium and, secondarily, calcium and iron. Classic examples include people experiencing fevers and those exposed to excessive environmental heat, such as athletes, manual laborers, or those living in hot climates.

Mineral Toxicity

Mineral toxicity syndromes resulting from excessive intake of copper, fluoride, iodine, iron, manganese, and selenium are well described. Examples of toxicity include the following:

- Iron overload in children can occur as a result of their taking supplements prescribed for their parents. Milk-alkali syndrome caused by excessive intake of calcium and absorbable alkali may develop in people treated for ulcers. Excessive intake of vitamin D can cause overabsorption of calcium. Lead poisoning may result from storing orange juice or other acidic juices in unglazed ceramic ware or wine in lead crystal carafes. More recently, containers made from these materials carry warning labels to this effect.

• Allergic reactions: Sulfite, used to prevent discoloration of salad bar vegetables and fruits and also as a reducing agent in some alcoholic beverages, can cause life-threatening pulmonary symptoms in people with asthma. A 1987 FDA mandate has restricted sulfite use in the United States and requires food labeling.

Free Radicals and Antioxidants

Free radicals are independent chemical species that have unpaired electrons. The medical importance of free radicals is due to their high reactivity, through which they can denature biomolecules such as proteins, lipids, and nucleic acids, resulting in tissue injury. Potentially harmful oxidative stresses may arise from exogenous sources, such as the diet or environmental pollution, including cigarette smoke and exhaust fumes, or as products of ionizing radiation. Many oxidants are also generated endogenously during normal physiologic processes such as mitochondrial respiration and activation of phagocytes during the immune response. An antioxidant is a natural or synthetic compound that is oxidized very readily and thus spares another compound from being oxidized. An extensive number of antioxidants serve as a defense against oxidative injury in vivo. Examples include enzymes such as superoxide dismutase, catalase, and peroxidases and vitamins such as beta-carotene, vitamin E, and vitamin C. Dietary sources of the antioxidant vitamins are listed in Table 2-7. Antioxidants are naturally present in foods and may also be added to processed foods.

The list of disorders in which free radical–mediated tissue injury has been implicated is extensive (Table 2-8). The direct association of free radicals with any specific toxicity or disease has been difficult to determine mainly due to the difficulty of measuring the ongoing process in vivo. Oxidative injury to nucleic acids, lipids, and proteins is thought to occur over time and may be a significant contributor to atherosclerosis, carcinogenesis, and degenerative diseases. The role of supplemental antioxidants in the prevention or treatment of these entities remains unclear. Antioxidant moieties have been shown in vivo to prevent oxidative damage by trapping or scavenging free radicals or by interrupting a free radical chain reaction. Clinical trials using supplemental antioxidants have shown mixed effects on oxidative damage and repair biomarkers. A major factor limiting progress in this area is the lack of consensus regarding the most appropriate biomarkers of oxidative damage and repair in humans, biologic tissue to be used, timing of sample collection, and variability in marker measures based on sample population.

Vitamin E

Alpha-tocopherol is a lipid-soluble molecule that exists in the lipid bilayer of cell membranes and lipoproteins. Apart from its other important biologic functions,

TABLE 2-7   Dietary sources of antioxidant vitamins.

	SOURCE	SERVING SIZE	AMOUNT (IU)		SOURCE	SERVING SIZE	AMOUNT (mg)
Vitamin A	Apricots, dried	1/2 cup	7085	**Vitamin C**	Acerola	1 cup	3872
	Bran, wheat	1 cup	1650		(Barbados		
	Broccoli, cooked	1 cup	3800		cherry juice)		
	Cantaloupe	1/4	3400		Black currants	1 cup	200
	Carrots, cooked	1 cup	15,750		Broccoli, cooked	1 cup	140
	Carrot, raw	1	11,000		Brussels sprouts	1 cup	135
	Cornflakes	1 cup	1180		Cauliflower	1 cup	69
	Endive, raw	1 cup	1650		Grapefruit	1	76
	Mango	1	11,090		Grapefruit juice	1 cup	95
	Parsley, chopped	1 cup	5100		Guava	1	242
	Peach	1	1330		Lettuce, loose	1 cup	75
	Prunes, dried	1 cup	2580		Mango	1	81
	Spinach, cooked	1 cup	14,580		Mustard greens	1 cup	117
	Squash, winter	1 cup	8610		Orange	1	66
	Tomato, raw	1	1350		Orange juice	6-oz glass	124
	Watermelon	1 slice	3540		Parsley, chopped	1 cup	103
Vitamin E	Almonds	100 g	41		Peppers, green	1 cup	102
	Margarine, hard	100 g	16		Strawberries	1 cup	88
	Margarine, soft	100 g	21		Tomato, raw	1	34
	Mayonnaise	100 g	19		Watermelon	1 slice	42
	Peanut oil	100 g	28				
	Safflower oil	100 g	59				
	Wheat germ oil	100 g	178				
	Soybean oil	100 g	12				
	Sunflower oil	100 g	73				
	Sunflower seeds	100 g	74				

Carotenoids (mcg/100 g portion)

	BETA-CAROTENE	ALPHA-CAROTENE	LUTEIN & ZEAXANTHIN	LYCOPENE	ß-CRYPTOXANTHIN
Orange, raw	51	16	36	—	15
Peaches, raw	97	1	57	0	24
Peas, canned	320	0	1350	0	0
Peppers red, raw	2379	59	—	—	2205
Sweet potato, baked	9488	0	0	0	0
Spinach, cooked	5242	0	7043	0	0
Tomato juice, canned	428	0	60	9318	0
Tomatoes, raw	393	112	130	3025	0
Watermelon	295	0	17	4868	103

Blank value indicates unreported data. Carotenoid contents of selected fruits and vegetables taken from Carotenoids Fact Book, VERIS Research Information Service, 1999.

TABLE 2-8   Clinical conditions in which free radicals are thought to play a role in pathogenesis.

SYSTEM/ORGAN	DISEASE PROCESS	
Cardiovascular	Atherosclerosis	Ethanol/doxorubicin-induced cardiomyopathy
	Reperfusion injury (postinfarct/transplant)	Keshan disease (selenium deficiency)
Brain	Hyperbaric oxygen	Ataxia-telangiectasia syndrome
	Neurotoxins	Aluminum overload
	Senile dementia	Neuronal ceroid lipofuscinosis
	Parkinson's disease	Demyelinating syndromes
	Hypertensive cerebrovascular injury/ cerebral trauma	
Kidney	Autoimmune nephrosis	Aminoglycoside nephrotoxicity
	Heavy metal nephrotoxicity	Renal graft rejection
Liver	Reperfusion injury	Hemochromatosis
	Endotoxin-induced liver injury	Wilson's disease
	CCl_4-induced toxicity	Acetaminophen-induced hepatitis
	Alcohol-induced liver disease	
Lung	Hyperoxic injury	Cigarette smoke
	Bronchopulmonary dysplasia	Asbestosis
	Oxidant pollutants	Emphysema
	Chemicals (paraquat, bleomycin)	ARDS
		Idiopathic pulmonary fibrosis
Skin	Solar/ionizing radiation	Porphyria
	Thermal injury	Contact dermatitis
	Bloom's syndrome	Photosensitive dyes/drugs (tetracyclines)
Eye	Retinopathy of prematurity	Photic retinopathy
	Cataracts	Macular degeneration
Blood	Malaria	Sickle cell disease
	Lead	Favism
	Fanconi's anemia	Drugs (primaquine, sulfonamides, phenylhydrazine)
Multiorgan diseases	Vasculitides	Aging
	Autoimmune diseases	Cancer
	Ischemia—reflow states	Radiation injury
	Drug- and toxin-induced reactions	Amyloid disease
	Nutritional deficiencies (kwashiorkor/ vitamins E and C deficiencies)	

ARDS, acute respiratory disease syndrome.

vitamin E is also considered to be nature's most effective lipid-soluble, chain-breaking antioxidant, protecting cell membranes from peroxidative damage. Inhibiting the propagating step, it is thought to be the first line of defense against lipid peroxidation. Results of clinical trials in patients with cardiovascular disease have varied, with some demonstrating a significant benefit and others showing no benefit, but all used different forms of vitamin E. Eight different forms of vitamin E exist, of which alpha-tocopherol is the form with the most prominent antioxidant activity.

Vitamin C (Ascorbic Acid)

Ascorbic acid is a water-soluble vitamin that provides the first line of defense against free radicals in plasma. It reacts directly with superoxide and hydroxyl radicals and reduces the tocopheroxyl radical back to alpha-tocopherol. The ease with which ascorbic acid can be oxidized has resulted in significant commercial utility, as it is used to prevent oxidation in a wide variety of food products. Its versatility as a free-radical scavenger has led to it being evaluated as an antioxidant in clinical trials. Vitamin C, however, may exhibit pro-oxidant properties in the presence of iron. The relevance of this effect in vivo is not clear, and no benefit has been seen in clinical trials with patients with cardiovascular disease.

Antioxidant Research—The Evidence

Early observations of an association between diet and cardiovascular disease and cancer were made in 1934. Since that time several observational studies have reported an inverse relationship between dietary antioxidant intake and the incidence of both of these entities. Few of these studies made any adjustment for concomitant changes in risk factors such as smoking, exercise, blood pressure, alcohol intake, cholesterol level, or family history. An overview of these studies is presented below.

Observational Studies—Cardiovascular Disease

The Nurses' Health Study is an observational study that addressed the association between vitamin E intake and the incidence of major coronary events over an 8-year period in 87,245 women aged 34 to 59 years. Adjusting for age and smoking status, the risk of a coronary event was significantly lower in the highest quintile of vitamin E intake as compared with those in the lowest quintile. The use of vitamin E supplements for 2 or more years was associated with a decrease in coronary heart disease (CHD) risk of 41%. The final conclusion of the observational study was that, although the data do not prove a cause-and-effect relationship, the use of vitamin E supplements in middle-aged women is associated with a reduced risk of CHD.

Intervention Studies—Cardiovascular Disease

Several studies have shown that dietary supplements of vitamin E inhibit the oxidative modification of LDL in vitro. Oxidation of the LDL cholesterol molecule is thought to be an essential step in the atherogenic process. The oxidizability of LDL cholesterol ex vivo is reportedly enhanced in men with an increased risk for development of atherosclerosis such as diabetics, smokers, and patients with CHD. Taken together, these data have suggested that vitamin E may play an important direct role in reducing the risk of developing atherosclerosis. However, the only definitive prospective data concerning a protective role for vitamin E in the prevention of atherosclerosis are from the Cambridge Heart Antioxidant

Study (CHAOS), in which administration of 400 IU vitamin E per day to 2002 men with known heart disease resulted in a 35% reduction in cardiovascular death and nonfatal myocardial infarction. In contrast, the Heart Outcomes Prevention Evaluation (HOPE) study found that 400 IU vitamin E did not affect cardiovascular outcomes in 10,000 subjects at high risk for coronary events. However, a different form of vitamin E was used, calling into question comparisons with the CHAOS study.

Observational Studies—Cancer

Carcinogenesis is considered to be a multistage process involving the steps of initiation, promotion, and progression of disease. The antitumorigenic effect of antioxidants was first described in 1934, when wheat germ oil was found to prevent tar carcinoma in mice, this effect being tentatively attributed to vitamin E in the oil. Subsequently, dietary vitamin E was shown to prevent artificially induced subcutaneous sarcomas. Several epidemiologic studies indicate that a diet rich in vegetables and fruits lowers the incidence of cancer in humans. In a review of 172 published studies, it was apparent that the quarter of the population with low dietary intake of fruits and vegetables had twice the cancer rate of those with high intake. A recent review by Van Poppel reported that 11 of 15 studies carried out in different countries around the world reported a significant inverse association of carotenoid intake and the risk of cancer. It is important to note that observational studies have generally focused on dietary sources of antioxidants, whereas interventional studies evaluated supplementation.

Intervention Studies—Cancer

The Nutrition Intervention Trial, designed to determine if antioxidant supplementation reduces the incidence of cancer, reported a 9% overall reduction in mortality in those subjects receiving (beta-)carotene, vitamin E, and selenium supplements. The risk reduction was significant after 2 years of supplementation. The mortality from stomach cancer was reduced by 41%, and for prostate cancer the reduction in incidence approached 60%. However, given that the primary endpoint for this research was skin cancer, a follow-up study to test the hypothesis that selenium supplementation may reduce prostate cancer risk is currently under way.

Summary

Oxygen free radicals have been implicated in a wide variety of disease processes. Targets for free-radical attack include lipids, protein, and deoxyribonucleic acid (DNA). The role of oxidant stress in the evolution of disease is unclear, in part due to the limitation of current methodology to assess free-radical generation in vivo. Despite the suggestion from observational studies that antioxidant vitamins play a beneficial role in cancer and cardiovascular disease, intervention data do not uniformly confirm this effect. It may be that the anticarcinogenic effect seen with some diets may be attributable to some active ingredient other than vitamins. Examples of such compounds include flavonoids, phenols, indoles, and isothiocyanates. The results from the observational studies may in fact reflect a healthier lifestyle in those who consume antioxidants. They may also reflect a very prolonged antioxidant intake, whereas the intervention trials to date have been no longer than 8 years. In addition, a consensus has yet to be reached on the optimum dose of antioxidant vitamins required to demonstrate maximum effect. The conflicting nature of the published data reinforces the need to avoid making premature recommendations with respect to the benefits of antioxidant supplementation in the prevention or treatment of disease, or both.

Phytochemicals

Phytochemicals are naturally occurring compounds found in foods of plant origin. Evidence has shown that those who consume a diet rich in fruits and vegetables, and thus phytochemicals, have a lower incidence of certain types of cancers and heart disease. Phytochemicals have been proposed to protect cells from cancer or coronary artery disease, or both, as well as other illnesses, such as urinary tract infections, rheumatoid arthritis, or immune suppressive states, through a variety of mechanisms. Table 2-9 provides a brief summary of some of the key phytochemicals under investigation, their food sources, and their potential protective role in health promotion and disease prevention. Encouraging data come from the study of the role of genistein isolated from soybeans. This compound has been shown to have antitumorigenic properties that prevent the formation of new capillaries that are necessary for tumor growth and metastasis. However, the presence of phytoestrogens in soy foods precludes advising their intake to patients previously treated for breast cancer, as they have been shown to stimulate the growth of breast tumors in animals. Other promising phytochemical-rich foods include but are not limited to fish rich in omega-3 fatty acids; cruciferous vegetables rich in isothiocyanates; garlic and onions, which are high in allylic sulfides; and grapes and most berries, which are rich in anthocyanines.

Further research needs to be completed to better understand how and to what extent these protective chemicals may reduce the incidence and prevalence of disease. The experimental and animal data for the chemopreventive and cardioprotective effects for many of the phytochemicals are impressive. However, well-designed clinical trials to determine the efficacy in humans remain scarce. Human studies need to be controlled for other variables, such as total fat consumption, alcohol use, dietary supplement use, and exercise. This growing area of research will be a significant focus for nutrition research as we continue to develop effective strategies for reducing the two leading causes of death in the United States—coronary artery disease and cancer. The best advice to give individuals is to eat a varied diet including the recommended five or more servings of fruits and vegetables daily that include a wide range of food colors in order to consume a variety of vitamins, minerals, and phytochemicals.

Conclusion

The debate on whether Americans should be taking supplements continues. Clearly, dietary supplements have a role in health maintenance and disease prevention for certain individuals as previously described. More is not necessarily

TABLE 2-9 Phytochemicals and disease prevention.

PHYTOCHEMICAL	FOOD SOURCE(S)	CLINICAL SIGNIFICANCE
Alpha-linoleic acid	Flaxseed, soy, walnuts	• Reduces inflammation • Lowers blood cholesterol • May protect against breast cancer • Enhanced immunity
Beta-carotene	Green and yellow fruits and vegetables	• Reduces risk of cataracts, coronary artery disease, lung and breast cancers • Enhanced immunity (elderly)
Capsaicin	Chili peppers	• Reduces risk for colon, gastric, and rectal cancer • Inhibits tumor promotion
Catechin (theaflavines, thearubigins)	Green and black tea, berries	• Reduces risk of gastric cancer • Antioxidant • Increased immune function • Decreased cholesterol production
Curcumin	Turmeric, curry, cumin	• Lowers cholesterol (?) • Reduces risk of skin cancer
Cynarin	Artichoke	• Decreases cholesterol levels
Ellagic acid	Wine, grapes, currants, nuts (pecans), berries (strawberries, blackberries, raspberries, seeds)	• Reduces cancer risk • Inhibits carcinogen binding to DNA • Reduces LDL cholesterol while increasing HDL cholesterol
Flavonols (polyphenols: catechin, theaflavin, EGCG)	Green and black tea	• Protection against chemically induced cancers, esophageal cancer (?), skin cancer • Antitumor promoters • Inhibit nitrosamine formation • Inhibit phase I and enhance phase II enzyme activity
Genistein	Soybean	• Reduces risk of hormone-dependent cancers • Alters hormone levels • Inhibits angiogenesis • Promotes differentiation • Reduces cholesterol levels • Reduces thrombi formation • Reduces osteoporosis • Reduces menopausal symptoms
Indoles	Cabbage, broccoli, Brussels sprouts, spinach, watercress, cauliflower, turnip, kohlrabi, kale, rutabaga, horseradish, mustard greens	• Reduce risk of hormone-related cancers • May "inactivate" estrogen • Increase glutathione-*S*-transferase activity • Inhibit growth of transformed cells

TABLE 2-9   (continued)

PHYTOCHEMICAL	FOOD SOURCE(S)	CLINICAL SIGNIFICANCE
Isothiocyanates Sulforaphane	Cabbage, cauliflower, broccoli and broccoli sprouts, Brussels sprouts, mustard greens, horseradish, radish	• Reduced risk of tobacco-induced tumors • Inhibit tobacco-related carcinogens from binding DNA • Induce phase II enzymes • Inhibit cP450 activation of carcinogens
Lignans	High-fiber foods, especially seeds	• Reduce risk of colon cancer • Reduce blood glucose and cholesterol • Antioxidant
Lycopene Carotenoid	Tomato sauce, catsup, red grapefruit, guava, dried apricots, watermelon, fresh tomato, red corn (?)	• Reduces risk of prostate cancer • May reduce cardiovascular disease
Monoterpene Limonene	Citrus (peel, membrane), mint, caraway, thyme, coriander	• Antioxidant • Reduces cancer risk (skin, breast) • Inhibits p21ras (G protein) • Suppresses HMG-CoA • Induces apoptosis (?) • Reduces cholesterol production • Reduces premenstrual symptoms
Organosulfur compounds Allylic acid	Garlic, onion, watercress, cruciferous vegetables, leeks	• Decrease lipid peroxidation • Reduce risk of gastric, colon, and lung cancers • Inhibit tumor promotion through inhibition of DNA adduct formation • Induce phase II enzymes • Antithrombotic • Reduce cholesterol • Reduce blood pressure • Antimicrobial
Polyacetylene	Parsley, carrots, celery	• Decreases risk for tobacco-induced tumors • Alters prostaglandin formation
Quercitrin	Pear skin, apple skin, bell pepper, kohlrabi, tomato leaves, onion, wine, grape juice	• Flavonoid • Anticancer • Antioxidant • Associated with reduced CHD • Decreases platelet aggregation
Phenolic acid	Cruciferous vegetables, eggplant, peppers, tomatoes, celery, parsley, soy, licorice root, flaxseed, citrus, whole grains, berries	• Inhibits cancer through inhibition of nitrosamine formation • Reduces risk for lung and skin cancers

DNA, deoxyribonucleic acid; LDL, low-density lipoprotein; HDL, high-density lipoprotein; HMG-CoA, 3-hydroxy-3-methylglutaryl–coenzyme A; CHD, coronary heart disease.
SOURCE: Reprinted with permission. Cyndi Thomson, PhD, RD, 1998.

better and, in fact, can be detrimental. Table 2-10 provides a list of populations at risk and the supplements that are of likely benefit. Several health care organizations such as the American Dietetic Association and the American Medical Association have practice guidelines for the use and sale of dietary supplements.

TABLE 2-10   Patient populations that benefit from supplements.

PATIENT POPULATION	SUPPLEMENT	DOSE
AIDS	Folic acid	400 μg
	Vitamin B$_{12}$	100–1000 μg
	Vitamin C	250–500 mg
	Selenium	200 μg
Anemia		
Iron deficiency	Iron	18 mg as tolerated
	Vitamin C	125–250 mg
Low B$_{12}$ and/or folate	B$_{12}$	10 μg
	Folic acid	400 μg
Alcohol abusers	Folic acid	400 μg
	Thiamine	100–400 mg
Coronary artery disease	Vitamin E	400–800 IU
Hyperhomocysteinemia	Folic acid	400–1000 μg
Elderly	Calcium	1200 mg
	Vitamin D	400 mg
Osteoporosis	Calcium	1200–1500 mg
	Vitamin D (low sun exposure)	400 IU
Chronic renal failure	Folic acid	1 g
	Vitamin C	100 mg
	Pyridoxine (B$_6$)	5–10 mg
Vegetarians	Calcium	800 mg
	Iron	10 mg
	Vitamin B$_{12}$	10 μg
	Zinc	10 mg
Wound healing	Vitamin A	800 μg
	Vitamin C	250–500 mg
	Zinc	10–25 mg

AIDS, acquired immunodeficiency syndrome.

For a list of references for this chapter, please visit the University of Pennsylvania School of Medicine's Nutrition Education and Prevention Program web site: *http://www.med.upenn.edu/nutrimed/articles.html*

Case 1

Iron Deficiency in Women

Elizabeth Ross and Lisa Hark

Objectives

- Describe the prevalence of and risk factors for iron deficiency in US women.
- Recognize signs and symptoms of iron deficiency.
- Evaluate and interpret laboratory values used to diagnose iron deficiency.
- Become familiar with methods for prevention and treatment of iron deficiency.

LH, a 36-year-old editor, presents to her family physician complaining of fatigue. She reports increasing fatigue over the past year and complains of "always being cold." One year ago, she gave birth to a full-term healthy baby. She initially assumed that her symptoms were due to the demands of caring for her infant but reports that her fatigue is much greater in severity than that experienced after delivering her first child 7 years ago. She had been an avid runner throughout her adult years but has been unable to run even a mile over the last few months due to overwhelming fatigue. She feels a lack of energy throughout the day and has difficulty focusing while at work.

LH has a history of heavy menses; she typically uses more than five sanitary pads on each of the first 2 days of her period, which lasts for 7 days. She resumed menstruating 4 months after giving birth. She occasionally has small amounts of blood in her stool from hemorrhoids but has not had any frank gastrointestinal (GI) bleeding and denies other sources of blood loss.

Past Medical History

LH has a recent history of iron-deficiency anemia. At 6 months' gestation, routine hemoglobin screening revealed a normal value of 12.5 g/L. One month after giving birth, LH's hemoglobin was tested by her gynecologist, revealing a significantly reduced level of 7.4 g/dL. Iron-deficiency anemia was suspected. Her laboratory results confirmed the diagnosis, and LH's gynecologist prescribed ferrous sulfate (325 mg three times per day) for 6 months. Unfortunately, LH found that the iron supplements caused constipation and abdominal pain. She discontinued them and began taking a multivitamin containing iron.

Diet History

LH avoids red meat due to its saturated fat content and eats chicken and fish about once a week each. In an effort to increase the calcium in her diet, she reports that she generally tries to eat a dairy food at each meal, milk with cereal for breakfast, yogurt and fruit at lunch, and cheese with pasta or in a casserole for dinner. She obtains most of her vegetable intake from salads containing lettuce, cucumbers, and tomatoes. She does not each much fruit.

Physical Examination

Vital Signs

Temperature: 98.6°F (37°C)
Heart rate: 80 beats per minute (BPM)
Respiration: 26 BPM
Blood pressure: 110/60 mm Hg
Height: 5'8" (173 cm)
Current weight: 145 lb (65.8 kg)
Body mass index (BMI): 24 kg/m^2

Examination

General: Pallor
Conjunctiva: Pale
Nails: No spoon nails

Laboratory Data

Current Laboratory Values	Normal Values
Hemoglobin: 9.5 mg/dL	12–16 g/dL
Hematocrit: 35%	37–48%
Reticulocyte count: 0.2%	0.5–1.5% of erythrocytes
Mean corpuscular volume (MCV): 82 fL	86–98 fL
Ferritin, serum: 7 ng/mL	Females: 12–150 ng/mL
Iron, serum: 40 μg/dL	50–150 μg/dL
TIBC: 425 μg/dL	250–370 μg/dL

Case Questions

1. What are the prevalence of and risk factors for iron-deficiency anemia in premenopausal women?

2. How was the diagnosis of iron-deficiency anemia confirmed in this patient?

3. What are the signs and symptoms of iron deficiency?

4. What questions should be asked of patients suspected of having iron deficiency? How would you counsel this patient to improve her dietary iron intake and absorption?

5. How should iron deficiency be treated?

Case Answers

1. **What are the prevalence of and risk factors for iron-deficiency anemia in premenopausal women?**

   Iron deficiency is a fairly prevalent problem in premenopausal women. According to the National Health and Nutrition Examination Survey (NHANES) III data (1994–1998), 5% of women aged 20 to 49 have iron-deficiency anemia and 11% have iron deficiency without anemia. The prevalence of iron deficiency among females of childbearing age has increased from 1979 to 1996.

   Risk for iron deficiency is a function of levels of iron loss, iron intake, iron absorption, and physiologic demands. Women in their childbearing years have greater iron needs than men because of menstrual blood losses, iron demands of the developing fetus during pregnancy, and blood loss during childbirth. Uterine fibroids may cause heavy and prolonged menses, leading to increased blood loss. In order to avoid the development of iron deficiency during this time, dietary iron intake must keep pace with increased demands. Those not consuming adequate quantities of iron-rich foods may be at risk for iron deficiency. According to the *USDA Survey of Food Intakes by Individuals* from 1994 to 1997, only one-fourth of all females of childbearing age (12 to 49 years) meet the US RDA for iron (15 mg) through their diets.

   Iron deficiency in women (and in men) may also be caused by other sources of blood loss, including frequent blood donation, gastrointestinal bleeding, neoplasms, inflammatory bowel disease, parasitic infections (more common in third-world populations than in developed countries), and hemorrhoids. Chronic blood loss may occur from the urinary tract as well.

   In this case, LH's heavy menstrual periods and aspects of her dietary intake (see answer to #4, below) increase her risk for iron deficiency. Occasional bleeding from hemorrhoids is most likely not a contributing factor.

2. **How was the diagnosis of iron-deficiency anemia confirmed in this patient?**

   Laboratory evaluation along with physical signs and symptoms can confirm a diagnosis of iron deficiency. Serum ferritin, iron, and total iron-binding capacity (TIBC) were outside the normal reference range. A complete blood count revealed a microcytic anemia with a low mean corpuscular volume (MCV) of 82 fL. Serum ferritin was low at 7 mg/mL. Serum iron was low at 40 μg/dL, and total TIBC was high at 425 μg/dL. In this patient, serum ferritin and iron levels were low, and

TIBC was high, confirming the diagnosis of iron deficiency. The patient's hemoglobin, hematocrit, and MCV were low, indicating a microcytic anemia, and reticulocyte count was low, indicating decreased red blood cell production.

Serum ferritin is the single best noninvasive measure of iron status. Serum ferritin concentrations reflect body iron stores (1 μg serum ferritin concentration is equivalent to approximately 10 mg stored iron). Compared to the gold standard of a bone marrow biopsy, serum ferritin is a sensitive and specific indicator of iron depletion. Levels below 15 mg/mL are 75% sensitive and 98% specific for iron deficiency. However, because serum ferritin is an acute-phase reactant, chronic infection, inflammation, or diseases causing tissue and organ damage can raise its concentration independent of iron status masking depleted tissue stores.

Transferrin saturation (which is equivalent to serum iron concentration divided by the TIBC × 100) reflects the extent to which iron-binding sites are vacant on transferring. It is another commonly used measure of iron deficiency. Overall, the measure does not perform as well as ferritin. Like ferritin, factors other than iron status can affect results of this test. Serum iron varies diurnally (higher in the a.m., lower in the p.m.), increases after meals, and is decreased by infection and inflammation. Inflammation, chronic infection, malignancies, liver disease, nephrotic syndrome, and malnutrition can reduce TIBC and oral contraceptive use, and pregnancy can increase it.

Iron deficiency often exists without anemia, but deficiency without anemia will progress to anemia if causes of deficiency are not corrected. Red blood cells are small, or microcytic, due to insufficient hemoglobin production, and numbers of new red blood cells, or reticulocyte counts, are low, indicating decreased bone marrow production of red blood cells.

In the presence of an inflammatory or infectious state when iron deficiency risk factors or symptoms of iron deficiency are present but ferritin is in the normal range, a complete blood count (CBC) and a reticulocyte count may be quite helpful. If iron deficiency is indeed present, erythrocyte indices should improve with iron administration, and a therapeutic trial of supplementation will help to confirm or rule out iron deficiency.

3. **What are the clinical signs and symptoms of iron deficiency?**

Fatigue is a common presentation of iron deficiency with or without anemia. Iron is necessary for hemoglobin synthesis in red blood cells, which functions in oxygen transport and delivery from the lungs to the tissues. Iron deficiency can lead to fatigue by interfering with this process. In addition, iron serves as a coenzyme for many physiologically important enzymes, including those involved in oxidative metabolism, dopamine and DNA synthesis, and free-radical formation in neutrophils.

Iron deficiency may cause a sensation of feeling cold and affect work capacity and exercise tolerance, neurotransmitter function, and immunologic and inflammatory defenses. Other symptoms of iron deficiency include cold intolerance, pica (compulsive eating of nonfood items), and pagophagia (compulsive eating of ice). Signs of iron deficiency on physical examination include pallor, pale conjunctiva, and spoon nails. Patients having any of these signs and symptoms should receive a laboratory evaluation for iron deficiency.

4. **What diet history questions should be asked of patients suspected of having iron deficiency? How would you counsel this patient to improve her dietary iron intake and absorption?**

In evaluating a patient for iron deficiency, the clinician should inquire about dietary intake of iron-rich foods, as well as dietary factors that may influence the absorption of iron (i.e., vitamin C intake). In American diets, major contributors to iron intakes are red meat, poultry, fish and shellfish, nuts and seeds, legumes and bean products, green leafy vegetables, raisins, whole grains, and fortified cereals.

Iron absorption is not directly correlated to iron intake. As physiologic iron levels decrease, gastrointestinal absorption of iron increases. The bioavailability of iron, or the percentage of dietary iron absorbed and ultimately physiologically available, also varies depending on the dietary source of the iron and other foods consumed at the same time as the iron-containing foods. Heme (dietary iron attached to hemoglobin) and nonheme iron are absorbed by different receptors on the intestinal mucosa. Iron bound to heme is highly absorbable, and 40% of iron from animal sources is in this form. The absorption of nonheme iron can be increased or decreased by various factors. Phytates, or inositol phosphate salts that store minerals in plant matter, bind iron in the lumen of the intestine and decrease its absorption. Polyphenols in tea, coffee, cocoa, spinach, and oregano inhibit iron absorption as well.

Iron is best absorbed in its ferrous form, and thus reducing substances, such as ascorbic acid in fruits, vegetables, and fortified cereals, increase iron absorption. Calcium inhibits the absorption of both heme and nonheme iron by an unknown mechanism, and epidemiologic studies show a correlation between intake of milk and prevalence of iron deficiency. Patients should also be asked about their dairy intakes. Those who eat dairy products or take calcium supplements or Tums at each meal may be at risk for iron deficiency.

In this case, dietary factors contributing to LH's ongoing iron deficiency include her avoidance of red meat and her intake of dairy products with each meal. One of the easiest ways for her to increase her dietary iron would be to add red meat to her diet at least on a weekly basis and to increase her consumption of chicken. She could also be counseled to eat iron-rich grains and vegetables at two meals a day with fruits and to eat iron-fortified foods, such as oatmeal and breakfast cereal.

5. **How should iron deficiency be treated?**

A ferritin of less than 15 mg/mL is indicative of suboptimal iron stores, and patients with levels in this range should receive a course of replacement therapy. Iron is best absorbed in its ferrous form, and ferrous salts of iron are generally used for oral supplementation. Ferrous sulfate, succinate, lactate, fumarate, glycine sulfate, glutamate, and gluconate are all about equally well absorbed and tolerated. Standard doses are 50 to 60 mg oral elemental iron twice a day. Vitamin C taken concurrently with the iron increases absorption. Constipation and gastrointestinal distress are common side effects of oral supplementation. In the event that these symptoms occur, the dose should be reduced by one half and oral supplementation continued. Enteric coated or delayed-release preparations should not be used; with these preparations iron is released distally in the small intestine or in the colon, where it is not well absorbed.

Parenteral administration is sometimes necessary in cases of intolerance of oral supplements. The most commonly used parenteral preparation is iron dextran (50 mg elemental iron per milliliter), which is most often given intravenously. Other intravenous preparations, such as iron sucrose, iron saccharate, and sodium ferric gluconate, are becoming more widely used and may be better tolerated than iron dextran. The most serious side effect of parenteral iron is anaphylaxis. For this reason, small test doses (25 mg iron dextran) should be administered and the patient observed in a controlled setting for 1 hour before full doses are administered for the first time. With iron dextran, a delayed reaction can be seen 24 to 48 hours after administration and can include symptoms such as arthralgias, backache, chills, dizziness, fevers, headache, malaise, myalgia, nausea, and vomiting. Symptoms generally subside within a week. This syndrome is most common in settings in which a total replacement dose is administered during a single infusion and is less likely if smaller doses are given on separate occasions.

Intramuscular administration of iron dextran may cause local skin site reactions and potentially carry a risk of carcinogenesis at the injection site. It is not recommended by these authors.

A 3-month course of oral therapy is recommended for the treatment of iron deficiency. In the presence of anemia, reticulocyte counts will begin to rise after a few days of supplementation and will peak in approximately 7 days. Hemoglobin will begin to rise after 10 to 14 days and will generally normalize in 2 months. Some hematologists recommend continuing supplementation for 6 to 12 months; however, as iron status improves, a lower proportion of the supplement dose is absorbed, and the benefits of supplementation are thus reduced as the course of therapy is lengthened. During therapy, patients should be monitored carefully for adherence because side effects are common.

During the course of supplementation, patients should be advised concerning diets higher in iron-containing foods and given advice to optimize absorption. Patients with sources of ongoing physiologic blood loss, such as heavy menses, may require continuous low-dose supplementation, such as an iron-containing multivitamin, after a full course of supplementation is complete.

Correctable causes of blood loss should be addressed while replacement therapy is administered. In settings such as this case, when heavy menses are a cause of iron deficiency, low-dose oral contraceptives may also be helpful to reduce menstrual flow.

See Chapter Review Questions, pages A-10 to A-12.

3

Herbal Medicine

Michael D. Cirigliano

> **Objectives***
>
> - List the most common herbal remedies used by patients seen in clinical practice.
> - Identify the potential drug-herb interactions and clinical toxicities associated with the use of popular herbal remedies.
> - Define common guidelines for the successful integration of herbal remedies into clinical practice.

Interest in the use of "natural" compounds, and herbal remedies in particular, has led to a renaissance of herbal use in the United States over the past decade despite concern within the medical community. Herbal sales during the first quarter of 1998 increased by more than 100% compared to the previous year. However, several recent scientific studies have failed to show statistically significant clinical benefit for a number of herbal remedies that were once held in high regard.

Integration of Herbal Remedies in Clinical Practice

The use of guidelines is necessary to assist the clinician in making rational decisions, especially in circumstances in which limited data are available, to assure patient safety. Basic guidelines do exist for using herbal treatments in the clinical setting (Table 3-1).

It is essential that health care professionals become knowledgeable regarding the use of "natural" products, especially herbal treatments. When herbal treatments are discussed in the office, the patient is less likely to rely on often

---

* SOURCE: Objectives for chapter and cases adapted from the *NIH Nutrition Curriculum Guide for Training Physicians* (*http://www.nhlbi.nih.gov/funding/training/naa*).

Table 3-1   Guidelines for the use of herbal remedies in clinical practice.

- All patients should be asked about use of herbal therapies and dietary supplements.
- "Natural" does not necessarily mean safe.
- Herbal/pharmaceutical interactions do occur; therefore know the literature and avoid interactions.
- Lack of standardization of herbal agents may result in variability among manufacturers in herbal content and efficacy.
- Lack of quality control and regulation may result in contamination during manufacture and potential misidentification of plant species.
- Herbal treatments should not be used if the patient is contemplating pregnancy or during pregnancy or lactation because of lack of long-term clinical trials proving safety.
- Herbal treatments should not be used in dosages higher than those recommended.
- Herbal treatments with known adverse effects and toxic effects should be avoided.
- Infants and children should not use herbal treatments. Elderly patients should exercise caution and be closely monitored.
- An accurate diagnosis and discussion of proven treatment options are essential before considering herbal treatments.
- Adverse effects should be documented in the patient's chart, therapy discontinued, and the Food and Drug Administration notified using MedWatch (FAX #1-800-FDA-0178).
- Clinicians should maintain Continuing Medical Education (CME) in herbal supplementation or develop professional relationships with competent health care providers to which patients can be referred.
- Maintain appropriate resources, including such items as *PDR for Herbal Medicine*, *German Commission E Report*, and *Pharmacist's Letter Natural Medicine's Comprehensive Database.*

SOURCE: Adapted from Cirigliano M, Sun A. Advising patients about herbal therapies. JAMA 1998;280:1565–1566.

erroneous information gleaned from friends, family, or the Internet. An environment that fosters open and candid discussions regarding alternative medicine, as well as other issues related to health, is central to ascertaining a complete understanding of the patient's medication use. Although randomized, controlled clinical trials for many herbal remedies are unfortunately lacking, scientific data are mounting in evidence-based medicine that can guide practitioners. Given the fact that many herbal treatments have the potential to interact with standard pharmaceutical agents resulting in untoward consequences, and the reality that providers will continue to be approached by patients for advice, dialogue with patients regarding use should be part of every office visit and hospital history and physical examination.

St. John's wort (SJW) in particular has been found to interact with many standard pharmaceutical agents, including oral contraceptives, antiretroviral agents such as indinavir, and immunosuppressants including cyclosporine. These reports may have contributed to a recent decrease in sales in the United States.

Herbal treatments are considered dietary supplements and not drugs; thus, premarket testing and studies on safety and efficacy are not required. Not only is there concern for patient safety, but medical and legal issues may arise. In many cases however, this decision is the patient's. The health care provider must then decide what to recommend to a patient who expressed the desire to use an herbal remedy in place of conventional pharmacologic agents. Eisenberg has published guidelines that serve as a valuable resource for practitioners. He advises patients and clinicians to be aware that, because of the lack of adequate information on efficacy and toxicity, advice about herbal products will remain imperfect and a matter of judgment. Advice based on available knowledge should be given in such a fashion that is congruent with the patient's personal needs and in the physician's best judgment. Responsible use of herbal treatments requires knowledge of the dosage, indications and contraindications, side effects, and potential drug-herb interactions. More studies of herbal treatments using sound investigational methodology are appearing in respected peer-reviewed journals. Although generally not applicable to acute care, herbal remedies add to the existing armamentarium of therapeutic options available to the clinician.

Many in the medical profession have likened herbal remedies to nothing more than placebos at best and potentially dangerous agents at worst. Despite sparse scientific data regarding many herbal treatments, patients may believe in the concept that "if it's natural, it must be safe."

Herbal Remedies: Patient Assessment

It is of utmost importance that all patients seen by health care providers be queried regarding the use of all forms of alternative or complementary therapies. This may prevent potential drug-herb interactions and allows the health care provider to assess whether supplements taken are beneficial. During these discussions, patients should also be made aware of the fact that just because something is natural, there is no guarantee of safety.

Drug-herb interactions do occur (Table 3-2), and recent evidence suggests that identifying such interactions will increase significantly over the next decade as patient use of herbal remedies and practitioner awareness of such use grows. One of the more significant interactions involves agents that have antiplatelet

Table 3-2   Selected drug-herb interactions.

HERB AND DRUG	RESULTS OF INTERACTION
Dong quai/warfarin	Increased INR and bruising
Siberian ginseng/digoxin	Raised digoxin concentrations
Garlic/warfarin	Increased INR
Ginkgo biloba/ASA/warfarin	Spontaneous bleeding
Ginseng/warfarin	Decreased INR
St. John's wort/SSRIs/OCPs/ indinavir/cyclosporine	Serotonin syndrome/Decreased serum drug levels
Yohimbine/tricyclic antidepressants	Hypertension

INR, International Normalized Ratio; ASA, acetylsalicylic acid;
SSRIs, serotonin reuptake inhibitors; OCPs, oral contraceptive pills.
SOURCE: Adapted from Fugh-Berman A. Herb-drug interactions.
Lancet 2000;355:134–138.

activity. These agents, when combined with warfarin (Coumadin) or nonsteroidal anti-inflammatory drugs (NSAIDs), have been associated with anticoagulation and delayed prothrombin and partial thromboplastin time (PT/PTT). Certainly, patients undergoing surgery should be counseled on the risks of these agents preoperatively, and they should be discontinued at least 2 weeks before surgery. Frequent measurements of the PT/PTT may be necessary for patients reporting use of these agents to avoid complications.

Standardization of Herbal Treatments

Although in traditional medicine we have become accustomed to using pharmaceutical agents that are continuously monitored to guarantee the same strength and high quality, unique problems with regard to herbal medicine exist. Herbs are unregulated complex entities that contain hundreds of constituents; therefore, it is difficult to find one particular component representing the active agent. In many cases, particular herbal treatments have been studied, with a focus on individual extracts and chemical entities. For instance, one ginkgo biloba extract in particular (Egb761) has been extensively studied. For this reason, patients should be counseled on the use of specific extracts if the majority of scientific evidence has been done using that extract. Manufacturers may or may not produce herbal products using extracts that have been the subject of scientific study. Other examples of this include LI160 for SJW (Quanterra) and black cohosh (Remifemin) (Table 3-3).

Whether or not there is benefit to standardizing an herbal treatment to one identifiable component is a matter of current debate. According to some, the goal of standardization, that is, to achieve a consistent level of the main therapeutically

Table 3-3   Selected formulations used in European controlled clinical trials.

HERB	USE/DOSE	US PRODUCT (IMPORTER)	EUROPEAN PRODUCT
Black cohosh	Menopause 40 mg bid	Remifemin	Remifemin
Ginkgo	Dementia 120–240 mg daily	Ginkgold (Nature's Way) Ginkoba (Pharmaton) Ginkai (Lichtwer)	Tebonin [Egb761] (Schwabe) Tebonin [Egb761] (Schwabe) Kaveri [LI1370] (Lichtwer)
Horse chestnut	Venous insufficiency 250 mg bid	Venostat (Pharmaton)	Venostasin (Klinge Pharma)
Saw palmetto	Benign prostatic enlargement 160 mg bid	ProstActive (Nature's Way)	Prostagutt (Schwabe) Permixon (Pierre Fabre)
St. John's wort	Depression 900 mg daily	Kira (Lichtwer Pharma) Movana (Pharmaton) Perika (Nature's Way)	Jarsin [LI-160] (Lichtwer Pharma) Neuroplant (Schwabe) Neuroplant (Schwabe)

SOURCE: Adapted from Rotblatt MD. Herbal medicine: a practical guide to safety and quality assurance. West J Med 1999;171:172–176.

effective active plant constituent, remains remote. Efforts to achieve this will require more characterization, bioactivity assessment, and stronger correlation with clinical endpoints. At this time, the standardization of phytomedicines serves primarily as an indicator of the quality of medicinal plant extracts. Other issues that should be discussed with patients who utilize or contemplate the use of herbal treatments is the lack of quality control and regulation, resulting in the potential for contamination and misidentification of plant species by individual manufacturers. For this reason, patients should be advised to use products from reputable manufacturers. Several large manufacturers of pharmaceuticals are now marketing their own lines of herbal treatments. Certainly, more federal regulation is needed, perhaps similar to agencies in Europe (i.e., German Commission E), to ensure the safe manufacture of herbal medicines. Herbal products currently manufactured in the United States are not required to undergo the rigors of Food and Drug Administration (FDA) drug approval.

Contraindications for the Use of Herbal Treatments in Special Populations

Herbal treatments should be taken only under the supervision of a physician or other qualified health care professional. Further research evaluating the safety and efficacy of the use of herbal treatments in special populations (elderly, children, etc.) is warranted.

Although herbal remedies are commonly used by the elderly, it is likely that the biologic changes associated with aging, such as decreased total body water, decreased muscle mass, and decreased renal and hepatic clearance, could significantly alter their bioavailability and clinical responsiveness in this population.

Based on a lack of studies related to product safety during pregnancy and lactation and the potential for harm to the fetus or infant, no women contemplating pregnancy, currently pregnant, or nursing should use herbal remedies. In one study with several methodologic flaws, SJW, along with several other herbal treatments, was implicated in decreasing fertility.

Most studies involving herbal treatments do not evaluate the long-term effects. Therefore, clinical monitoring is advised. As with any pharmaceutical agent, as dosage is increased, an increase in the risk of side effects may occur. It is, therefore, wise to recommend using the lowest dosages of herbal treatments initially and monitor side effects. As with other standard medications, idiosyncratic reactions may occur.

Herbal remedies are not without risks. One example is herbal remedies containing tannins. Although found throughout nature in teas and certain vegetables, repeated exposure to high levels has been documented to increase the risk of certain oropharyngeal cancers with long-term exposure. Additionally, several herbal remedies have been theoretically thought to possess carcinogenic components that over time may be problematic. Herbal remedies should only be recommended when sufficient clinical data are available regarding efficacy, side effects, and long-term safety. Patients wishing to remain on herbal remedies

Table 3-4   Selected potentially toxic herbals.

HERB	POTENIAL TOXICITY
Pheasant's eye	Cardiac arrest
Arnica	GI/muscle toxicity
Pennyroyal	Hepatotoxicity
Yohimbine	Hypertension
Mistletoe	GI bleeding/CNS toxicity

SOURCE: Adapted from Yarnell E, Meserole L. Toxic botanicals: is the poison in the plant or its regulation? Alternative & Complementary Therapies 1997; 3(1):13–19.

should be monitored periodically for specific signs of toxicity and potential adverse effects. Periodic measurements of liver function tests and renal function may be prudent. Ultimately, all patients should be advised not to take herbal treatments that have been identified to cause specific harm on a long-term basis without the supervision of a physician (Table 3-4).

Reported or Potential Toxicity with the Use of Herbal Products

A number of herbal remedies have documented liver toxicity. Table 3-5 lists a selected compendium of compounds that should not be consumed due to toxicity. Herbal remedies have been known to cause toxicity to a variety of organ systems. However, the liver appears to be the most common target organ for serious herbal toxicity. Chaparral, for example, has been implicated in acute hepatitis, causing subacute hepatocellular necrosis leading to cholestatic hepatitis and eventually liver failure requiring transplantation. Germander has also been implicated in causing hepatotoxicity with a marked increase in serum aminotransferase levels and may lead to death. Several Chinese herbal treatments have also been found to cause liver toxicity; these include Jin Bu Huan, which contains the alkaloid levotetrahydropalmitine. It is believed that this herbal remedy contains structural similarities to hepatotoxic pyrrolizidine alkaloids, which were previously documented to cause hepatic veno-occlusive disease leading to portal hypertension (Table 3-5). Clinically, exposure to this compound leads to hepatomegaly and ascites caused by hepatic central vein dilatation and fibrosis. Several case reports have documented this association with a variety of herbal treatments. In addition, it appears that infants and young children are particularly susceptible to this effect. In utero exposure has been linked with hepatic veno-occlusive disease and death in a newborn infant.

Other organ systems have also been documented to suffer damage from the ingestion of toxic herbal remedies. Of note, cardiotoxicity and nephrotoxicity are documented in the literature. Cardiotoxicity has been associated with ingestion of herbal products that contain aconite alkaloids. It is hypothesized that these agents activate sodium channels and have widespread effects on the excitable membranes of cardiac, neural, and muscle tissue. In case reports this has led to fatal arrythmias and even death.

Table 3-5 Herbal supplements associated with hepatic injury.

HERB	CLINICAL MANIFESTATIONS	PATHOLOGIC FINDINGS
Chaparral	ALT/AST elevations	Acute and chronic liver injury Portal inflammation
Jin Bu Huan	ALT/AST elevations	Acute and chronic liver injury
Germander	ALT/AST elevations	Acute and chronic liver injury
Mistletoe	ALT/AST elevations	Acute and chronic hepatitis
Comfrey	ALT/AST elevations	Hepatic veno-occlusive disease
Pennyroyal	ALT/AST elevations	Acute liver injury

ALT, alanine aminotransferase; AST, aspartate aminotransferase.
SOURCE: Adapted from Bashir RM, Lewis JH. Hepatotoxicity of drugs used in the treatment of gastrointestinal disorders. Gastroenterol Clin North Am 1995;24:937–967.

In general, although herbal remedies do possess the potential for harm, the widespread use among the population to date has not led to large numbers of adverse events, albeit that underreporting of acute herbal reactions may occur. With common sense and, more importantly, knowledge of potential side effects and toxicities of herbs, the physician can integrate herbal remedies into practice safely. Herbal remedies have the potential to add a great deal to the existing treatment options available for patients. Further study and long-term trials are needed to assess safety and efficacy.

Patients who wish to use herbal remedies may want to seek the advice of an herbalist or traditional Chinese medicine practitioner. Unfortunately, current regulations with regard to licensing may make referral to a reputable practitioner difficult, and the physician may be left relying solely on "word of mouth" reputation. This is clearly not a satisfactory situation. Once again, it behooves the health care provider to become knowledgeable enough regarding herbal treatments that sound advice can be given to patients who wish to undergo this form of therapy.

Reporting Adverse Events

Manufacturers of herbal supplements are not required by law to report adverse events. MedWatch, the Food and Drug Administration's (FDA's) medical products reporting program, was designed to enable health care professionals to voluntarily report adverse events and product problems (*http://www.fda.gov/medwatch*). Its purpose is to identify problems associated with herbal remedies and communicate this information to the medical community. This program can help to remove unsafe products from distribution quickly.

Once a potential problem or adverse event is identified, the FDA can initiate one of the following:

- Labeling change
- Boxed warning

- Product recalls and withdrawals
- Medical and safety alerts

Popular Herbal Remedies

A number of herbal remedies are commonly self-prescribed by patients. The most popular and well researched of these are presented as a basic primer with regard to use, potential toxicity, and efficacy based on scientific analysis below.

American Ginseng (Panax quinquefolius)

Indications

Most ginseng consumption in the United States is for increasing energy and as an "adaptogenic" agent. This concept comes from the theory that ginseng increases the body's ability to adapt to both emotional and physical stress. In traditional Chinese medicine, ginseng is used to restore vital energy (qi or chi). American ginseng, however, is thought to be a "calming" herbal, as compared to the very popular Asian ginseng (Panax ginseng) that is much more stimulating.

Pharmacology

Ginsenosides are thought to be the most important chemical entities responsible for American ginseng's effects.

Scientific Analysis

Several studies have revealed a hypoglycemic effect along with a decrease in prolactin levels. A number of studies have shown facilitation in task behavior in memory-compromised animals with anticholinergic-induced amnesia. Additionally, several studies have shown American ginseng to possess antioxidant properties.

Adverse Effects

No significant adverse effects have been reported.

Summary

American ginseng, like Asian and Siberian ginseng, is used as an adaptogenic agent. Mixed results in a large number of trials make recommendations difficult. Its use, however, has continued for thousands of years.

Asian Ginseng (Panax ginseng)

Indications

As with American ginseng, Asian ginseng is used mainly as an adaptogenic agent. It also is used to boost energy and stamina. Asian ginseng is more "stimulating" than American ginseng and has been used for thousands of years in Chinese traditional medicine.

Pharmacology

Asian ginseng has been shown to have antiplatelet, vasodilatory, and cytoprotective effects against ischemia and toxins.

Scientific Analysis

A large number of randomized controlled trials have been performed, yielding mixed results. Although touted as being able to enhance physical performance, evaluation of the literature does not suggest any significant benefit. In addition, no significant benefits in memory, concentration, and cognitive function have been noted.

Adverse Effects

Minimal side effects have been reported. Asian ginseng has the potential to interact with warfarin.

Summary

The efficacy of Asian ginseng has not been established beyond a reasonable doubt for any indication.

Black Cohosh (Cimicifuga racemosa)

Indications

Black cohosh is most commonly used for menopausal symptoms and as an alternative to hormone replacement therapy.

Pharmacology

Active ingredients include the triterpene glycosides. Although originally thought to possess estrogenic properties, more recent studies have failed to show these effects.

Scientific Analysis

A number of clinical trials have revealed contradictory results with regard to treatment and efficacy of menopausal symptoms.

Adverse Effects

Minimal gastric distress occurs, but black cohosh is usually well tolerated.

Summary

Several studies show benefit in the treatment of menopausal symptoms. However, data are contradictory, and no impact on bone density has been found.

Soy Protein/Phytoestrogens

Indications

Soy isoflavones are most commonly used as a treatment for hot flashes and as an alternative to hormone replacement therapy. Soy protein has been shown to modestly lower total cholesterol and low-density lipoprotein (LDL) cholesterol levels in both hypercholesterolemic and normocholesterolemic men and women.

Pharmacology

Soy isoflavones are nonsteroidal molecules that have structural similarity to estradiol-17β.

Scientific Analysis

A number of studies have noted statistically significant reduction of menopausal hot flashes and serum cholesterol. Several have also shown a modest increase in bone density. Data regarding efficacy in reducing cholesterol levels is strong with intake of greater than or equal to 25 g soy protein per day.

Adverse Effects

The safety of large doses of isoflavones is currently being debated. Studies conducted using rats with low levels of endogenous estrogen have shown a higher incidence of breast cancer risk with long-term isoflavone use. Other animal studies suggest a protective effect in animals with normal levels of endogenous estrogen. Unfortunately, very few human studies to date have been performed to assess the actual risk.

Summary

Although few data exist on safety, most experts believe that increased dietary soy is safe in patients who wish not to take hormone replacement therapy for hot flashes. More data are needed regarding the use of isoflavone supplements. Soy protein is indicated for use in reducing cholesterol levels. The FDA has approved a health claim for products containing 6.25 g soy protein per serving.

Chamomile (Matricaria recutita)

Indications

Chamomile is most often used as an anti-inflammatory, antispasmodic, and calming agent. It is also used topically to treat inflammatory skin and mucous membrane disorders.

Pharmacology

Active ingredients include the terpenoids. These constituents can inhibit the inflammatory mediators of the arachidonic acid cascade such as 5-lipoxygenase and cyclo-oxygenase.

Scientific Analysis

A number of clinical trials have shown benefit as an antispasmodic and for colic. One small study showed sedative effects.

Adverse Effects

Chamomile is generally regarded as a mild and safe herb. Allergic reactions can occur in patients who are allergic to ragweed.

Summary

Chamomile appears to be a mild and generally safe herbal for the treatment of colic and anxiety. It is most often used topically for skin disorders.

Echinacea [Echinacea species (spp)]

Indications

Echinacea is used for the treatment of mild upper respiratory infections.

Pharmacology

Alkylamides, caffeic acid derivatives, and echinacosides are thought to be the most important constituents. Oral preparations appear to enhance nonspecific phagocytosis by stimulating leukocyte function and enhancing T-cell function.

Scientific Analysis

Several well-designed studies have shown that echinacea has no role in the prevention of the common cold. On the other hand, data do exist that support the notion that echinacea shortens the length of flu-like illness.

Adverse Effects

Echinacea preparations are generally well tolerated. Use in patients with autoimmune illness is contraindicated due to its immune stimulating effects.

Summary

Although the use of echinacea to prevent colds has not been proven, a number of studies do show a shortened length of illness while taking it.

Ephedra (Ma Huang)

Indications

Ephedra is most commonly used for asthma and nasal congestion. It also has become very popular as a stimulant and energizer for weight loss. Most recently, it has been combined with guarana (which contains high levels of caffeine) for weight loss.

Pharmacology

The most important constituents of ephedra are the alkaloids pseudoephedrine and ephedrine.

Scientific Analysis

Clinical trials involving the benefits of ephedrine and pseudoephedrine are well established. Most recently, herbal weight-loss preparations have used the combination of Ma Huang with guarana, leading to modest weight loss through the mechanism of increased thermogenesis. A number of studies do show modest weight loss; however, this is minimal at best and is only effective when combined with diet and exercise.

Adverse Effects

Adverse effects are well documented with use. High doses of ephedra can induce hypertension, arrhythmias, nervousness, tremor, insomnia, and tachycardia. Several deaths have been reported, and this product has been banned in several international markets.

Summary

Data show benefit for weight loss when combined with a reduced-calorie diet and exercise. Potential serious side effects can occur, and deaths have been reported. The use of ephedra is not recommended.

Ginger (Zingiber officinale)

Indications

Ginger root is widely used as a digestive aid for mild dyspepsia and is used to treat and prevent nausea and motion sickness.

Pharmacology

Active compounds in ginger include the phenolic compounds gingerol and shogaol. Ginger is thought to act as an antioxidant, prostaglandin, and leukotriene inhibitor and to inhibit platelet aggregation.

Scientific Analysis

In human pharmacologic studies, oral administration has produced variable results. Results of a number of human trials have shown statistically significant effects in the treatment of motion sickness and as an antiemetic. In one study, ginger was more effective than placebo and dimenhydrinate (Dramamine) for motion sickness.

Adverse Effects

Ginger has no known clinical adverse effects other than heartburn, which occurs rarely.

Summary

Ginger has been shown in a number of clinical studies to be of benefit in the treatment of nausea and motion sickness. It is not unreasonable to have patients use ginger for mild nausea and motion sickness as long as a proper diagnosis has been made before treatment.

Garlic (Allium sativum)

Indications

Garlic has been used extensively throughout history in various cultures. It is used to treat infections, heart disease, and diabetes and is currently used most often as an antithrombotic agent and antioxidant. It is widely used to reduce abnormal cholesterol and blood pressure.

Pharmacology

Garlic contains pharmacologically active sulfur compounds including alliin and allicin. Allicin stimulates fibrinolysis, inhibits arachidonic acid conversion, and reduces platelet aggregation. Epidemiologic studies have suggested that people who eat garlic and onions have lower lipid and cholesterol levels.

Scientific Analysis

A large body of data exists regarding garlic and its use for hypercholesterolemia and hypertension. Unfortunately, despite common claims and advertising, the evidence for garlic's beneficial effects on cholesterol and blood pressure is inconsistent, and many studies have shown positive as well as negative effects.

Adverse Effects

Garlic can cause malodorous breath or body odor. In addition, dyspepsia, flatulence, anorexia, and dermatitis have occurred. Allergic reactions have also been noted in the literature. Garlic supplementation should be considered a possible risk factor for bleeding.

Summary

Garlic supplementation appears safe for most patients who wish to use a "natural" product for cardiovascular health. However, long-term beneficial effects have not been well established.

Ginkgo Leaf Extract (Ginkgo biloba)

Indications

Ginkgo leaf is commonly used to improve cognitive function in the elderly. It is used for treating dementia, including Alzheimer's, and for conditions associated with vascular insufficiency, including intermittent claudication. It is also used to treat premenstrual syndrome (PMS).

Pharmacology

The mechanism of action of ginkgo is not completely understood. It is thought that the flavonoids in the gingko leaf have antioxidant properties that protect tissues from oxidative damage.

Scientific Analysis

Much of the scientific evidence indicates that ginkgo may be modestly effective in improving cognitive function, particularly short-term visual memory in nondemented patients. However, a recent report, published in the *Journal of the American Medical Association* (*JAMA*), found no significantly measurable benefit from this herb.

The National Center for Complementary and Alternative Medicine (NCCAM) is beginning a 5-year study of 3000 people aged 75 and older (the largest study ever of dementia) to determine if daily ginkgo ingestion can prevent dementia or Alzheimer's disease.

Adverse Effects

Ginkgo has been used safely in clinical trials up to 1 year. Reported adverse effects include mild gastrointestinal symptoms, such as constipation, stomach upset, and allergic skin reactions.

Summary

The ginkgo tree is the oldest living tree species in the world. Ginkgo is the most commonly prescribed herb in Germany, where it is the preferred treatment for dementia. More research is needed to confirm the use of ginkgo to improve memory and cognitive function in otherwise healthy older adults.

Milk Thistle (Silybum marianum)

Indications

Milk thistle is typically used as a hepatoprotectant in patients with viral hepatitis as well as alcoholic cirrhosis. It is also commonly used in Europe as a treatment for Amanita mushroom poisoning.

Pharmacology

Milk thistle contains silybin. Silybin acts as an antioxidant and inhibits the enzyme 5-lipoxygenase. As a result of this inhibition, silybin reduces the formation of inflammatory leukotrienes and limits the activity of Kupffer cells in vitro, which may slow the progression of chronic liver disease.

Scientific Analysis

At least 14 randomized, controlled trials involving milk thistle have evaluated its efficacy and safety. Unfortunately, most were of poor methodologic quality. Many showed some improvement in liver function tests and biopsy-proven cirrhosis.

Adverse Effects

No major side effects have been reported for patients using milk thistle. Loose stools and other mild gastrointestinal effects may develop in some, but these occur rarely.

Summary

Although clinically relevant benefits have not been clearly established, it may be reasonable to have patients with cirrhosis and viral hepatitis take milk thistle given its safety record and significant lack of drug interactions.

Conclusion

The use of botanical and herbal remedies to reduce the symptoms, treat, or prevent chronic disease is on the rise. It is clear that herbal remedies have potential for interactions with standard pharmaceutical agents as well as inherent toxicities. These negative attributes, however, should be tempered with the fact that, in most cases, herbal remedies are safe and many demonstrate clinical efficacy when used in the appropriate settings and in the proper dosages. As more clinical data become available, patients stand to gain from the use of herbal remedies, especially in the setting of mild illness in which more potent pharmaceutical medications may not be indicated. It is hoped that studies of the cost effectiveness of herbal therapy will justify the use of these remedies because of the fact that they are easily obtained by patients and in most cases are less expensive than standard medications.

With time, a number of herbal remedies may stand the test of scientific study and will add to the clinician's existing armamentarium of medicinal agents available for use in treatment. Certainly, these agents require careful scrutiny and analysis. Health care professionals are uniquely positioned to provide patients with reliable, scientifically sound advice on the use of herbal remedies in the context of a varied, nutritionally balanced diet. Therefore, they must expand their knowledge and understanding of the growing body of scientific evidence so that optimal medical and nutritional care can be provided to all patients.

Herbal remedies will add to the overall care of patients and will enhance the practice of medicine in the coming years. It is important for health professionals to be informed and open minded in order to provide needed guidance to their patients regarding herbal supplements.

For a list of references for this chapter, please visit the University of Pennsylvania School of Medicine's Nutrition Education and Prevention Program web site: *http://www.med.upenn.edu/nutrimed/articles.html*

Case 1

Drug-Herb Interaction

Philippe Szapary and Ara DerMarderosian

Objectives

- Describe the hypothesized mechanism of action and metabolism of St. John's wort.
- Evaluate the safety and efficacy of St. John's wort for the treatment of depression.
- Provide effective dietary counseling for patients on warfarin therapy.
- Recognize the importance of quality control when recommending over-the-counter dietary and herbal supplements.
- Recognize the potential for toxicity and drug-herb interaction of St. John's wort and other commonly used botanicals.

LB is a 54 year-old woman who was in good health until 2 weeks ago, when acute shortness of breath and palpitations developed while she was driving to work. On arrival in the emergency room, she was found to have atrial fibrillation with a rapid ventricular response. She was admitted to the cardiac intensive care unit and treated medically with beta-blockers to slow down her heart rate along with intravenous and then oral anticoagulants to reduce her risk of stroke. She was discharged on the fourth hospital day and now comes to see her physician for management of her warfarin anticoagulation 1 week later, after hospital discharge. LB has been stable on a warfarin dose of 3 mg per day with an International Normalized Ratio (INR) in the appropriate therapeutic range of 2.0 to 3.0. At today's visit, it is noted that her INR is subtherapeutic at 1.2. She denied any changes in medication compliance or diet and denied starting any recent antibiotics.

On further questioning, LB admits to taking some over-the-counter dietary supplements. She currently takes vitamin E, 400 IU once a day, as a "cardioprotective antioxidant"; calcium carbonate, 500 mg twice a day for bone health; and St. John's wort, 300 mg twice a day, which she buys from her local health food store. She states that she started St. John's wort 3 weeks ago because a friend told her it might help "lift her spirits." She has no known food or drug allergies.

Past Medical History

LB has a history of mild hypertension, which has been primarily managed with a sodium-restricted diet. She also has a history of mild depression, which she attributes to being perimenopausal. She has never had an episode of major depression or psychiatric hospitalization and has never been treated with prescription antidepressants. She denies any thoughts of suicide.

Medications

Her medications include warfarin, 3 mg at bedtime, and atenolol, 50 mg per day in the morning.

Social History

LB lives with her husband and their two cats. Her children are grown and in college. She explains that she has not been feeling like her usual self since the hospitalization. She often awakens during the night and has a difficult time going back to sleep. She still enjoys playing bridge and gardening but describes herself as frequently distracted and occasionally "blue." She avoids alcohol and tobacco and drinks one cup of coffee daily.

Review of Systems

General: She reports losing approximately 5 lb since her admission.

Gastrointestinal (GI): Her appetite is poor.

Physical Examination

Vital Signs

Temperature: 98.6°F (37°C)

Heart rate: 72 beats per minute (BPM)

Respiration: 16 BPM

Blood pressure: 138/84 mm Hg

Height: 5'4" (152.4 cm)

Current weight: 150 lb (68.04 kg)

Usual weight: 155 lb (70.31 kg)

Body mass index (BMI): 25.7 kg/m^2

Examination

General: No apparent distress

Skin: Warm and dry

Head, ears, eyes, nose, throat (HEENT): Within normal limits

Cardiac: Irregularly irregular radial pulse; normal S1 and S2 without S3 or S4

Abdomen: Soft, nontender, nondistended

Extremities: No clubbing, cyanosis, or edema

Neurologic mental status examination: Alert and oriented to person, place, and time with slightly depressed affect; sensory and motor examinations grossly intact

Laboratory Data

Patient's Laboratory Values	Normal Values
Prothrombin time = 13.4 seconds	<13 seconds
INR = 1.2	*
Thyroid-stimulating hormone (TSH) = 3.1 μU/mL	0.5–5.0 μU/mL

*Target therapeutic range for patients being anticoagulated with warfarin therapy = 2–3.

Case Questions

1. What is known about the mechanism of action and metabolism of St. John's wort?

2. What safety issues are of concern for patients taking St. John's wort alone or in combination with other drugs?

3. Is St. John's wort effective in the treatment of depression?

4. What issues related to the product quality are important to consider when assessing over-the-counter dietary supplements?

5. Based on LB's medical history, what treatment recommendations for depression would be appropriate at this time?

6. What dietary advice should be provided to all patients on warfarin (anticoagulant) therapy?

Case Answers

1. **What is known about the mechanism of action and metabolism of St. John's wort?**

    SJW, also known as *Hypericum perforatum*, is one of the most commonly used herbal remedies in the Western world. Extracts of this popular botanical have been used since the early nineteenth century to treat mood disorders. The exact mechanism of action of SJW remains unknown, but, like many herbs, it likely involves multiple pathways. A number of early studies suggested that *Hypericum* inhibits monoamine oxidase (MAO), an enzyme involved with the breakdown of some neurotransmitters that influence mood. Other postulated mechanisms from animal studies include the inhibition of serotonin reuptake, the downregulation of serotonin receptors, and inhibition of gamma–aminobutyric acid (GABA) pathways.

    Metabolism of SJW constituents is especially relevant when one considers the potential for toxicity and drug-herb interaction. In a study of the action of *Hypericum* on human cytochrome P450 activity, it was found that long-term administration in humans resulted in a significant and selective induction of CYP3A activity in the intestinal wall. CYP3A is one subtype of the many cytochrome P450 enzymes that help to detoxify and metabolize drugs. If an herbal supplement induces one of these enzymes, other drugs may be metabolized faster. If an herbal supplement inhibits this enzyme, the functional level of other drugs may rise and cause toxicity. In this case, blood levels of drugs metabolized by this enzyme, such as cyclosporine, digoxin, warfarin, theophylline, and protease inhibitors, can be expected to fall during chronic administration of SJW.

2. **What safety issues are of concern for patients taking St. John's wort alone or in combination with other drugs?**

   When used in monotherapy at doses up to 900 mg per day, SJW has been shown to be safe, with a better side-effect profile than prescription antidepressant agents. One study found that 3% of SJW-treated patients dropped out secondary to side effects (GI irritation, tiredness, and restlessness), compared to a 16% dropout rate in the imipramine group. In the most recently published multicenter trial involving 340 subjects, 900 mg SJW caused more anorgasmia and frequent urination than placebo, but SJW resulted in fewer side effects than did 50 to 100 mg sertraline.

   Relevant to this case, SJW can reduce the efficacy of warfarin and thus lead to underanticoagulation. This might increase the risk of thromboembolic complications in patients with atrial fibrillation. Thus, although LB was previously therapeutically anticoagulated on her 3-mg dose of warfarin, her recent daily use of SJW has likely caused her INR to be subtherapeutic, thereby possibly increasing her risk of stroke.

   When used in combination with other drugs, SJW can cause clinically significant toxicities related to the upregulation of CYP3A. As a result, there are several reports of transplanted organ rejection related to concomitant use of SJW and cyclosporine. Additionally, SJW can reduce the levels of the antiarrhythmic digoxin used to treat patients with heart failure or atrial fibrillation. These are just some of the examples of possible drug-herb interactions. Table 3-6 lists other drug-herb interactions for commonly used botanicals.

3. **Is St. John's wort effective in the treatment of depression?**

   Well over 20 randomized, placebo-controlled studies have evaluated the safety and efficacy of SJW in treating mild to moderate depression. St. John's wort has also been compared with tricyclic antidepressants (amitriptyline, imipramine) and more recently with two selective serotonin reuptake inhibitors (SSRIs), fluoxetine and sertraline. The majority of placebo-controlled studies has shown that standardized extracts of SJW in the dose range of 300 to 900 mg daily are moderately effective in the treatment of mild to moderate depressive symptoms. Some studies have shown equivalence of 900 mg SJW to low-dose imipramine and low-dose fluoxetine. A recent study of patients with major depression failed to show improvement over both placebo and standard doses of sertraline. Differences in study design (lack of active control and placebo), study

Table 3-6   Selected drug-herb interactions.

BOTANICAL	COMMON USAGE	DRUG/DRUG CLASS	POTENTIAL INTERACTION
Green tea extract	Antioxidant	Warfarin	Decreased drug activity
Kava	Anxiety	Benzodiazepines	Additive sedative effect
Valerian	Insomnia	Barbiturates	Additive sedative effect
St. John's wort	Depression	Cyclosporine, digoxin, warfarin, indinavir, oral contraceptives, amitriptyline, theophylline	Decreased drug activity
St. John's wort	Depression	SSRIs	Increased drug activity
St. John's wort	Depression	Oral contraceptives	Intermenstrual bleeding
Echinacea	Immune stimulant	Immunomodulatory Drugs (prednisone, methotrexate, cyclosporine)	Decreased drug activity
Garlic	Hypercholesterolemia	Warfarin	Decreased drug activity
Ginkgo	Memory enhancement	Warfarin, aspirin	Increased risk of bleeding
Panax ginseng	Increases well-being	Warfarin	Decreased drug activity
Panax ginseng	Increases well-being	Hypoglycemic drugs	Enhanced drug activity
Yohimbine	Increases libido	TCA	Hypertension
Ephedra	Weight loss/energy	Antihypertensives	Decreased drug activity

SSRIs, selective serotonin reuptake inhibitors; TCA, tricyclic antidepressant.
SOURCE: Adapted with permission from DerMarderosian A, ed. Guide to Natural Products.
2nd ed. St. Louis: Facts & Comparisons, 2001.

populations (major vs. mild/moderate depression), and dosing of SJW or comparator agents is likely responsible for some variance in results.

4. **What issues related to the product quality are important to consider when assessing over-the-counter dietary supplements?**

    The Dietary Supplement and Health Education Act (DSHEA) of 1994 created a new class of compounds called "dietary supplements" that do not need to meet the same regulatory scrutiny as prescription pharmacologic agents. As a result of DSHEA, herbal remedies marketed as dietary supplements cannot make claims that their products can be used to "diagnose, prevent, mitigate, treat, or cure a specific disease." DSHEA thus led to a marked increase in the availability and popularity of dietary supplements in the United States. Although DSHEA required that botanicals be labeled with the parts of the plant used and the strength of the ingredients it is represented as having, many herbal products have been found to contain less or none of the proposed active compounds. This stems in part from the complexity of herbal preparations, which can contain several potentially bioactive constituents. The strength and potency of an herbal extract can depend, among other things, on the time of year the plant was cultivated, the quality of the soil, the parts of the plant that are used, and variations in processing of the herb.

    The problems of quality control can be illustrated with the case of SJW. The most common analytical "marker" compound used in standardizing

SJW extracts is hypericin, even though it is not the only active principle. SJW also contains, among other substances, pseudohypericin and protohypericin, as well as flavonoids and volatile oils. The majority of the American products are standardized to contain at least 0.3% hypericin. Some more recent products are standardized to what is believed to be the major antidepressive agent, hyperforin, at a level range of 3% to 5%. Some products are sold as capsules, whereas others are alcoholic liquid extracts. Finally, many products contain SJW as one of several possibly active compounds. Of note, the majority of the European clinical studies used a specific extract called *LI-160*, delivering 900 mg per day of the aerial parts (leaves and flowers) of the dried herb. Even when products are standardized, batch-to-batch variability can also lead to inconsistent therapeutic effects. Thus, the quality of a dietary supplement is difficult to ascertain for consumers, who must rely on independent testing of products (*http://www.consumerlabs.com*) or use products specifically tested in clinical trials.

5. **Based on LB's medical history, what treatment recommendations for depression would be appropriate for her at this time?**

By taking a thorough medication and supplement history, the astute clinician recognized that the recent addition of SJW may have reduced the effectiveness of warfarin. LB was counseled to stop the SJW and increase the dose of warfarin for 3 days before returning to her stable dose of 3 mg. A more in-depth psychosocial history did not reveal evidence for major depression. LB was diagnosed with adjustment disorder and will follow up in 1 week's time for a re-evaluation of her INR.

6. **What dietary advice should be provided to all patients on warfarin therapy?**

It is widely believed that vitamin K intake inversely influences the efficacy of warfarin-based anticoagulant therapy. Therefore, the most important dietary advice to give patients is to maintain their intake of vitamin K–containing foods fairly constantly from day to day. Phylloquinone is the predominant dietary form of vitamin K. An understanding of the dietary vitamin K–warfarin interaction and knowledge of high, medium, and low dietary sources of vitamin K are necessary for successful anticoagulation.

Higher concentrations of vitamin K are found in dark-green leafy vegetables, such as spinach, kale, and collard greens, and in the outer peels of certain fruits, such as apples and grapes. Other significant dietary sources of vitamin K are found in certain oils, including soybean, canola, cottonseed, and olive, although values fluctuate since these oils are highly susceptible to both daylight and fluorescent light (see Appendix).

See Chapter Review Questions, pages A-12 to A-15.

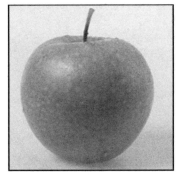

PART II

Nutrition Throughout the Life-Cycle

4

Nutrition in Pregnancy and Lactation

Carine Lenders and Peter Cherouny

Objectives*

- Understand the metabolic and physiologic consequences of pregnancy and lactation.
- Determine the appropriate weight gain during pregnancy for normal-weight, underweight, and overweight pregnant women.
- Recommend dietary modifications to help alleviate common nutritional problems during pregnancy.
- Recognize the additional nutritional requirements for women during pregnancy and lactation.
- Recognize the importance of incorporating nutrition into the history, review of systems, and physical examinations of prepregnant and pregnant women.

Nutrition plays a key role in both normal and high-risk pregnancies (e.g., twins, adolescent pregnancies, and gestational diabetes). Pregnancy is an anabolic condition requiring additional energy and nutrients. These increased demands put pregnant women and their fetuses at risk for nutritional deficiencies. Nutritional status may be further compromised by disease and genetic conditions, such as diabetes, sickle cell disease, phenylketonuria (PKU), cardiovascular disease, infections, thyroid disorders, sexually transmitted disease, obesity, psychological conditions, and eating disorders.

---

* SOURCE: Objectives for chapter and cases adapted from the *NIH Nutrition Curriculum Guide for Training Physicians* (*http://www.nhlbi.nih.gov/funding/training/naa*).

Metabolic and Physiologic Consequences of Pregnancy

The metabolic and physiologic changes that occur during pregnancy accommodate the growth and development of the fetus and the alterations in maternal body composition. These changes include the growth of the fetoplacental unit, increased maternal blood volume, initial increased maternal fat stores, changes in gastrointestinal (GI) motility, and breast development to prepare for lactation. An increase in fetoplacental hormones is associated with both maternal insulin resistance and the increased uptake of fatty acids by extrauterine tissues, which favors glucose delivery to the fetus. In addition to energy, other nutrients required by the fetus must be supplied by the maternal diet.

Integrating Nutrition into the Obstetric History

Ideally, every woman should meet with a health care provider for a prepregnancy physical and nutrition assessment; however, according to the March of Dimes, 50% of pregnancies are unplanned. A major objective of the obstetric health care team is to collect sufficient information to evaluate the pregnant woman's nutritional status and identify risk factors for the pregnancy.

A detailed obstetric history should include the following: 1) total number and dates of prior pregnancies (parity) with maternal and fetal outcomes and complications; 2) prior deliveries involving low-birth-weight (<2500 g) or small-for-gestational-age (less than tenth percentile for gestational age) neonates, stillbirths (≥20 weeks), abortions (<20 weeks), and neonatal deaths; 3) previous weight-gain patterns and total weight gain during pregnancies; 4) prior history of significant nausea, vomiting, or hyperemesis associated with pregnancy; 5) past history of gestational diabetes; and 6) a history of contraceptive use.

The medical history should also probe for maternal risk factors and chronic diseases, such as disorders of absorption or metabolism, infections, diabetes mellitus, PKU, sickle cell disease, hypertension, renal disease, anorexia, and bulimia. Lifestyle risk factors, such as pregnancy at the younger or older age ranges, previous nutritional deficiencies, and caffeine, tobacco, illicit drug, and alcohol use, also should be identified. Complementary and Alternative Medicine (CAM) options, including herbal medicines, alternative pharmacologic and biologic treatments, or other therapies need to be specifically explored, as their use may not be volunteered and they may be inappropriate or even dangerous during pregnancy.

Additional questions regarding social, economic, and emotional stresses; religious practices (including dietary restrictions and fasting); and drug, alcohol, and tobacco use are important because they may influence a pregnant woman's dietary practices and can negatively affect the health of the mother and fetus. If appropriate, specific questions should address availability of food and ability to store and prepare food, including participation in medical and food assistance programs. The woman's working environment, both inside and outside the home, should be reviewed with concern toward the identification of conditions that may limit nutritional intake.

Clinical signs and symptoms, such as hyperemesis gravidarum (excessive vomiting), poor weight gain, weight loss, dehydration, and constipation during pregnancy also have nutritional implications.

Nutrition Assessment in Pregnancy

The purpose of a nutrition assessment is to identify those women with nutritional risk factors that could jeopardize their health or the health of a fetus. Thorough evaluation of a woman's nutritional status before or during pregnancy includes clinical, dietary, and laboratory components.

Both patient interview and written questionnaire formats are appropriate for gathering information about current and past dietary practices. Pertinent dietary information includes appetite, meal patterns, dieting regimens, cultural or religious dietary practices, vegetarianism, food allergies, and cravings or aversions, or both. Information about abnormal eating practices, such as following food fads, bingeing, purging, laxative or diuretic use, or pica (eating nonfood items: ice, detergent, starch, chalk, clay, rocks, and so on), is also essential. Other relevant information includes the habitual use of caffeine-containing beverages (>200 mg per day), sugar substitutes and other special "diet" foods, alcohol, tobacco, prescription and over-the-counter medications, and vitamin, mineral, and herbal supplements, as dietary supplements may not be volunteered and their use may be inappropriate or dangerous during pregnancy. A woman's current dietary practice can be assessed using the 24-hour recall, usual intake, or a food frequency questionnaire.

Some women are receptive to nutrition counseling just before or during pregnancy, making this an opportune time to encourage the development of good nutritional and physical activity practices aimed at preventing medical problems, such as obesity, diabetes, hypertension, and osteoporosis. Prepregnant and pregnant women who are found to have nutritional risk factors may benefit from a referral to a registered dietitian for nutrition education.

Physical Examination

An essential part of the clinical evaluation is assessing prepregnancy weight for height by calculating the body mass index (BMI) or using BMI tables (see Figure 1-2). The BMI is used to evaluate weight status and should be explained to the patient to help her set appropriate weight-gain goals. Whenever possible, prepregnancy weight should be ascertained from clinical records obtained just before pregnancy. Current weight should also be measured and rate of weight gain assessed at each visit.

Laboratory Evaluation

Routine tests related to the nutritional status of pregnant women should be performed at the beginning of pregnancy and intermittently as appropriate including screening for anemia (hemoglobin, hematocrit) and for gestational diabetes, the latter at 24 to 28 weeks' gestation. When iron stores are low, serum ferritin and mean corpuscular volume (MCV) levels should be checked. The clinician must be aware of ethnic or racial differences when interpreting these laboratory studies. For example, African-American women are more likely to have higher levels of ferritin than are white women. Patients of African-American, Southeast Asian, and Mediterranean descent are also at increased risk for having sickle cell disease, sickle cell trait, and/or one of the thalassemias. They should be evaluated for these inherited disorders if their initial screen shows anemia in the presence of normal iron stores. Urinary screening for the presence of glucose and protein as a screen for diabetes and renal disease, respectively, and infection should also be conducted (Table 4-1).

Maternal Weight-Gain Recommendations

Maternal weight gain is attributable both to increases in maternal weight (increased circulating blood volume, breast mass, uterine size) and fetoplacental growth within the uterus (increased size of the fetus, placenta, and amniotic fluid volume) during pregnancy. During the first half of gestation, weight gain primarily reflects changes in maternal stores and fluid status. In the second half of gestation, weight gain is the result of a continued increase in maternal stores and fluid as well as fetal growth. Rapid weight gain near the end of gestation, after approximately 32 weeks, usually represents the accumulation of tissue edema.

Because the relationship between maternal weight gain and infant birth weight is closely correlated, the rate of weight gain during pregnancy is important. Most weight gain should occur in the second and early third trimesters (18 to 30 weeks). Adequate weight gain in the second trimester of pregnancy appears to be protective of fetal and neonatal weight even if weight gain is inadequate during the remainder of the pregnancy.

Low prepregnancy weight and low maternal weight gain are risk factors for low birth weight, both intrauterine growth restriction and preterm birth, and an increased incidence of perinatal death. Weight-gain goals vary depending on the prepregnancy BMI of the woman, the number of fetuses (twins, triplets, etc.), and the mother's age. The impact of maternal weight gain on birth weight (decreased incidence of low birth weight with increased weight gain during pregnancy) decreases as prepregnancy BMI increases. The current weight-gain recommendations set by the Institute of Medicine (IOM) for a normal pregnancy are the same as those from the American College of Obstetricians and Gynecologists (Table 4-2).

Racial and Ethnic Minorities

Although these guidelines serve as a starting point for evaluating weight gain, specific recommendations for individuals vary with individual needs. Data from national studies suggest that fetal birth weight and maternal weight gain are lower

Table 4-1   Nutrition-related issues on the obstetric workup.

Present illness

General: Chronic disease states, recent weight change, weight gain during the pregnancy, edema, and dehydration.

GI complaints: Diarrhea, nausea, vomiting, heartburn, and constipation.

Medical history

Is the woman taking prenatal vitamins, other dietary supplements, herbs, teas or, alternative therapies? How often does she take them?

Does the woman take any additional iron supplements?

Does the woman have any food allergies or sensitivities? If yes, which ones?

Does the woman have any nonfood cravings (pica: ice, dirt, cornstarch, clay, detergent)?

Social history

Does the woman drink alcohol? If so, what type, quantity, frequency, duration?

How many meals does the woman eat daily? How many snacks?

Does the woman avoid any specific food groups, such as fruits, vegetables, starches, milk, or meats?

What type of milk (whole, 2%, 1%, skim, lactose free) does the woman drink, if any?

Was the woman following any special diet before becoming pregnant? Is she a strict vegetarian (vegan)?

Family history

A three-generation pedigree should be identified and the ages and general health or cause of death for each family member noted. Familial occurrences of any specific disease with nutritional significance (genetic storage diseases) and a history of children in the family born with anomalies are noted.

Review of systems

General: Fatigue, weight change (how much and over what period of time?).

Mouth: Dentition and condition of gums, lips, tongue.

GI/abdomen: Appetite, food intolerance, nausea, vomiting, constipation, or diarrhea.

Physical examination

Blood pressure, prepregnancy weight, body mass index, weight gain during pregnancy so far (per week or month), goal for appropriate weight gain during pregnancy.

Laboratory evaluation

Glucose: normal: 70–110 mg/dL

Hematocrit: female normal: 36–46%

Hemoglobin: female normal: 12–16 g/dL

Others as indicated in high-risk patients

SOURCE: Lisa Hark, PhD, RD, University of Pennsylvania School of Medicine. Used with permission.

for African-American women than for white women, even when controlling for gestational age and other factors. The incidence of low birth weight is higher in African-American infants than in infants of other racial and ethnic origin. In an attempt to improve fetal growth, the IOM recommends that these women gain toward the higher end of the recommended weight gain for their BMI. No weight gain recommendations have been made for pregnant women from other minorities, as there has been little research into their specific needs.

Table 4-2   Recommended total weight gain ranges* for pregnant women by prepregnancy body mass index.

PREPREGNANT BMI CATEGORY	TOTAL WEIGHT (kg)	(kg)/ 4 WEEKS	TOTAL WEIGHT (lb)	(lb)/ 4 WEEKS
Underweight (BMI: 19.8)	12.7–18.2	2.3	28–40	5.0
Normal (BMI: 19.8–26.0)	11.4–15.9	1.8	25–35	4.0
Overweight (BMI: 26.1–29.0)	6.8–11.4	1.2	15–25	2.6
Obese (BMI >29.0)	6.8	0.9	15	2.0
Twin gestation	15.9–20.4	2.7	35–45	6.0

BMI, body mass index = weight (kg)/height (m^2).

* Applies to the second and third trimesters only.

SOURCE: Reprinted with permission from the National Academy of Sciences. Nutrition during pregnancy. Washington, DC: National Academy Press, 1990.

Adolescence

It is helpful for the health care team to stress to the adolescent patient the importance of good lifelong nutritional habits, as well as the nutritional changes necessary for optimal pregnancy outcome. Young adolescents, in particular, may still be growing and may need to gain additional weight to accommodate normal growth during the 40 weeks of the average pregnancy.

The pattern of weight gain, as well as the total weight gain, has been shown to be particularly important in the adolescent population. Inadequate weight gain before 24 weeks, even if total pregnancy weight gain is adequate, is associated with low-birth-weight deliveries in the adolescent population. Recent research on adolescents suggests that the components of the diet are also important determinants of birth weight. Adolescents whose diets are higher in total carbohydrates and lower in protein and fat appear to have lower overall risks of delivering a lower-birth-weight baby and having a preterm delivery compared to adolescents with diets lower in carbohydrates. Adolescents are more likely to consume diets that are low in micronutrients, such as iron, zinc, folate, calcium, and vitamin A, B_6, and C, and higher in energy from macronutrients, including total fat, saturated fat, and sugar.

Maternal Nutrient Needs: Current Recommendations

The recommended dietary allowances (RDAs), dietary reference intakes (DRIs), and estimated safe and adequate daily dietary intakes (ESADDIs) for pregnant and lactating women are listed in Table 4-3. These recommendations are based on estimates derived from accretion rates of nutrients measured in fetuses, as well as from clinical and epidemiologic data. These recommendations are not

Table 4-3 Dietary reference intakes: recommended daily allowances and adequate intakes for women 19 to 50 years of age.

NUTRIENT	NONPREGNANT	PREGNANT	LACTATING
Protein (g)	46	60	65
Vitamin A (RE)[a]	700	770	1300
Vitamin D (mg)	5[b]	5[b]	5[b]
Vitamin E (mg)	15	15	19
Vitamin K (mg)	90[b]	90[b]	90[b]
Vitamin C (mg)	75	85	120
Thiamine (mg)	1.1	1.4	1.4
Riboflavin (mg)	1.1	1.4	1.6
Niacin (mg NE)[c]	14	18	17
Vitamin B_6 (mg)	1.3	1.9	2.0
Folic acid (μg)	400	600	500
Vitamin B_{12} (mg)	2.4	2.6	2.8
Calcium (mg)	1000[b]	1000[b]	1000[b]
Phosphorus (mg)	700	700	700
Magnesium (mg)	310–320	350–360	310–320
Iron (elem) (mg)	18	27	9
Zinc (mg)	8	11	12
Iodine (μg)	150	220	290
Selenium (μg)	55	60	70

[a] Retinol equivalents (REs).

[b] Adequate intake (AIs).

[c] Niacin equivalents (NEs).

SOURCES: National Academy of Sciences, Institute of Medicine, Dietary Reference Intakes 1997, 1998, 2000, 2001, 2002.

Table 4-4 Recommended servings per day by food groups.

PYRAMID FOOD GROUP	SERVINGS/DAY
Bread and cereals	6–11 servings
Vegetables	3–5
Fruits	2–4
Low-fat dairy products	3–5 (1 cup/serving)
Meat or meat substitutes	2–3 (3 to 4 oz/serving)
Alcohol	Not recommended

specific for individuals but were developed to evaluate groups for epidemiologic purposes. Recommended servings per day by food group are listed in Table 4-4.

The most significant increases in nutrient needs are for protein, vitamins, and minerals. Protein needs increase by approximately 30%, folic acid by 200%, calcium and phosphorus by 50%, magnesium by 15%, and iron by at least 100%. Therefore, it is vital that pregnant women not only consume the extra energy, or calories, required but that the energy is coming from high-quality or nutrient-dense food.

Dietary Characteristics of Pregnant Women

Anna Siega-Ritz reviewed the food patterns of pregnant women in the United States and stratified her findings by race. In the pregnant population, she found that low nutrient-dense foods were major contributors to total energy, carbohydrate, and fat intake. Dietary carbohydrates were mostly refined and included soft drinks and other fruit juices, biscuits and muffins, and white bread. Dietary fat intake higher than 30% was observed for more than half of the women and was mainly of animal origin. When milk consumption was examined, women were twice as likely to consume whole milk as reduced-fat milk.

In this study, the most important sources of folate and iron were fortified foods, such as ready-to-eat cereals, grains (white bread, bagels, crackers, biscuits, muffins), and rice. Nearly 60% of the women had an adequate folate intake. Both plant and animal food sources contributed to iron intake, with ground beef representing the most commonly consumed food. Only one-third of all women were able to get enough iron from their diet, and two-thirds reported taking iron supplements.

Energy

The total maternal energy requirement for a full-term pregnancy is estimated at 80,000 calories. An additional 300 calories per day is recommended during the second and third trimester of pregnancy. This represents a 15% to 17% increase in energy requirements for a 25- to 35-lb (11 to 14 kg) weight gain. Little to no additional energy is required during the first trimester in otherwise healthy pregnant women. However, increased energy needs are required in early pregnancy for women who have depleted nutrient reserves due to conditions such as hyperemesis gravidarum, eating disorders and low BMI, chronic disease states, or famine.

Protein

Diets in the United States generally contain at least adequate, if not excessive, protein intake. It is recommended that pregnant woman consume 60 g protein per day. This represents a 30% or 15 g per day increase over the 46 g per day recommended for nonpregnant women. This recommended intake provides the protein necessary for the increased protein deposition that occurs in maternal, fetal, and placental tissues.

Vitamin and Mineral Supplementation Guidelines

Routine vitamin/mineral supplementation for women reporting appropriate dietary intake and demonstrating adequate weight gain (without edema) is not mandatory. However, most childbirth providers prescribe a prenatal vitamin and mineral supplement because many women do not consume enough food to meet their increased nutritional requirements, especially with regard to folic acid, during the first trimester of pregnancy.

Supplementation with a prenatal vitamin, and possibly referral to a registered dietitian, is advised for women with the following conditions or complications in association with pregnancy:

- Pregnancy involving multiple gestations (twins, triplets)
- Frequent gestations (less than a 3-month interpregnancy interval)
- Use of tobacco, alcohol, or chronic medicinal or illicit drug use
- Severe nausea and vomiting of pregnancy or hyperemesis gravidarum
- Eating disorders, including anorexia, bulimia, and compulsive eating; over- or undernutrition
- Inadequate weight gain during pregnancy: adolescence
- Eating restrictions including strict vegetarianism (avoidance of all animal products, including dairy) and food allergies or intolerances
- Chronic illness
- Prior history of low-birth-weight babies or other obstetric complications, possibly associated with nutritional abnormalities; social (e.g., religion, poverty) factors that may limit appropriate intake.

Calcium

In 1998, the DRIs for calcium were increased in the adolescent population to 1300 mg per day, compared with the 1000 mg per day recommendation for women from 19 to 50 years old. During pregnancy, DRIs were increased to 1200 mg per day (see Table 4-3). As nonpregnant women generally consume only 75% of their recommended calcium intake, pregnant women should be encouraged to add calcium-rich foods or take a supplement to achieve the DRI. Adequate calcium intake is critical for young women, whose bones continue to increase in bone density until they are about 25 years of age. Furthermore, pregnancy poses the potential risk of maternal bone demineralization, which can lead to osteoporosis. Additional calcium is believed to be stored in the maternal skeleton as a reserve for lactation. Although controversial, studies of maternal calcium supplementation with 1000 to 2000 mg per day have shown a reduction in pregnancy complications, such as pregnancy-induced hypertension, pre-eclampsia, low birth weight, and premature delivery rates.

Vitamin D

Vitamin D supplementation (10 to 25 mg per day) has been associated with higher serum values in women with vitamin D deficiency, increased fetal birth weight, and decreased incidence of neonatal hypocalcemia, neonatal seizures, and maternal osteomalacia. Conversely, there is some evidence that excessive vitamin D intake during pregnancy may cause fetal hypercalcemia, which can lead to fetal growth retardation, aortic stenosis, and deposition of calcium in the brain and other organs.

Vitamin A

In Western countries, vitamin A supplements are generally not required because of the adequate amounts found in the food supply. However, low-income adolescents may consume a diet low in vitamin A. Excessive vitamin A intake has been reported to be teratogenic. Patients should be aware that some over-the-counter vitamin supplements may contain more than the RDA for vitamin A [700 mg retinol equivalents (REs) per day] and should be discontinued during pregnancy. Pregnant women should also discontinue use of topical creams containing retinol derivatives to treat acne. Upper tolerable limit has been set at 3000 mg RE per day.

Folic Acid

Folic acid supplementation before and during early pregnancy decreases the risk of fetal and neonatal neural tube defects (NTD). To be effective in lowering the incidence of fetal NTD, folic acid supplementation should be started before conception and continued during the first 4 weeks after conception, until closure of the neural tube. As half of all pregnancies in the United States are unintended, it is important that folic acid supplementation be discussed with women of childbearing age.

The current DRI recommendation for folate throughout pregnancy is 600 μg per day. Almost all prenatal vitamins are now supplemented with at least 800 μg folic acid. The recommended maximum daily intake of folic acid is 1000 μg because higher doses may mask a vitamin B_{12} deficiency. Up to 4000 μg per day may be recommended for women, under the supervision of a physician, who have a history of a child born with an NTD (see Case 1).

Iron

During pregnancy, iron is necessary for the production of red blood cells in both the mother and fetus and for fetoplacental growth. Maternal blood volume increases by up to 50%, requiring 500 mg elemental iron. The fetus requires an additional 300 mg elemental iron, accumulating most of its iron stores during the third trimester; this may help to explain why iron-deficiency anemia is most prevalent in this trimester.

According to the Centers for Disease Control and Prevention (CDC), screening for anemia should take place before pregnancy, as well as during the first, second, and third trimesters in high-risk individuals. Hemoglobin levels less than 11 g/dL or hematocrit levels less than 33% in the first and third trimesters indicate anemia. Hemoglobin levels less than 10.5 g/dL or hematocrit levels less than 32% during the second trimester indicate anemia. Since hemoglobin levels normally decline during pregnancy because of the significant increase in maternal blood volume, ferritin and MCV should also be measured as diagnostic criteria, since these values remain constant.

Iron-deficiency anemia during pregnancy has been associated with an increased risk of maternal and infant death, preterm delivery, and low-weight babies and has negative consequences for normal infant brain development and function. The prevalence of iron deficiency in pregnancy is higher in African-American women, low-income women, teenagers, women with less than a high school education, and women who have had two or three prior pregnancies. *Healthy People 2010* goals include reducing anemia among pregnant females in their third trimester from 29% to 20% and reducing ethnic and income disparities. Women, Infant, and Children's (WIC) programs have been successful in reducing the prevalence of iron-deficiency anemia during pregnancy and postpartum.

The DRI for elemental iron is 27 mg per day during the second and third trimester of pregnancy. For treatment of iron-deficiency anemia during pregnancy, therapeutic iron doses of 60 to 120 mg per day can be prescribed. However, because iron may constipate some pregnant women, advising tolerance levels of insoluble fiber, fluids, and regular physical activity is important (see Chapter 2, Case 1). Benefits have also been seen from supplementing women with iron for at least 3 months postpartum.

Dietary Fiber

No specific recommendations have been made for dietary fiber intake during pregnancy. However, increased intake of high-fiber foods, such as vegetables, whole grains, and fruits, is recommended for the prevention and treatment of constipation, a common problem during pregnancy. One should always advocate adequate fluid intake when increasing dietary fiber.

Fluids

Pregnancy represents a unique state in which circulating blood volume increases by 50%. Tissue fluid also increases, whereas blood pressure generally decreases in the second trimester before recovering to prepregnant levels near term. This is the result of vasodilation of the capacitance venous blood vessels, requiring substantial fluid intake during pregnancy in order to maintain blood pressure and blood flow to vital organs. The increase in circulating blood volume begins in the early part of pregnancy, and the failure of this to occur has been associated with preterm delivery, intrauterine growth restriction, and the hypertensive disorders of pregnancy. General recommendations are to drink at least 64 oz (1920 mL) water per day. In areas where the water supply is suspected to contain lead, women should be encouraged to drink bottled water. Excessive lead intakes may result in spontaneous abortion, decreased stature, and impaired neurocognitive development of the baby.

Food Contamination

Food contaminated by contact with heavy metals or pathogenic bacteria can produce devastating results in the developing fetus. Most heavy metals are considered teratogenic. In particular, cases of teratogenicity or embryotoxicity have been reported involving methyl mercury, lead, cadmium, nickel, and selenium. Mercury can be removed from vegetables by washing with soap and water or by removing the skins. Eating raw fish products (sushi, clams, oysters) should probably be avoided during pregnancy due to the risk of hepatitis or intestinal parasites. Bacterial contamination of food supplies must also be avoided. Appropriate handling and cooking of uncooked meats can minimize the risk of food poisoning from bacteria such as *Escherichia coli*. All dairy foods and juices should be pasteurized. *Listeria monocytogenes* contamination causes food poisoning both during and outside of pregnancy but can create a blood-borne, transplacental infection that can be fatal to the developing fetus. Although the incidence of listeriosis is low, it can be prevented by avoidance of risky foods that include cold, precooked meats (luncheon meats) and soft cheeses or cheese products.

Alcohol

Alcohol is a known teratogen. Excessive consumption of alcohol by pregnant women can result in fetal alcohol syndrome (FAS). Although there is little evidence to suggest that drinking small amounts of alcohol can cause birth defects, there is no known safe level of alcohol consumption during pregnancy. Therefore, it is currently recommended that alcohol intake be avoided by pregnant women and women attempting to become pregnant.

Caffeine

It is not clear whether there is an acceptable level of caffeine intake during pregnancy. Recent studies indicate an association between the equivalent of two cups of coffee a day and spontaneous pregnancy loss in the first trimester. The US Food and Drug Administration's recommendation is for pregnant women to reduce their caffeine intake from all sources: coffee, tea, cocoa, and cola drinks.

Common Nutritional Problems during Pregnancy

Discomforts of pregnancy, such as nausea and vomiting, constipation, and heartburn, can generally be alleviated by implementation of the guidelines summarized below.

Nausea and Vomiting

Nausea and vomiting appear to be associated with increased levels of the pregnancy hormone human chorionic gonadotropin (hCG). HCG doubles every 48 hours in early pregnancy and peaks at about 12 weeks' gestation. Nausea is experienced by 60% of pregnant women, and, of these, a small percentage require hospitalization for severe hyperemesis gravidarum. Strategies for managing nausea and vomiting are the following:

- Eat small, low-fat meals and snacks (fruits, pretzels, crackers, nonfat yogurt) slowly and frequently.
- Avoid strong food odors by eating room temperature or cold foods and using good ventilation while cooking.
- Drink fluids between meals rather than with meals.
- Avoid foods that may cause stomach irritation, such as spearmint, peppermint, caffeine, citrus fruits, spicy foods, high-fat foods, or tomato products.
- Avoid eating or drinking for 1 to 2 hours before lying down.
- Take a walk after meals.
- Wear loose-fitting clothes.
- Avoid fragrances, such as perfume, household cleaners, and air fresheners.

Constipation

Constipation during pregnancy is associated with an increase in water reabsorption from the large bowel. In addition, smooth muscle relaxation with resultant slower gastrointestinal tract motility occurs during pregnancy. The pregnant woman often notes overall GI discomfort, a bloated sensation, an increase in hemorrhoids and heartburn, and decreased appetite. Strategies for managing constipation include the following:

- Increase fluid intake to 2 or 3 qt per day, including water, juice, milk, and soup.
- Increase daily dietary fiber intake through ingestion of high-fiber cereals, whole grains, legumes, fruits, and vegetables.
- Participate in moderate physical activity, such as walking, low-impact aerobics, and swimming.

Heartburn and Indigestion

Heartburn and indigestion are usually caused by gastric content reflux that results from both lower esophageal pressure and decreased motility. Limited gastric capacity, secondary to a shift of organs to accommodate the growing fetus, contributes to these symptoms in the third trimester of pregnancy. Strategies for managing heartburn or indigestion are the same as those suggested previously for managing nausea.

Gestational Diabetes Mellitus

Gestational diabetes mellitus (GDM) is defined as any degree of glucose intolerance with onset or first recognition during pregnancy. It occurs in approximately 4% of all pregnancies, resulting in more than 200,000 cases annually. GDM is usually diagnosed during the second or third trimester of pregnancy, at which time insulin-antagonist hormone levels increase and insulin resistance normally occurs. After delivery, approximately 90% of all women with GDM become normoglycemic but are at increased risk of developing type 2 diabetes.

Because fetal morbidity may be increased, it is currently recommended that all pregnant patients be screened for GDM at 24 to 28 weeks of gestational age, as the use of risk factors alone may fail to identify up to 50% of patients with GDM. For high-risk patients, earlier screening is recommended by 16 weeks. High-risk patients are those with a personal history of abnormal glucose tolerance, certain ethnic groups with high prevalence of gestational diabetes (African-American, Native American, Southeast Asian, Pacific Islander, Hispanic), obesity, a first-degree relative with type 2 diabetes, glucosuria, or prior poor obstetric history consistent with diabetes (e.g., macrosomic infant, fetal anomalies, neonatal hypoglycemia).

The main screening tool for GDM is the standardized 150-mL, 50 g glucose load 1-hour serum glucose screen. A threshold level greater than or equal to 130 to 140 mg/dL for the 1-hour screen should be chosen based on the population studied. For the roughly 20% of patients who test positive, a 3-hour 100 g glucose load test is performed. Two criteria are currently used for the diagnosis of GDM, and either appears acceptable. The diagnosis of GDM is made when two or more serum glucose values are met or exceeded.

Medical Nutrition Therapy for Gestational Diabetes

The goals of medical nutrition therapy for GDM are to provide energy levels for appropriate gestational weight gain, achievement and maintenance of normoglycemia, and absence of ketones. Individualization of the meal plan is recommended, as the ideal percentage and type of carbohydrate are controversial. Monitoring blood glucose, urine or blood ketones, appetite, and weight gain is essential for individualizing the meal plan and in adjusting the meal plan throughout pregnancy.

Generally, 40% to 45% of total energy intake will be from carbohydrate, which is distributed throughout the day into three small to moderate-sized meals and two to four snacks. An evening snack is usually needed to prevent accelerated ketosis overnight. Carbohydrate is not as well tolerated at breakfast as it is at other meals, possibly due to the associated increased levels of cortisol and growth hormones. Therefore, the initial meal plan may limit carbohydrate to 30 g at breakfast, with adjustments made later based on blood glucose monitoring results. Protein containing food can be added to satisfy hunger because they do not affect blood glucose levels, can be added.

Patients with serum glucose values persistently above the thresholds require the addition of insulin therapy in order to achieve adequate glycemic control. Recent data evaluating the use of second-generation sulfonylureas, like glyburide, are encouraging but require more study.

The goal of therapy is to prevent the maternal and fetal complications that have been associated with GDM. Maternal complications include fetal macrosomia and its attendant fetal and maternal injury associated with delivery (increased risk of cesarean section, operative vaginal delivery, and shoulder dystocia). Fetal complications include a possible increased incidence of fetal death and ketonemia, which has been associated with lower intelligence scores at 2 to 5 years of age. Overall, the data are inconclusive as to whether these goals are attainable.

The diagnosis of GDM is an excellent predictor of type 2 diabetes developing later in life. This risk is at least 50% over the 15 to 20 years following the pregnancy. It is recommended that a patient with GDM be rescreened for type 2 diabetes after pregnancy.

Lactation (Breastfeeding)

Metabolic and Physiologic Changes during Lactation

Breast enlargement begins early in pregnancy as a result of the hormones generated by the pituitary gland and the corpus luteum. The lacteal cells also differentiate in preparation for milk production that begins when the infant is born. As the breast undergoes these preparatory changes, the areola (the pigmented area surrounding the nipple) becomes darker and more prominent, and the skin over the nipple becomes more elastic and more erect in order to facilitate suckling.

Lactogenesis is believed to be initiated by the abrupt decrease in progesterone and estrogen following parturition (giving birth). As the infant begins to suckle, stimulating the receptors in the nipple and areola, nerve impulses are sent to the hypothalamus. The hypothalamus, in turn, stimulates the release of the hormones oxytocin and prolactin from the posterior pituitary gland. Prolactin stimulates milk production in the breast, and oxytocin stimulates myoepithelial cells around ducts to contract and eject milk from the alveolus. Milk accumulates in the lactiferous sinuses under the areola and is released when the areola is compressed between the baby's tongue and palate. Factors that may influence milk production and composition include the following:

- How soon the mother and infant begin nursing. Nursing within the first hour after birth is optimal.
- Breastfeeding schedule: feeding on demand without interruption, at least 10 minutes on each breast.
- Infant weight and maturity.
- Infant illness.
- Maternal age and parity (number of children previously borne).
- Maternal stress.
- Maternal fluid intake (recommend drinking to thirst at least 3 qt per day).
- Maternal use of cigarettes, alcohol, and oral contraceptives.

Benefits of Breastfeeding

Breastfeeding has been recommended as the "gold standard" for infant feeding by all professional groups from the World Health Organization to the American Academy of Pediatrics. The current *Healthy People 2010* goals are to have 75%

of mothers breastfeeding their infants at discharge and continuing through the first year of the baby's life. Table 4-5 outlines what health professionals can do to promote breastfeeding.

Table 4-5   What health professionals can do to promote breastfeeding.

- Encourage education about the benefits of breastfeeding in medical school curriculum, during residency, and in continuing medical education courses.
- Give patients preconception and prenatal guidance and preparation.
- Refer women to mother-to-mother support groups in the community.
- Become familiar with initiation of lactation and management of common problems.
- Give patients educational materials that promote breastfeeding, written by lactation experts rather than formula companies.
- Help patients start breastfeeding within 1 hour of delivery and ensure that healthy infants are not separated from their mothers.
- Give patients postpartum support and encouragement to maintain breastfeeding.
- Seek information to help resolve problems; do not automatically suggest formulas.
- Support hospital initiatives to encourage breastfeeding, such as establishing the Baby Friendly Hospital Initiative.
- Work with hospitals to employ International Board-Certified Lactation Consultants and to eliminate formula in discharge packs.
- Encourage hospital nursery policy that avoids all supplemental feedings and bottles, particularly at the initiation of lactation.
- Avoid medications that are unsafe during lactation, and choose alternatives with less distribution in the milk.

SOURCE: Reprinted with permission from Lawrence RA, Lawrence RM. Breastfeeding, the Guide for the Medical Profession. 5th ed. St. Louis: Mosby, 1999.

Bioactive and Immunologic Benefits

Breast milk contains leukocytes (macrophages), immunoglobulins (Ig; secretory IgA, IgG, IgM, and antiviral antibodies), bifidus factor (to support *Lactobacillus bifidus*), lysozymes (promotes lysis of bacteria), interferon, lactoferrin (binds whey protein and inhibits growth of *E. coli*), lactadherin (protects against symptomatic rotavirus infections), growth factors and cytokines (bFGF, EGF, NGF, TGF, G-CSF, interleukins, TNF-alpha, among others), prostaglandins, hormones (pituitary, hypothalamic, and steroid), GI peptides (VIP, gastrin, GIP), and others (complement factors, glutamine, oligosaccharides, nucleotides, long-chain polyunsaturated fatty acids). Some of these agents help individually or in groups to minimize the infectious risk of the newborn.

Health and Social Benefits

Breastfed infants are hospitalized less often than formula-fed infants during the first 6 months of life. Significant health care cost savings from the decreased incidences of lower respiratory infection, otitis media, and gastroenteritis are noted in the human milk–fed infant. Strong evidence has shown that human milk also decreases the incidence and severity of diarrhea, bacteremia, bacterial meningitis, urinary tract infection, and necrotizing enterocolitis. Studies describe the protective effect of human milk for immune- or autoimmune-related diseases such as chronic and inflammatory bowel diseases, type 1 diabetes mellitus, and allergic diseases. Human milk may also be helpful against sudden infant death syndrome (SIDS) and lymphoma. Breastfeeding promotes good jaw and tooth development in the infant and also fosters mother-infant bonding.

Maternal benefits include accelerated weight loss, decreased accumulation of adipose tissue, delayed return of ovulation with increased child spacing, improved bone remineralization with resumption of menses postpartum, and reduced ovarian and premenopausal breast cancer risk. Breast milk is convenient because it is at the proper temperature and it does not require heating or special preparation such as mixing with sterilized water, or storage.

Types of Breast Milk

The human breast produces three types of breast milk. Colostrum, produced during pregnancy and present in highest concentration during the first few days of lactation, is high in protein, immunoglobulins, beta-carotene, sodium, potassium, chloride, fat-soluble vitamins, minerals and unique hormones. These substances encourage the growth of bifidus flora, maturation of the GI tract, and the passage of the meconium or first stools. Transitional milk is produced during days 6 through 15 as the volume increases and is higher in concentration of fat and lactose and lower in protein and minerals than colostrum. Mature milk, produced from day 15 through weaning, is basically an emulsion of fat in sugared (lactose) water and provides 20 to 22 calories per ounce (30 mL) and optimal nutrition.

Breast Milk Composition

Breast milk is rich in most nutrients and other substances required to sustain the newborn's appropriate growth during the first 6 months of life. The nutrient components present in breast milk are the following:

Fat

The total amount of fat in breast milk is constant, but its composition varies. Initially, breast milk is similar to skim milk, with a relatively low fat content. As the infant continues to suckle and a period of letdown occurs, breast milk becomes higher in fat and calories. Therefore, it is essential that the infant be allowed to nurse on each breast until he or she is satisfied to derive the full fat from the feeding. Encouraging the infant to suckle on each breast for 10 minutes or more ensures adequate calorie consumption. The emptying time of breast milk from the infant's stomach is, on average, $1^{1}/_{2}$ hours, compared with 3 hours for formula-fed infants. The fat content of breast milk provides 50% of the infant's total energy requirements in readily absorbable form.

Protein

Breast milk contains whey and casein. Whey protein accounts for 60% to 80% of the total protein in breast milk and is present mainly in the form of alpha-lactalbumin, lactoferrin, and secretory IgA. Casein accounts for 20% to 40% of breast milk's total protein and forms micelles that enhance the infant's ability to absorb calcium, phosphorus, iron, zinc, and copper. The protein concentration is low but optimal.

Carbohydrates

The primary carbohydrate source in breast milk is lactose. Small amounts of glucose, oligosaccharides, and glycoproteins are also present. The last two have immunologic functions.

Fluoride

Fluoride supplements are most appropriate for infants who are breastfeeding for at least 1 year where there is no fluoride in the water supply.

Vitamin D

Some breastfed infants are at risk for rickets caused by vitamin D deficiency because breast milk contains only small quantities of this nutrient. This is especially true of dark-skinned infants of mothers with poor vitamin D status due to poor diet, lack of sun exposure, or both, such as certain women, who, for religious reasons, remain heavily clothed. These infants may benefit from vitamin D supplementation (400 IU per day).

Vitamin K

Breast milk contains a small amount of vitamin K, but supplementation after delivery generally is not necessary, as most newborns receive vitamin K intramuscularly immediately after delivery to prevent hemorrhagic disease of the newborn.

Nutritional Recommendations for Lactating Women

Energy

Approximately 85 kcal is required to produce 100 mL breast milk. Stored energy from maternal fat reserves provides 100 to 150 kcal per day, but this may not be sufficient. Therefore, current recommendations advise that the daily caloric intake of lactating women be increased by 500 kcal per day. This may not be necessary for all women. Postpartum women should avoid diets and medications that promise rapid weight loss. Weight loss should always be gradual, and this is particularly true for lactating women, who burn more calories than nonlactating women in support of breast milk production.

Calcium

Normally, 2% to 8% of total body calcium is mobilized for breast milk production during lactation but will be restored after the onset of menses. Among adults of low socioeconomic status, diets are often low in calcium and vitamin A. A recent revision of guidelines for breastfeeding women has been provided for selective nutrients (see Table 4-3).

Iron

Iron requirements are lower during lactation (9 mg per day) than during pregnancy (27 mg per day) until menstruation resumes (18 mg per day). In the United

Table 4-6 Common problems experienced while breastfeeding.

PROBLEMS*	TREATMENT
Nipple	
Inverted nipples	Identify before delivery; recommend nipple shells. Shells may discourage women from breastfeeding at all. Sometimes best to discuss during pregnancy and treat after delivery with breast pump.
Sore nipples	Advise patients to avoid soaps and ointments; demonstrate proper latch on and positioning of the infant.
Breast	
Engorgement	Recommend hand expression or pumping; mild heat may soften the areolar mound before a feed. Cold is best treatment after a feed.
Milk duct stasis	Recommend rest, heat, massage, alternate feeding positions, frequent nursing. Distinguish from galactocele or mastitis.
Mastitis	Recommend rest, heat, massage, alternate feeding positions, frequent nursing; give antibiotics that cover *Staphylococcus aureus* for a minimum of 10 days.
Abscess	Abscess is a rare event usually due to inadequate treatment of mastitis. Consider needle aspiration or incision and drainage.
Infant	
Baby sleeps during feeding	Teach the mother to watch for feeding cues or signs of feeding interest, such as facial movements, opening mouth indicating hunger. Baby should not have to cry to get the mother's attention. When baby is sleepy, changing the diaper, massage, and visual stimulation may be helpful.
Hungry baby	Increase frequency or length of feedings for growth spurt; milk production will increase.
Jaundice	Identify cause, which is usually inadequate caloric intake, and allow the baby to nurse much more frequently; if it is a breast-milk jaundice, continue feedings unless bilirubin is approaching 20 mg/dL (see Table 4-8). Breast-milk jaundice is rare; develops after 5th day, peaks 10th to 14th day and may persist, and is improved by more aggressive feeding and stimulation of stooling.
Poor weight gain	Recommend frequent nursing (every 2 to 3 hours), express breast milk and feed by cup, allow/encourage unrestricted nursing, and ensure adequate length of time for nursing; consider supplemental nursing system with expressed milk or, if other efforts fail, use formula in the supplemental system.
Other	
Inhibited letdown	Warm shower, privacy, local heat, soft music, low lighting, relaxation techniques, gentle breast massage.
Medications	Assess need, choose drugs safe for lactation.
Monilial infections	Treat with topical antifungals on breast and oral nystatin for infant.
Work-related	Educate patient about various breast pumps and devices; support and encourage using the pump at work.

* Mothers having problems should be referred to an International Board-Certified Lactation Consultant (IBCLC) if they are not resolved.

SOURCE: Reprinted with permission from Lawrence RA, Lawrence RM. Breastfeeding, a guide for the Medical Profession. 5th ed. St. Louis: Mosby, 1999.

States, studies of lactating women consuming a 2700 kcal daily diet suggest that they are not likely to meet the RDAs for calcium and zinc. Diets that contain less than 2700 kcal per day may also be low in magnesium, vitamin B_6, and folate. Adolescent mothers' diets may be particularly low in iron.

Vitamin Supplements

Prenatal vitamin supplements are routinely prescribed to lactating women to ensure adequate intake. However, lactating women should also be encouraged to obtain their nutrients from a well-balanced, varied diet. Also, they should continue to drink to thirst or approximately 2 to 3 qt fluids per day to prevent dehydration while breastfeeding.

Common Problems Experienced While Breastfeeding

Informed physicians and nurses can readily manage most of the common problems associated with breastfeeding; however, referral to a mother-to-mother support group can be very helpful for most common problems, and referral to a Certified Lactation Consultant can ensure continued lactation when problems are more complex. Table 4-6 lists the most common problems and the suggested treatments. Breastfeeding is only contraindicated in the following conditions:

Maternal Infections

Tuberculosis, typhoid, active herpes in the area of the breast, rubella, mumps, human immunodeficiency virus (HIV), and, in some cases, cytomegalovirus (CMV)

Table 4-7   Commonly prescribed drugs considered compatible with breastfeeding (Committee on Drugs, American Academy of Pediatrics).

ANTIBIOTICS	ANTIHYPERTENSIVES	ANTICONVULSANTS
Ampicillin	Captopril	Carbamazepine
Amoxicillin	Hydrochlorothiazide	Phenobarbital
Ciprofloxacin	Methyldopa	Phenytoin
Clindamycin	Nadolol	Valproic acid
Cloxacillin	Propranolol	
Dicloxacillin sodium		
Erythromycin		
Gentamicin		
Ketoconazole	ANALGESICS	OTHER
Penicillin	Acetaminophen	Digoxin
Rifampin	Aspirin	Heparin
	Codeine	Magnesium sulfate
	Ibuprofen	Immune globulin (human; RhoGAM)
		Rubella vaccine
		Warfarin sodium

SOURCE: Adapted from American Academy of Pediatrics statement on drugs: the transfer of drugs and other chemicals into human breast milk. Pediatrics 2001;108:776–789.

are all contraindications for breastfeeding in the United States. In some countries, the infant mortality risks of not breastfeeding may override the morbidity and mortality risks associated with the possible acquisition of such maternal infections.

Medications

Commonly prescribed drugs that are compatible with breastfeeding are listed in Table 4-7. As in pregnancy, some medications, herbal remedies, nutritional supplements, and alternative therapies are not appropriate during lactation. Illegal substances, such as amphetamines, cocaine, heroin, or marijuana, as well as nicotine, pass into breast milk when ingested by the mother, who should be discouraged from using these drugs while breastfeeding. Several drugs, including nicotine and estrogen-containing oral contraceptives, can decrease milk supply and interfere with milk production.

Specific drugs that are contraindicated in the treatment of breastfeeding women are bromocriptine, tetracycline, cyclophosphamide, cyclosporine, doxorubicin, ergotamine, lithium, methotrexate, phencyclidine (PCP), and phenindione.

Table 4-8   Managing breastfeeding jaundice.

Early-onset (before 5 days postpartum)

- Leave infant with the mother; provide couplet care for mother and infant so they are not separated.
- Encourage/allow mothers to nurse for longer periods and more frequently (minimum of 8 times a day in first week or two).
- Avoid formula supplementation, which interferes with lactation stimulation.
- Do not give glucose water or sterile water supplementation.
- Monitor serum bilirubin concentrations daily on an outpatient basis until they plateau or drop below 10 mg/dL. Initiate phototherapy according to American Academy of Pediatrics (AAP) guidelines.

Late-onset (5–15 days postpartum)

- If bilirubin concentration reaches 17 to 20 mg/dL, breast should be pumped to maintain lactation, and human milk feeding should be interrupted for 24 to 48 hours as a diagnostic test.
- Instruct mothers to maintain milk production by regularly expressing their milk during the interruption.
- Monitor serum bilirubin levels every 12 to 24 hours and initiate phototherapy according to AAP guidelines.
- *Resume breastfeeding after a decrease in serum bilirubin concentration to check for rebound. May be able to continue breastfeeding if bilirubin stays low.*

SOURCE: Reprinted with permission from Lawrence RA, Lawrence RM. Breastfeeding, a Guide for the Medical Profession. 5th ed. St. Louis: Mosby, 1999

For a list of references for this chapter, please visit the University of Pennsylvania School of Medicine's Nutrition Education and Prevention Program web site: *http://www.med.upenn.edu/nutrimed/articles.html*

Case 1

Prevention of Neural Tube Defects

Ann Honebrink and Frances Burke

Objectives

- Define the prevalence, etiology, and pathogenesis of neural tube defects.
- Describe the association between folate levels and prevention of neural tube defects in the developing fetus.
- Given a prepregnant woman's detailed medical, obstetric, dietary, and social history, evaluate the risk of having a child with a neural tube defect.
- Evaluate the nutritional adequacy of a prepregnant woman's diet.

PL, a 32-year-old married woman, has missed her period and discovers that she is pregnant. This was an unplanned pregnancy, and PL presents for her first prenatal visit at 5 weeks of gestation (normal gestation period is 40 weeks). She is a gravida 3 para 1011.

> The term *para* has four components that describe the number of pregnancies: n full-term births; n preterm births; n early pregnancy losses, including miscarriages, elective terminations, and ectopic pregnancies; and n live children. Thus, as a para 1011, PL has had one full-term birth, no preterm births, one miscarriage, and one living child.

Past Medical/Surgical and Obstetric History

PL's previous delivery was by cesarean section. This was performed for arrest of the normal progress of labor at 39 weeks' gestation. Her infant weighed 7.5 lb (3.4 kg) at birth. She is not hypertensive and has no history of pregnancy-induced hypertension during her previous gestation. Her 1-hour glucose tolerance test at 28 weeks was normal in her prior pregnancy. She has no chronic medical problems and has had no surgeries other than the cesarean section and a dilation and evacuation at the time of her miscarriage. PL currently takes no medications, vitamins, minerals, or herbal supplements. She denies any allergies or food sensitivities to medications or foods.

Social History

PL stays at home to care for her 2-year-old daughter. She reports having little free time to exercise. She does not smoke or drink alcohol. She denies any history of sexual abuse or domestic violence. She lives at home with her husband and daughter.

Family History

PL has a sister-in-law (her husband's sister) who had a 24-week loss of a baby found to have anencephaly. Her parents, siblings, and other nieces and nephews are all in good health and free from chronic diseases. Both of her paternal grandparents had heart disease before their deaths in their mid-sixties. Her maternal grandmother has type 2 diabetes mellitus controlled on a sulfonylurea agent, and her maternal grandfather had a myocardial infarction and died at 54 years of age.

Physical Examination

Vital Signs

Temperature: 98.4°F (37°C)
Heart rate: 80 beats per minute (BPM)
Respiration: 18 BPM
Blood pressure: 120/70 mm Hg
Height: 5'6" (168 cm)
Current/usual weight: 145 lb (66 kg)
BMI: 23.5 kg/m^2

General: Tired-looking, pale, in no acute distress
Heart: Regular rate and rhythm with no murmurs, rubs, or gallops
Respiration: Lungs clear to auscultation and percussion
Abdomen: Soft and nontender without any masses
Pelvic: External genitalia normal, cervix clear on speculum examination, uterus soft and top-normal size (consistent with 5-week pregnancy) with no adenexal masses on bimanual examination, no tenderness
Extremities: Varicose veins with no clubbing, cyanosis, or edema; veins nontender and not inflamed

PL's 24-Hour Dietary Recall

Breakfast (home)	Bagel	1
	Cream cheese	1 Tbsp.
	Coffee	1 cup
	2% Low-fat milk	1 oz (30 mL)

Lunch (home)	Turkey breast lunchmeat	3 oz (85 g)
	Potato bread	2 slices
	Mayonnaise	1 Tbsp.
	Diet Coke	12 oz (360 mL)
Snack (home)	Pretzels	1 oz (28 g)
Dinner (home)	Fried flounder	5 oz (142 g)
	Corn on the cob	1 ear
	Margarine	1 Tbsp.
	Diet Coke	12 oz (360 mL)
	Low-fat frozen yogurt	1 cup

Total Calories: 1521 kcal
Protein: 80 g (21% of total calories)
Carbohydrate: 179 g (47% of total calories)
Fat: 54 g (32% of total calories)
Folate: 238 μg
DRI for folate during pregnancy: 600 μg
Calcium: 608 mg
Iron: 10 mg

Case Questions

1. What is the physiologic basis for the increased folate requirements for normal neural tube development during pregnancy?
2. What is the incidence of NTDs in the United States and who is at higher risk of having a child with an NTD?
3. What is the evidence that folate supplementation reduces the risk of neural tube defects?
4. How can an individual develop a folate deficiency? Which populations are at risk for low folate intake?
5. Describe the rationale for the food fortification program and its potential benefits.
6. List food sources high in folate. Based on the nutrition assessment of PL's diet history, what dietary modifications would you suggest?
7. Should a vitamin and mineral supplement be considered for this patient? Why or why not?

Case Answers

1. **What is the physiologic basis for the increased folate requirements for normal neural tube development during pregnancy?**

   Folate, and its metabolically active form tetrahydrofolate, is a cofactor for the enzymes involved in one-carbon transfers that include the synthesis of nucleic acids and several amino acids (see Chapter 8, Case 1, on alcohol and vitamin deficiencies). Therefore, adequate levels are particularly important at times of rapid cell growth, such as in fetal and placental development. Women are thought to have pregnancies affected by NTDs for two reasons, and frequently for a combination of these two reasons. The first is a dietary deficiency of folate, and the second is a genetic defect in the production of enzymes involved in folate metabolism.

   The neural tube is formed very early in pregnancy, between 18 and 30 days after conception. This means that formation is initiated even before the woman may know she is pregnant, since the missed period would generally occur at 14 days after conception. Since the neural tube goes on to form the spine and brain, defects in the formation of the neural tube can include the absence of formation of most of the brain (anencephaly) as well as defects in the closure of the lower tube (spina bifida to the open neural tube defects, meningoceles, and myoceles). This early formation, and the detrimental effects of folate deficiency on neural tube formation, form the basis for the recommendation that folic acid supplementation should begin before conception and continued at least through the first trimester of pregnancy.

2. **What is the incidence of NTD in the United States and who is at risk of having a child with an NTD?**

   Approximately 1 in 1000 pregnancies in the United States are affected by NTDs, resulting in about 4000 affected pregnancies per year. Of these, approximately 1500 fetuses are either electively or spontaneously terminated and 2500 fetuses result in affected live births. Women who have had a previous pregnancy affected by an NTD or who are personally affected by an NTD are at the highest risk (2% to 3%) in a current pregnancy. A family history of a close family member (sibling, niece, or nephew) with an NTD raises a woman's risk of an affected pregnancy to approximately 1%, as does a maternal history of diabetes or the consumption of certain antiseizure medications such as valproic acid or carbamazepine. Since PL's sister-in-law lost a baby with anencephaly at 24 weeks' gestation, her risk increases. However, 95% of children with NTDs are born to couples without any family history of these defects.

   In women with a history of a previously affected pregnancy, it has been shown that supplementation with 4 mg (4000 μg) folic acid per day initiated 1 month before attempting to conceive and continued throughout the first 3 months of pregnancy reduced the risk of a repeat NTD by 72%. Although there is not yet definitive evidence that other high-risk groups (such as close family members of affected individuals, diabetics, or women on antiseizure medications) will benefit from higher levels of supplementation, many experts believe that women in these groups should be prescribed a higher dose of a folic acid supplement, at least 1000 μg per day, before conception and in early pregnancy. When recommending higher levels of supplementation to patients, it is important to emphasize that a separate folic acid supplement and *not* multiple doses of multivitamins (MVI) be used. Additional daily MVI consumption could lead to toxicity of other vitamins, particularly vitamin A, which is teratogenic to the developing fetus.

3. **What is the evidence that folate supplementation reduces the risk of NTD?**

   An analysis of multiple randomized clinical trials compiled in the Cochrane database has shown that periconceptual and early pregnancy consumption of folate supplements decreases the occurrence of children born with NTDs. In addition, recent comparison of US birth certificate data shows a 19% drop in the prevalence of reported NTDs from October 1998 to December 1999 (since mandatory folic acid fortification of enriched grain products) compared to October 1995 to December 1996. Higher-risk reductions (up to 75%) have been seen in studies using higher levels of daily folate supplementation compared to the folate intake estimated to be consumed in the average American postfortification diet. In addition, observational studies of populations with a higher baseline rate of NTDs compared to the United States also show a greater risk reduction.

4. **How can an individual develop a folate deficiency? Which populations are at risk for low folate intake?**

   The term *folate* includes all compounds that have the vitamin properties of folic acid, including folic acid and naturally occurring compounds in food. Folate deficiency in humans is attributed to suboptimal dietary intake of folate, behavioral and environmental factors, and genetic defects. Humans cannot synthesize folate from other sources and are therefore entirely dependent on dietary sources or supplements to meet their folate requirements. Folate deficiency is common today since most adults frequently consume diets high in fat and processed foods, with less than the daily recommended servings of fresh fruit and vegetables. Minority women from low socioeconomic and educational backgrounds have been found to have poor folate intakes due to limited use of folate-rich foods.

   Folate functions as a methyl donor for the enzyme methylenetetrahydrofolate reductase (MTHFR), which is involved in the conversion of homocysteine to methionine. Folate deficiency results in an elevated serum homocysteine level. It is estimated that two-thirds of hyperhomocysteinemia is due to a folate deficiency. Mutations in the MTHFR gene that have been linked to an increased risk of NTD increase the metabolic requirement for folate and also result in elevated serum homocysteine levels. These levels can be normalized by additional folate intake. However, genetic defects appear to account for only a small percentage of cases of folate deficiency.

5. **Describe the rationale for the food fortification program and its potential benefits.**

In September 1992, the US Public Health Service (PHS) recommended that all women of childbearing age consume 400 μg folate daily to lower their risk of having a child with an NTD. The PHS made recommendations as to how this could be achieved, which included 1) improving dietary habits, 2) fortification of the US food supply, and 3) daily consumption of a folate supplement. However, most women were not getting this amount from their diets and were not taking folate supplements. According to the National Health and Nutrition Examination Survey (NHANES III), folate intake was 230 ± 7.8 μg per day for nonpregnant women ages 20 to 29 and 237 ± 9.0 μg per day for ages 30 to 39, levels below the DRIs, which have been increased to 400 μg per day for nonpregnant women and 600 μg per day during pregnancy.

The March of Dimes has conducted public education campaigns encouraging women of childbearing age to consume an adequate daily intake of folate. Surveys were conducted from 1995 to 2001 on a national sample of women aged 18 to 45 by the Gallup organization to measure changes in behavior and awareness relative to folate consumption. However, despite public health campaigns, only 19%, or approximately one in five women, are aware that adequate folate could help prevent birth defects (Figures 4-1 and 4-2).

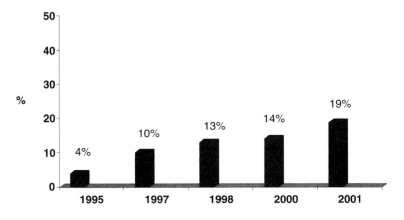

Source: *March of Dimes Survey*

Figure 4-1   Knowledge that folic acid prevents birth defects (based on all women aged 18 to 45).

SOURCE: Reprinted with permission from the March of Dimes. Folic Acid and the Prevention of Birth Defects. A National Survey of Pre-pregnancy awareness and behavior among women of child-bearing age. 1995–2001. Executive summary.

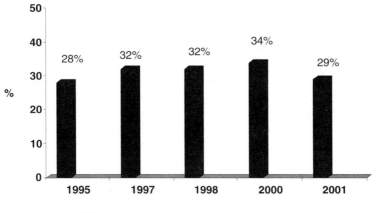

Source: *March of Dimes Survey*

Figure 4-2   Women taking a daily multivitamin containing folic acid (based on all women aged 18 to 45).

SOURCE: Reprinted with permission from the March of Dimes. Folic Acid and the Prevention of Birth Defects. A National Survey of Pre-pregnancy awareness and behavior among women of child-bearing age. 1995–2001. Executive summary.

Folic acid, also known as *pteroylmonoglutamic acid*, is the synthetic compound used in dietary supplements and fortified foods. Since January 1, 1998, the Food and Drug Administration (FDA) has required that manufacturers fortify all enriched grain products (flour, breads, rolls and buns, corn, grits, cornmeal, farina, rice and noodle products) with 140 μg folic acid per 100 g (3.5 oz) of grain product. Even though folic acid is a water-soluble vitamin with no known toxicity, the FDA set this limit because of the concern that higher doses of folic acid might mask a vitamin B_{12} deficiency. Folic acid would correct the anemia (pernicious, megaloblastic, or macrocytic anemia) but does not prevent the neurologic consequences associated with a vitamin B_{12} deficiency.

6. **List food sources high in folate. Based on the nutrition assessment of PL's diet history, what dietary modifications would you suggest?**

    Major sources of dietary folate include dark-green leafy vegetables, dried beans, citrus fruits, and fortified cereals. Orange juice is the largest single source of folate consumed by Americans, and it is estimated that it contributes approximately 10% of one's daily intake of dietary folate.

    Folate occurs mainly in the diet in the conjugated form (polyglutamate). Foods containing 55 μg folate per serving are considered to be excellent sources of folate. When assessing dietary folate intake, it is important to ask very specific questions since there are wide variations in folate content within each food group. For example, 8 oz of orange juice contains approximately 100 μg folate, as compared to negligible amounts in apple juice.

An analysis of PL's intake shows that she is only consuming 238 μg folate, well below her recommended intake. An individual can easily consume 400 to 500 μg folate daily by following the Food Guide Pyramid guidelines that suggest 3 to 5 servings of vegetables, 2 to 4 servings of fruits, and 6 to 11 servings of grain daily. PL's diet is deficient in fruits and vegetables. Recommended dietary modifications could include either adding orange juice or a fresh orange or grapefruit to breakfast, carrots sticks to lunch, and a green vegetable, such as broccoli or asparagus, to dinner. In addition to these naturally occurring sources of folate, a ready-to-eat fortified breakfast cereal could contribute significantly to PL's folate intake. Folate is also contained in whole grains such as oatmeal or oat bran cereals, wheat germ, whole-grain breads, and brown rice that could easily be incorporated into PL's diet (see Appendix).

7. **Should a vitamin and mineral supplement be considered for this patient? Why or why not?**

Because at least 50% of pregnancies in the United States are not planned and folate-containing supplements have greater bioavailablity than dietary folate, it is recommended that all women of childbearing age consume supplemental folate. The results of two randomized controlled clinical studies conducted in the early 1990s showed that 50% or more of NTDs could be prevented if women consumed a folic acid–containing supplement before and during the early weeks of pregnancy in addition to a high-folate diet. Therefore, to reduce the risk of bearing a child with an NTD, the American Academy of Pediatrics, along with the US PHS, recommends that women of childbearing age consume 400 μg folic acid per day. This is the amount of folate contained in an over-the-counter multivitamin supplement.

Currently, evidence is insufficient to provide a recommendation to use food folate as the method to reduce the risk of NTD. If a woman has previously given birth to a baby with an NTD, she should consult her doctor before her next pregnancy to discuss the amount of supplemental folate that she should take.

When synthetic folate (a monoglutamate) is consumed as a supplement in the fasting state, it is nearly 100% bioavailable. In contrast, when folate is consumed with food, as in fortified cereal grain products, its absorption is reduced to approximately 85%. Naturally occurring food folate is less well absorbed by the body than synthetic folate because the polyglutamate side chain of food folate must be cleaved before absorption can occur. This converts food folate to the monoglutamate form, which is taken up by a specific carrier in the cell membrane of the small intestine. Sauberlich and associates found that food folate is approximately 50% bioavailable. Thus, supplemental folate taken when a person is fasting is two times more bioavailable than food folate, and folate taken with food (including folate-fortified foods) is 1.7 times more bioavailable than food folate. These are only estimates and may be revised over time as more data are analyzed.

Case 2

Encouraging Breastfeeding

Judith B. Roepke and Ruth Lawrence

Objectives

• Identify the documented advantages of breastfeeding for both mothers and infants.

• Effectively encourage pregnant women to initiate and continue breastfeeding their infants during the first year of life.

• Effectively counsel women regarding techniques and positioning in order to successfully breastfeed their infants.

• Provide appropriate nutritional recommendations for breastfeeding women.

• Compare and contrast the growth patterns of breastfed and formula-fed infants.

LW is a 26-year-old woman who is gravida 1, para 0, in her thirty-seventh week of gestation. She is 5'6" (168 cm) tall and weighed 130 lb (59 kg) before becoming pregnant (prepregnancy BMI: 21.0 kg/m^2). She now weighs 160 lb (73 kg), and her pregnancy has been uncomplicated. LW is considering breastfeeding and questions her childbirth provider about it and whether she can continue after she returns to work 3 months postpartum. LW also plans to lose her pregnancy weight quickly and fears that dieting will keep her from producing enough breast milk to feed the baby adequately.

Go to questions 1–4.

Follow-Up

LW, who has been breastfeeding her infant, returns at 6 weeks postpartum for her checkup. She has lost 20 lb (9 kg) and currently weighs 140 lb (63.5 kg; BMI = 22.6 kg/m^2). She reports that she is even hungrier than she was during her pregnancy but cannot find time to eat. She is afraid that she is not producing enough milk because the baby always appears hungry and is not as chubby as her friend's formula-fed baby. She reports that her mother told her she should avoid eating vegetables and chocolate because they will upset the baby's stomach and produce gas. LW is also concerned about how to feed the baby when she returns to work in 2 months.

LW's 24-Hour Dietary Recall

Breakfast (home)	Cornflakes	1 cup
	Skim milk	$^1/_2$ cup
Lunch (home)	Whole-wheat bread	2 slices
	Peanut butter	2 Tbsp.
	Jelly	1 Tbsp.
	Orange juice	8 oz (240 mL)
Snack (home)	Snickers candy bar	1–2 oz (57 g)
	Water	1 cup
Dinner (home)	Baked chicken	2 thighs (6 oz; 170 g)
	Baked potato	1 medium
	Margarine	2 Tbsp.
	Applesauce	$^1/_2$ cup
	Diet cola	12 oz (360 mL)
Snack (home)	Ice cream	1 cup

Total calories: 2035 kcal
Protein: 78 g (15% of calories)
Carbohydrate: 228 g (44% of calories)
Fat: 95 g (41% of calories)
Calcium: 505 mg
Iron: 8.4 mg

Case Questions

1. What advice can be given to LW to help her decide to breastfeed her infant?
2. How quickly can a postpartum woman expect to lose weight?
3. What dietary recommendations should be given to LW to ensure that her baby will receive adequate nutrition?
4. What are the guidelines regarding frequency and length of time to breastfeed an infant?
5. How will LW know if her breastfed baby is getting enough to eat? Compare the growth patterns of breastfed and formula-fed infants.
6. How should LW's weight loss and dietary intake be assessed?
7. How can breastfeeding women prepare to return to work?

Case Answers

Part 1: Encouraging Breastfeeding

1. **What advice can be given to LW to help her decide whether to breastfeed her infant?**

    According to the Subcommittee on Nutrition during Lactation, the Committee on Nutritional Status during Pregnancy and Lactation, the Food and Nutrition Board of the Institute of Medicine, and the National Academy of Sciences, breastfeeding is recommended for all infants in the United States. Exclusive breastfeeding is the preferred method for normal full-term infants from birth to 6 months because of the documented advantages for both the baby and the mother. Breastfeeding, complemented by appropriate introduction of solid foods after 6 months of age, is recommended for the remainder of the first year, or longer if desired. To achieve this goal, it is important to learn how to breastfeed during the early months and after returning to work. For that reason LW should be encouraged to contact a leader from a mother-to-mother support group such as La Leche League.

    It is important that a mother receive social and emotional support for her decision to breastfeed. Women are most likely to succeed at breastfeeding when encouraged by their health care provider(s) during pregnancy and outside sources for support and assistance [husband, patient's mother or mother-in-law, mother-to-mother support groups, and an International Board-Certified Lactation Consultant (IBCLC) (see Table 4-5)].

2. **How quickly can a postpartum woman expect to lose weight?**

    A woman should not expect to return to her prepregnancy weight immediately after delivery. On average, a new mother loses 15 lb (6.8 kg) within the first week after delivery. Many mothers are concerned about their weight gain during pregnancy and worry that they may not return to their prepregnancy weight since most women retain 5 to 10 lb (2.3 to 4.5 kg) per pregnancy. Lactating women who eat nutritionally balanced diets typically lose 1 to 2 lb (0.45 to 0.9 kg) per month during the first 4 to 6 months of lactation, a rate more rapid than if they were bottlefeeding their infants. A weight loss of more than 1.5 lb (0.68 kg) per week, even in women with excess fat stores, can decrease breast milk production and jeopardize the nutritional status of both the mother and the baby. However, not all women lose weight during lactation. Some studies suggest that approximately 20% of women maintain or gain weight during this time and may lose the additional weight after they wean their infants.

3. **What dietary recommendations should be given to LW to ensure that her baby will receive adequate nutrition?**

    The Institute of Medicine makes the point that breast milk will be ideal even if the diet is not ideal. Lactating women should be encouraged to obtain their nutrients from a well-balanced, varied diet to meet their nutritional needs while lactating. Lactating women have an increased need for essentially all nutrients, especially protein, calcium, and vitamins A and C compared with nonlactating women. The specific needs of individual women vary depending on the volume of milk produced daily, the age and size of their infants, their individual metabolism, and their postpartum nutritional status.

During pregnancy, most women store approximately 2 to 4 kg body fat, which can be mobilized to supply a portion of the additional calories used for lactation. Body fat supplies an estimated 200 to 300 kcal per day during the first 3 months of lactation. An additional 500 kcal per day, which is needed for lactation, must come from the diet.

4. **What are the guidelines regarding frequency and length of time to breastfeed an infant?**

Breastfeeding should be initiated within the first 2 hours after birth. Feeding the baby on demand, frequent suckling, and completely emptying milk from the breasts help to increase the mother's milk supply. The duration of a feeding should not be limited during the first few days. In the beginning, it may take 2 to 3 minutes of suckling to stimulate the release of oxytocin (hypothalamic hormone stored in the posterior pituitary gland). Oxytocin initiates "letdown," the term for the process by which the milk begins to empty from the breast due to the contraction of myoepithelial cells. Prolactin, a hormone released from the anterior pituitary gland, also stimulates milk production. Early and frequent feeding reduces the risk of engorgement. Removing the infant before letdown does not stimulate milk supply and may frustrate both the mother and infant.

The infant should be encouraged to suckle the first breast until the milk flows. When the infant stops suckling and pulls away from the breast, the baby should be placed on the other breast for as long as the infant suckles. Although the duration of feeding may vary among infants, feeding should be infant led and not clock led.

The composition and volume of breast milk change during each feeding. The milk provided after approximately 5 to 10 minutes is the richest in fat and, therefore, caloric content. It is called the "hind milk." Infants need to nurse long enough to become satiated and to obtain sufficient calories from the breast milk for appropriate growth and development. Mothers should be instructed that the infant will get 75% of the milk volume in the first 5 to 10 minutes after the letdown but only 50% of the calories because breast milk becomes higher in fat and calories the longer the milk is produced/removed.

Once lactation is established, an infant who suckles vigorously usually empties the breast in 10 to 20 minutes after letdown has occurred. It may take up to an hour to "empty" both breasts. Infants will suckle until satisfied and should alternate starting breasts with each feeding in order to ensure even milk production. A full-term newborn infant should feed

8 to 12 times during 24 hours. Human milk is easily digested and empties from the infant's stomach in 90 minutes, whereas formula empties in 3 to 4 hours.

Read Follow-Up at beginning of case.

5. **How will LW know if her breastfed baby is getting enough to eat? Compare the growth patterns of breastfed and formula-fed infants.**

The best way to be sure that babies are receiving adequate amounts of breast milk is to monitor their growth and development. Milk production generally works on the principle of supply and demand. That is, the more a baby feeds, the more milk is produced. In the first few days of life, it is not uncommon for a full-term newborn to feed every 1 to 3 hours during each 24-hour period; this helps to stimulate initial milk production. Once the milk supply is established approximately 6 weeks postpartum, feeding frequency will diminish. A baby who has at least six wet diapers and a minimum of three stools per day and is gaining weight appropriately (at least 7 oz per week) is usually consuming enough milk. Breastfed and formula-fed infants have slightly different growth patterns. In the first 2 to 3 months, human milk-fed infants gain weight more rapidly. After the first few months of life, the weight gain is similar to that of formula-fed infants and then begins to slow down.

Although breast-fed infants consume less milk over the 24-hour period and therefore have a lower energy intake, they are more energy efficient than formula-fed infants. By their third birthday, breast-fed infants have a lower percentage of body fat and are rarely obese. Data from the Darling study has shown that breastfed infants cannot be overfed and have a decreased risk of becoming overweight or obese, which may be because they learn to stop eating when they are satisfied.

Part 2: Follow-Up

6. **How should LW's weight loss and dietary patterns be assessed?**

According to her diet history, she is not consuming adequate calories to maintain her weight and simultaneously produce adequate amounts of breast milk to feed her baby. Her calorie requirements for lactation are estimated to be 2700 kcal per day, calculated on the basis of 30 kcal per kg per day plus an additional 500 kcal per day for lactation. Her diet does not provide adequate amounts of iron, calcium, vitamin A, vitamin B_{12}, folate, and zinc. To enhance her nutrient intake, she should be encouraged to follow the Pyramid Guide and to increase her intake of whole-grain or enriched breads and cereals, fruit and vegetables, and 2% low-fat milk or yogurt and include an iron-rich snack, such as raisins or dried fruit in the morning. She should also be advised to continue to take her prenatal vitamin. In addition, her fluid intake is low, and she should be encouraged to drink more nutritious fluids (up to 2 liters per day), such as skim milk, 100% juices, and water.

7. **How can breastfeeding women prepare to return to work?**

   A mother returning to work can continue to breastfeed by renting or purchasing a breast pump to remove milk during the day for use at home while she is working. The advantages of pumping the breast at least every 4 hours are to ensure that the baby will receive breast milk when the mother is at work and to promote the continued supply of breast milk even though the baby is not feeding during the day. Breastfeeding exclusively whenever the woman is not working will help milk production to continue. Breast milk can be stored in the refrigerator for up to 8 days and in the freezer for 1 month.

   The father or a caretaker should offer the bottle because the baby may expect to breastfeed when the mother is present. Offering one bottle of expressed breast milk about once a day, starting approximately 2 weeks before the mother returns to work, may help the infant learn how to suck from a bottle, which is different from breastfeeding. Once the mother returns to work, the baby should be given expressed breast milk from a bottle or cup during the day. When the mother returns from work, she should breastfeed as soon as possible.

See Chapter Review Questions, pages A-15 to A-17.

5

Infants, Children, and Adolescents

Andrew M. Tershakovec and Linda Van Horn

Objectives*

- Differentiate the changing nutritional needs of developing children from infancy to adolescence.
- Identify differences in nutritional recommendations for children by age, stage of development, and gender.
- Explain how nutritional and dietary behaviors learned in childhood, such as obesity and hypercholesterolemia, can have significant impact on adult health concerns.
- Specify the effects of undernutrition on growth and development.

Childhood Growth and Development Patterns

Energy and nutrient requirements of children are proportional to their resting energy expenditure plus the energy needed for activity and normal growth. These requirements vary dramatically depending on the general stages of growth and on the child's individual developmental pattern. Growth curves derived from observations of large numbers of normal healthy children have been developed to establish expected ranges of weight, height, and head circumference growth for purposes of comparison. The most commonly used of these curves are age and gender specific.

The new growth charts that have been developed by the Centers for Disease Control and Prevention (CDC) are based on National Health and Nutrition Examination Survey (NHANES) data collected from 1971 to 1994

* SOURCE: Objectives for chapter and cases adapted from the *NIH Nutrition Curriculum Guide for Training Physicians* (*http://www.nhlbi.nih.gov/funding/training/naa*).

(*http://www.cdc.gov/growthcharts*). These charts more appropriately represent the combined growth patterns of breastfed and formula-fed infants, including all racial and ethnic groups, and include body mass index (BMI)-for-age and gender values. BMI provides a guideline based on weight and height to assess the degree of undernutrition, overweight, and obesity. Since the development of body fat varies according to age and gender, BMI should be plotted on age- and gender-specific charts.

Children undergo two rapid growth spurts: the first during infancy and early childhood, followed by a period of steady, slower growth, and the second in adolescence. Rapid body growth (especially during the first 3 years of life, and again in adolescence) and brain development require adequate calories and nutrients to support appropriate passage through all the developmental stages that characterize this period.

Children may be underweight if their BMI-for-age and gender fall below the fifth percentile. From the fifth up to the eighty-fifth percentile, they have an acceptable weight. Greater than the eighty-fifth percentile, they are at risk of being overweight, since excess adipose tissue is not easily assessed in overweight children. Greater than the ninety-fifth percentile and above is used to diagnose overweight in children and adolescents. In addition to evaluating single points on the growth curve, the pattern of change over time should be evaluated.

Individual Variability

Consideration of individual differences is also important when assessing the nutritional needs of children. Population growth curves may mask such individual differences. Thus, it is necessary to evaluate each child's stage of growth and development to assess that child's nutritional needs.

Mechanisms of Growth

Cell Division

In utero and early in life, much of an individual's growth is attributable to cell division. This consideration is important because undernutrition early in life may block cell division. Later, some cells lose the ability to divide. At this point, the total number of cells and the individual's potential future growth may be diminished. Providing the optimal environment, including adequate nutrition, for dividing cells to achieve their growth potential is therefore crucial to prevent permanent stunting.

Differential Growth Patterns

Different organ systems develop at different times and at different rates (Figure 5-1). The general growth pattern parallels the height growth curve, showing rapid early growth, a subsequent period of steady, slower growth, and the final growth spurt during adolescence. Key differences in specific organ systems that depart from that general pattern are the topic of this section.

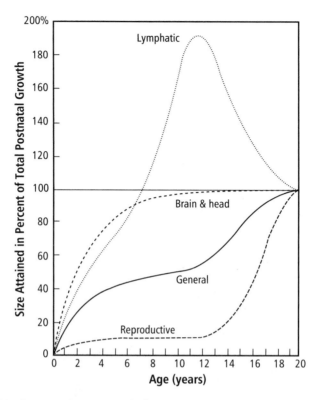

Figure 5-1   **Yearly organ system growth chart.**

(SOURCE: Reprinted with permission from Abraham M, ed. Rudolph's Pediatrics. 20th ed. Norwalk, CT: Appleton & Lange, 1996.)

Brain and Central Nervous System   All children should have their head circumference measured until age 2 years. In the central nervous system (CNS) and the brain, rapid growth is seen in the first few years of life. The human brain reaches 70% of its adult size by age 3 years and 90% by age 7. Accordingly, the CNS of a malnourished child under age 4 may be susceptible to permanent damage. Thus, the consequences of famines are perpetuated for many years by affecting the development of young children.

Lymphatic System   The lymphatic system undergoes rapid growth until puberty, when it actually surpasses its ultimate adult size and then regresses to adult size.

Reproductive System   The reproductive system is largely dormant until puberty, when it undergoes rapid growth. The profound effects of undernutrition on the reproductive system during adolescence are commonly demonstrated in anorexic girls with delayed sexual development or amenorrhea. This is also observed with adolescent female athletes with very low body fat. Knowing the sequence of pubertal changes and their appropriate timing, as outlined in the Tanner stages, is important in evaluating pubertal delay and growth arrest.

Determining Pediatric Nutrient Requirements

Children's body composition changes as they grow. It is important to consider body composition when assessing nutritional needs because metabolic and nutrient needs are dependent on lean body mass. The percentage of body weight attributable to fat, or fat mass, is high for infants and toddlers and decreases as children enter their elementary school years. In puberty, fat mass increases again. The development of body composition in boys and girls is basically parallel until puberty. At the end of adolescence, boys proportionately lose some body fat as they become adults, whereas females deposit more body fat during adolescence and maintain this proportionate increase in fat through adulthood. Differences between boys and girls also occur with respect to lean body mass (LBM). Again, the percentage of LBM is very similar in both sexes until puberty. Then boys triple their LBM, while girls double theirs. This helps define the increased caloric needs of adolescent boys and men, as opposed to adolescent girls and women. As they enter adulthood, females manifest a higher percentage of total body fat and a lower percentage of muscle mass than males.

Various recommended energy and nutrient allowances have been formulated for growing children based on these body composition changes and the changing nutritional needs with growth and development. These recommended allowances are thought to fulfill children's energy and nutrient needs in proportion to the metabolically active tissue at various stages of development. As shown in Table 5-1, the basal metabolic rate (BMR) is the same for girls and boys until they enter puberty, when it increases more rapidly for boys because of their higher percentage of muscle mass.

Adjustments for Activity and Illness

To estimate an individual's true energy needs, adjustments are necessary for special circumstances such as differing activity levels, illnesses, and other factors. For example, fever raises energy needs 12% for each degree above 98.6°F (37°C) of body temperature. Illness, trauma, recovery from undernutrition, and serious burns can almost double energy requirements. On the other hand, chronic undernutrition can decrease energy needs by 20% to 30%. Decreased growth and activity during severe illness also decrease energy needs considerably.

Evaluating Dietary Adequacy in Children

It is very difficult to accurately assess dietary intake. When dietary assessments are attempted, it is common to observe differences between reported intake and estimated caloric needs due to underreporting of actual intake. Thus, specific assessment of dietary intake should only be undertaken when necessary, such as when evaluating a child for abnormal growth or development. When tracking a child's growth over time, it is important to pay attention to the curve the child follows in relation to the age- and gender-specific growth percentiles from the standard CDC growth charts. In most cases, a child's growth rate will remain stable along a percentile curve. A child who has been growing steadily at the fifth percentile for

Table 5-1   Standard basal metabolic rate chart.

	MALE	FEMALE
WEIGHT (kg)	Kcal/24 hr	
3	140	140
5	270	270
7	400	400
9	500	500
11	600	600
13	650	650
15	710	710
17	780	780
19	830	830
21	880	880
25	1020	960
29	1120	1040
33	1210	1120
37	1300	1190
41	1350	1260
45	1410	1320
49	1470	1380
53	1530	1440
57	1590	1500
61	1640	1560

SOURCE: Tsang RC, Nichols BL, eds. Nutrition during infancy.
Philadelphia: C. V. Mosby, 1988. Reprinted with permission.

his or her age and sex is less of a concern than one who has measured consistently in the fiftieth percentile on the growth curve and subsequently drops to the fifth.

According to the *Healthy People 2010* goals, growth retardation is not a problem for the majority of young children in the United States. However, up to 15% of low-income African-American children are below the fifth percentile for their height-for-age.

Infant Feeding: Breast Milk Versus Formula

Except for special formulas, manufacturers of infant formulas generally try to approximate the composition of human breast milk. The specifics of infant formulas are discussed in Table 5-2. Table 5-3 compares the nutrient content of breast milk with that of infant formula. (See Chapter 4 for additional information on lactation.)

Weaning Babies from Breast Milk or Formulas

Most health care providers believe that cow's milk is an important source of calories, protein, and calcium for children over the age of 1. The American Academy

Table 5-2   Indications and types of infant formulas.

FORMULA	INDICATIONS	UNIQUE PROPERTIES	EXAMPLES
Milk-based	Breast milk substitute for term infants	$+/-$ Iron Ready to feed, powder, or liquid concentrate Variable whey: casein 20 kcal/oz	Enfamil, Similac, Gerber, Good Start, Lactofree
Soy-based	Breast milk substitute for infants with lactose intolerance or milk protein allergy*	Lactose-free, some sucrose, or corn-free 20 kcal/oz May contain fiber	Prosobee, Isomil, Soyalac, I-Soyalac, Isomil-DF
Premature	Breast milk substitute for infants <38 weeks' gestational age	Low lactose Whey: casein 60:40 Higher calcium and phosphorus 24 kcal/oz	Enfamil, Premature, Similac Special Care, Similac Natural Care, Enfamil HMF, Similac Neocare
Older infant	Transition to whole milk	16 kcal/oz	Advantage, Good Nature
Hypoallergenic	Milk or soy protein allergy	Hydrolyzed protein Sucrose-free Lactose-free	Nutramigen
Predigested	Malabsorption Short bowel syndrome Allergy	Lactose-free Hydrolyzed protein or free amino acids	Alimentum, Pregestamil, Neocate
Fat-modified	Defects in digestion, absorption, or transport of fat	Contains increased % of kcals as MCT	Portagen, Alimentum, Pregestamil
Carbohydrate-modified	Simple sugar intolerance	Requires addition of complex carbohydrate to be complete	RCF 3232 A
Amino acid-modified	Inborn errors of metabolism	Low or devoid of specific amino acids that cannot be metabolized	Multiple products
Electrolyte-modified	Renal or cardiac disease or other disease state requiring low renal solute load	Decreased sodium content	Similac PM 60/40 SMA

*Children allergic to milk protein may also be allergic to soy protein.
SOURCE: Department of Clinical Nutrition, Children's Hospital of Philadelphia. 1997.

of Pediatrics (AAP) recommends that cow's milk not be given to children under 1 year of age. When cow's milk is introduced earlier, it may cause the following problems.

Gastrointestinal Blood Loss

The protein in cow's milk may induce a reaction with the small bowel mucosa, causing chronic gastrointestinal (GI) blood loss and subsequently iron-deficiency anemia.

Table 5-3   Comparison of breast milk and infant formulas (nutrients per 100 calories).

	BREAST MILK	SIMILAC	ENFAMIL	ISOMIL
Protein (g)	1.54	2.14	2.10	2.45
% of calories	6	9	8	11
Source	Mature term human milk	Cow's milk	Reduced mineral/ whey/nonfat milk	Soy Protein isolate
Fat (g)	5.74	5.40	5.3	5.46
% of calories	52	48	47	49
Source	Mature term human milk	Soy and coconut oils	Palm olean/soy/ coconut/sunflower	Soy and coconut oils
Cholesterol (mg)	22	1.6	<1	0
Carbohydrate (g)	10.6	10.7	10.9	10.3
% of calories	42	43	43	41
Source	Lactose	Lactose	Lactose	Corn syrup
Vitamins				
Vitamin D (IU)	3.0	60	60	60
Vitamin K (μg)	0.3	8.0	8.0	15
Minerals				
Calcium (mg)	41	73	78	105
Phosphorus (mg)	21	56	53	75
Iron (mg)	0.04	1.8	1.8	1.8
Renal solute load				
(mOsm)	11.1	14.3	14.2	16.3

SOURCE: Department of Clinical Nutrition, Children's Hospital of Philadelphia. 1997.

Excessive Renal Solute Load

Infants' kidneys are relatively immature and have difficulty handling the extra renal solute load occasioned by the higher protein and phosphorus content of cow's milk.

Iron-Deficiency Anemia

Infants who are fed cow's milk before 1 year of age are at risk for iron deficiency due to the low iron content of cow's milk and its potential for inducing blood loss. Altered behavior and cognitive function have been reported in iron-deficient infants and toddlers. The data concerning the reversibility of these alterations are conflicting; however, an increasing body of evidence suggests that these effects may be long-term and possibly permanent.

Even though breast milk is lower in iron than cow's milk, the iron in breast milk is more bioavailable and therefore readily absorbed. Babies born prematurely are at higher risk for iron deficiency than full-term infants and should have supplemental iron or an iron-fortified formula from birth. Encouraging consumption of iron-fortified solid foods or foods naturally high in iron is further recommended. Sources of dietary iron appropriate for infants and children include iron-fortified formula and infant cereals, red meat, dark-green leafy vegetables, and dried fruit such as raisins. (Note: Raisins may be a choking risk for children <3 years of age.)

The prevalence of iron deficiency in the United States has decreased significantly over the last 20 years. *Healthy People 2010* reported that 9% of children aged 1 to 2 years and 4% of children aged 3 to 4 years have iron-deficiency anemia. Previously, the highest rates of iron deficiency were encountered in children under 3 years of age. This group was thought to be at risk for iron deficiency due to rapid growth rates, high iron requirements, and diets that were frequently low in iron. The current lower prevalence may be due to supplemental food programs for low-income families, such as the Women, Infants, and Children (WIC) program, as well as increased iron supplementation in infant cereals and formulas.

Other population groups in the United States are still at risk for iron deficiency, particularly adolescent female athletes. These girls have increased iron requirements once they begin menstruating, superimposed by the increased needs associated with the pubertal growth spurt. The association of iron deficiency with exercise is not well understood (see Case 3).

Introducing Solid Food

Recommendations concerning the introduction of solid food have changed considerably over the years. In the past, many children ate a wide variety of foods as early as the first month of life. Now the consensus among health care providers is to delay the introduction of solid foods until the child is at least 4 months old. The AAP recommends breast milk as the sole nutrient source until 6 months of age.

Introducing solid foods earlier in the infant's life may stimulate the development of food allergies. Furthermore, infants are not physiologically ready to accept solid foods from a spoon until approximately 4 months of age, when the oral extrusion reflex becomes extinguished. Other important considerations are the development of head and neck control and coordination of the oral musculature, both of which occur at roughly 3 to 4 months of age.

The introduction of solid foods marks the beginning of a critical period during which the infant learns to master eating from a spoon and accepts different tastes and textures. Not coincidentally, an infant's readiness for these experiences generally corresponds to a physiologic need to supplement the amounts of calories and nutrients available from breast milk or formula. However, breast milk, formula, or a combination should still continue to be the major source of calories and nutrients during the remainder of the infant's first year. The common belief that solid food can help to "fatten up" or help the baby to sleep better are misconceptions. As Table 5-4 shows, most solid foods are calorically less dense than breast milk or formula and therefore should not be the sole nutrient source.

Table 5-4   Comparison of the relative caloric densities of common infant food sources.

FOOD	CALORIC DENSITY
Cow's milk	20 kcal/oz
Infant formula	20 kcal/oz
Human milk	22 kcal/oz
Baby food vegetables	9–19 kcal/oz
Baby food fruits	14–20 kcal/oz

General Guidelines for Introducing Solid Foods

Although no real consensus exists among the experts regarding when and how to introduce solid foods, parents may find the following guidelines helpful, which are summarized in Table 5-5.

Introducing New Foods

New foods should not be introduced too often—generally not more frequently than every 3 days—and more than one new food should not be introduced at a time. Following this procedure makes it easier to detect a child's inability to tolerate a newly introduced food.

Cereals

In the United States, the most common initial solid food is rice cereal. Generally offered first at 4 to 6 months of age, rice cereal is fortified with iron, nonallergenic, and usually well tolerated. One should begin with 1 to 2 Tbsp. in the morning, mixed with formula or breast milk. The cereal should be mixed to a consistency similar to that of applesauce. It can be thinned or thickened as preferred by the child. Cereal can be thickened as the child grows older. Feeding cereal from a spoon helps the baby learn this new skill, which takes a few weeks. Parents should be advised to avoid putting cereal in a bottle. This does not help children sleep through the night and may lead to overfeeding and potentially choking as a result of the need to make a larger nipple hole to prevent clogging.

Fruits

Cooked and strained or pureed fruits, either homemade or purchased baby food without added sugar, can be started after rice cereal. Fresh, mashed bananas also can be introduced at this time. Peeled, soft fruits such as peaches and pears can be cut into small pieces and started at 8 to 10 months of age. Foods that are harder to chew, such as apples, should be deferred until the child has a greater capacity to chew. Juices, such as apple juice, can also be offered at this time, although in limited amounts.

Vegetables

Cooked, strained vegetables without added salt or spices, either homemade or purchased baby food, are appropriate to start at 6 to 8 months of age. The

Table 5-5 How to feed your infant.

AGE	BREAST MILK OR IRON-FORTIFIED INFANT FORMULA[a]	CEREALS AND BREADS	FRUITS AND FRUIT JUICES[b]	VEGETABLES	PROTEIN FOODS	DAIRY PRODUCTS
0–6 mo	5–10 feedings/d 17–24 fl oz/d (510–720 mL)	None	None	None	None	None
6–7 mo	4–7 feedings/d 24–32 fl oz/d (720–960 mL)	Rice or barley infant cereals (iron fortified) Mix cereal with formula or breast milk until thin Start with 1 Tbsp. at each feeding for a few days, and increase to 3–4 Tbsp./d Feed with small baby spoon (don't expect baby to eat much at first)	No fruits No fruits juice	None	None	None
7–8 mo	4–5 feedings/d 24–32 fl oz/d (720–960 mL)	Single-grain infant cereals–rice, oatmeal, barley (iron fortified) in the morning 3–9 Tbsp./d, mixed with breast milk or infant formula; 2 feedings/d Oven-dried toast or teething biscuits, crackers, or toast strips	Strained or mashed fruits (fresh or cooked), mashed bananas, applesauce Infant 100% fruit juices <4 oz/d mixed with water and served in a cup	Strained or mashed, well-cooked: dark yellow or orange (not corn), dark-green vegetables Start with mild vegetables such as green beans, peas, or squash 1/2–1 jar or 1/4–1/2 cup/d	None	Cottage cheese, yogurt

Table 5-5 (continued)

AGE	BREAST MILK OR IRON-FORTIFIED INFANT FORMULA[a]	CEREALS AND BREADS	FRUITS AND FRUIT JUICES[b]	VEGETABLES	PROTEIN FOODS	DAIRY PRODUCTS
8–9 mo	3–4 feedings/d 24–32 fl oz/d (720–960 mL)	Infant cereals or plain hot cereals mixed with breast milk or formula Toast, bagels, crackers, teething biscuits Small pieces of cooked noodles, potatoes	Peeled soft fruit wedges: bananas, peaches, pears, oranges, apples (skin removed) 100% fruit juices including orange and tomato juices 4–6 oz/d (120–180 mL)	Cooked, mashed vegetables	Well-cooked, strained, ground, or finely chopped chicken, fish, and lean meats: 2–3 Tbsps/d (remove all bones, fat, skin); no peanut butter until 1 yr; cooked dried beans; egg yolk	Cottage cheese, yogurt, bite-size cheese strips
10–12 mo	3–4 feedings/d 24–32 fl oz/d by cup or bottle (720–960 mL)	Infant or cooked cereals mixed with breast milk or formula Unsweetened cereals, white/ wheat breads Mashed potatoes, rice, noodles, spaghetti	All fresh fruits peeled and seeded or canned fruits packed in water All 100% fruit juices 4–6 oz/d (120–180 mL)	Cooked vegetable pieces Some raw vegetables: tomatoes, cucumbers	Small tender pieces of chicken, fish or lean meat Cooked beans No peanut butter until 1 yr	Cottage cheese, yogurt, bite-size cheese strips

[a] These are general guidelines. Feeding schedules vary somewhat between children.

[b] Infants have no specific need for juice.

SOURCE: Lisa Hark, PhD, RD, and Diane Barsky, MD, University of Pennsylvania School of Medicine. Healthy Eating for Kids and Teens web site: *http://www.uphs.upenn.edu/nutrimed/healthykids*. Used with permission.

importance of avoiding salt and spices should be stressed. Infants do not require extra sodium, and adding salt may encourage a greater salt intake later in life. Raw vegetables—such as cucumbers and tomatoes—and corn can be introduced at 1 year of age. Hard vegetables such as raw carrots should not be introduced until the child's top and bottom molars have erupted to allow adequate chewing and help prevent choking.

Eggs

Cooked egg yolks can be introduced to infants over the age of 6 months, but the introduction of egg whites should be delayed until they reach 1 year of age because of the potential risk of inducing an allergy to eggs in younger infants. (Egg allergies are important, as they may delay or limit the administration of vaccines that are produced in eggs.)

Meat

Ground or finely chopped chicken, fish, and meats, either homemade or purchased baby food, are generally given after fruits and vegetables have been introduced and are tolerated. They should be well pureed to avoid the risk of choking.

Starch/Carbohydrates

Children tend to like pasta, spaghetti, noodles, and dry cereal. However, other essential foods with a higher nutrient density should be introduced first during the meal to ensure that the child's diet is complete and balanced.

Fat

Children under age 2 years need a high-calorie diet to help ensure normal brain development and to support rapid growth. Because fat is the most calorically dense food, and because young children have a limited volume capacity for food intake, limiting fat intake in young children's diets may jeopardize normal growth and brain development. Therefore, the AAP recommends that dietary fat should not be limited before age 2 years. On the other hand, children need not eat high-fat foods such as whole milk, French fries, chicken nuggets, pizza, macaroni and cheese, hot dogs, fried foods, and ice cream every day, especially if they are at risk of overweight (greater than eighty-fifth percentile) or overweight for weight-for-age (greater than ninety-fifth percentile).

Psychosocial and Behavioral Implications and Recommendations

Eating habits formed in the first 2 years of life are thought to persist for several years, if not for a lifetime. Therefore, healthy eating patterns should be established as early as possible. Children's appetites vary with their growth rate, which may fluctuate from day to day. Studies have shown that when children are allowed to determine on their own how much they eat, their intake may vary considerably from meal to meal, but over a period of days and weeks, it remains stable and appropriate to their needs.

Potential Problems

Children begin expressing personal preferences at an early age and simultaneously develop mechanisms for self-control. Parents must therefore take care to strike a balance between helping guide a child's food choices to develop healthy eating habits and providing sufficient opportunities for experimentation and control. Overcontrolling parental behaviors have been associated with a child's decreased ability to appropriately control his or her own caloric intake. Parents should provide children with a healthy selection of food, and children should be allowed to determine how much food they need to eat. Children who consume a variety of foods over time and demonstrate appropriate growth are likely to be consuming an adequately balanced diet. Parents who worry that their child is not eating enough and allow the child to eat anything, and at any time of the day, simply to ensure that he or she eats something may be promoting the development of poor eating habits.

Problems also surface when parents get into prolonged power struggles with their children over eating issues. Two-year-old children may want to eat the same food for days at a time. Meeting their request may be a better response than turning mealtime into a battle. Left on their own, children eventually will tire of the same food, but if winning each mealtime struggle is in the balance, these episodes may worsen. Confusion and rushing at mealtimes may also disrupt the formation of appropriate eating habits.

Nutritional Recommendations for Adolescents

Adolescents undergo major physical and psychological changes that affect their behavior and nutritional status. Issues of autonomy and rebellion, testing and searching behaviors, and the development of formal operational thought (logical reasoning) are all normal characteristics of adolescence that must be considered when addressing their nutritional needs and behavior.

Requirements for Growth

Adolescents' energy and nutrient needs increase as they enter their pubertal growth spurt. Although infants, children, and adolescents all grow rapidly, the energy needs of adolescents, on a per-kilogram basis, are much lower than those of infants and children. Infants double their body weight over a few months, whereas older children and adolescents may double their weight over a period of 5 to 10 years.

Sexual Development

Previously described body composition changes that occur in adolescence also influence energy and nutrient needs. Furthermore, these needs differ in men and women. As girls go through puberty and start menstruating, their iron and protein needs increase to replace their losses. Adolescent girl athletes may be at high risk of iron-deficiency anemia as well. As boys enter puberty, their percentage of lean body mass increases relative to that of girls, thus increasing their protein, calorie, and overall nutrient requirements more than those of adolescent girls.

Nutritional Factors in Preventing Cardiovascular Disease

The association between elevated cholesterol levels and heart disease has been well documented in adults. Several studies suggest that adult atherosclerosis has its roots in childhood. Furthermore, lifestyle factors, such as dietary intake, have been linked to lipoprotein levels and other cardiovascular disease (CVD) risk factors in children and adults. The epidemiology of childhood and adult hypercholesterolemia is described below.

Autopsy Studies

Young victims of accidental death and some American soldiers killed in the Korean and Vietnam Wars were found to have significant atherosclerosis of their coronary arteries. The presence of these lesions at their young ages suggested the early onset of the atherosclerotic process.

Bogalusa Study

The natural history of CVD risk factors in children has been studied for over 20 years as part of the Bogalusa Heart Study. Autopsy studies of those children and young adults who have died of unrelated causes have shown a correlation between premorbid cholesterol levels and early atherosclerotic changes. Similar studies have demonstrated an association between atherosclerotic disease and other risk factors, such as smoking.

Tracking

Children with high cholesterol levels tend to become adults with high cholesterol levels. However, as tracking is not perfect, some have argued that treating all hypercholesterolemic children is inappropriate, as not all the children will become hypercholesterolemic adults. Others believe that the initial dietary treatment is safe and healthy for all children and therefore will not harm those who do not eventually become hypercholesterolemic adults.

Issues in Hypercholesterolemia Screening

The current recommendations for identifying hypercholesterolemic children suggest screening only those with a positive family history of early heart disease or hypercholesterolemia in first-degree relatives. A positive family history of early heart disease is defined as a parent or grandparent with a heart attack, angina, angioplasty, or other evidence of cardiovascular disease before age 55 in men and 65 in women. The following issues underlie these recommendations.

Failure to Thrive

Very-low-fat diets may be too low in calories or nutrients to support normal growth and development for a child. Concern over the possibility of placing children on inappropriate diets, together with the potential for misdiagnosis, has led many to question the safety of screening and intervention for hypercholesterolemia in children. However, studies have shown that children can grow appropriately when receiving a balanced, low-fat diet.

Current Recommendations

Recommendations from the National Cholesterol Education Panel, and confirmed by the AAP and the American Heart Association, recommend that children with a positive family history of heart disease be screened. A diet that contains less than 30% of calories as fat (but more than 20%), less than 10% of calories as saturated fat, and less than 300 mg cholesterol per day is recommended for all children older than 2 years and as initial therapy for those who are hypercholesterolemic (see Chapter 7). Children under the age of 2 are believed to require a higher-fat diet to maintain normal growth and central nervous system development. Greater dietary modification should be considered for hypercholesterolemic children who do not respond adequately to this dietary modification (e.g., <7% saturated fat and 200 mg cholesterol per day). However, it must be remembered that many low-fat foods are not low in calories and thus should not be eaten with impunity, especially given the current epidemic of obesity in childhood.

Dietary intervention must be viewed as one component of a comprehensive program to reduce cardiovascular disease risk. Exercise, controlling elevated blood pressure, avoiding excessive sedentary activities, avoiding smoking, and avoiding excessive weight gain and obesity are all factors that should be assessed in hyperlipidemic adolescents.

Obesity in Childhood and Adolescence

According to the NHANES III (1988 to 1994), the prevalence of childhood obesity is rising among the US population. The NHANES III indicated that the percentage of overweight children (6 to 11 years of age) increased from 4% in 1965 to 13% in 1999 and the percentage of overweight adolescents (12 to 19 years of age) increased from 5% in 1970 to 14% in 1999, based on the assessment of BMI. This increased incidence of childhood obesity is thought to be due to the development of an environment (easy access to calorically dense food, decreased opportunity for exercise, increased opportunity for sedentary activity) that supports excessive weight gain in predisposed individuals.

Numerous tracking studies have demonstrated that an obese child runs an increased risk of becoming an obese adult. Obese children may be even more obese as adults than they would have been if they had first become overweight in adulthood. Thus, preventing or treating childhood obesity should significantly decrease adult obesity and its accompanying medical problems. Obese children are at increased risk for sleep apnea, hypertension, hyperlipidemia, type 2 diabetes, orthopedic problems (such as slipped capital femoral epiphysis), pseudotumor cerebri, and psychosocial problems. A study from Cincinnati suggested that the prevalence of type 2 diabetes has increased 10-fold in children over a 12- year period (1982 to 1994). This increase is thought to be largely due to the increased rate of obesity (see Case 1).

Etiology of Obesity: Genetics and Environment

According to current estimates, a child with two obese parents has an 80% chance of becoming obese, whereas the proportion drops to 40% of children with only one obese parent. Studies comparing the relative body weights of adopted children with their biologic and adoptive parents' weight suggests a major genetic component in the incidence of obesity.

Despite this seemingly indisputable evidence of genetic influence on the development of obesity, however, multiple environmental influences also have been well documented. A higher prevalence of obesity exists in only children, children of older parents, and children whose parents are separated. Children who watch many hours of television are also more likely to be obese. Decreased physical activity and increased snacking while watching TV most likely contribute to this phenomenon. The large number of food commercials aimed at children during children's shows may also be a factor, as well as the dramatic increase in portion sizes, fast food, soda, and soft drink consumption.

Treatment of Overweight Children and Adolescents

Comprehensive treatment programs, including a major behavior modification component, have been shown to be moderately effective in the treatment of childhood obesity. Active participation of parents and the family also are strongly recommended. In addition to dietary modification, intervention programs should aim to increase physical activity and minimize sedentary behavior, specifically television viewing (see Case 1).

Nutrition and Dental Health

Nutrition has an obvious impact on the development of teeth and ongoing dental health. To develop dental caries, cariogenic bacteria and an appropriate food source for the bacteria are necessary. Different foods have varying effects on the development of caries according to the food's sugar content and potential to adhere to the teeth. Eating frequently and consuming foods that adhere to the teeth provide the cariogenic bacteria with a readily available food source that promotes cavity formation. Factors affecting dental health include tooth development and eruption, cariogenic bacteria, sugar intake (sucrose, maltose, lactose, and fructose), frequency of eating, adherence of food, and fluoride.

Fluoride, either in fluoridated water or in a supplement, helps prevent cavity formation. However, care must be taken to avoid administering too much fluoride because it may stain the teeth. Discoloration occurs most commonly in children who receive an inappropriately high fluoride supplement and also drink fluoridated water. The Committee on Nutrition of the AAP has developed recommendations concerning fluoride supplementation based on the fluoride content of the local water supply. The committee also suggests that infants under 6 months of age should not receive fluoride supplementation. Test kits are now available, since fluoride levels in rural areas can vary dramatically even in short distances.

Parents should also be advised not to put infants to sleep with a bottle. Bacteria that colonize the plaque covering teeth metabolize carbohydrates, producing acid, which in turn demineralizes teeth. If this demineralization is allowed to proceed, cavities are formed. Children who are allowed to sleep with a bottle bathe their teeth in formula, supporting demineralization. In severe cases, the incisors can be eroded to the gum line.

As soon as teeth erupt, they should be cleaned with a washcloth or baby toothbrush. Toothpaste should not be used until 2 years of age, with a pea-sized amount being sufficient. Brushing children's teeth on a regular basis should be strongly encouraged by health care providers.

Calcium Requirements and Bone Density

Recent evidence suggests that bone mineral content peaks in adolescents or young adults and then begins to decrease as a person ages. Maximizing peak bone mineral content early in life may help prevent osteoporosis with advancing age. Enhancing calcium intake in childhood and adolescence has been recommended to help increase bone mineral content. Surveys show that many American children and adolescents have suboptimal calcium intake. For example, one study showed that only 29.5% of girls and 42.5% of boys were meeting the daily recommended intake for calcium. Dairy products are the most efficient food source of calcium. Low-fat milk and cheese should be recommended to avoid excessive fat, saturated fat, and cholesterol intakes. Calcium can also be increased with calcium supplementation. In addition, weight-bearing exercise promotes increased bone mineral density. Unfortunately, many adolescent girls, who as elderly women have a relatively high risk of osteoporosis, have a poor calcium intake and are relatively sedentary, limiting attainment of a healthy bone density.

Certain considerations (such as anorexia, intestinal malabsorption, chronic renal failure, and chronic use of certain medications, such as steroids and diuretics) are associated with reduced bone density. Children with these conditions should have their bone density evaluated. In addition, children with a history of recurring fractures should be evaluated.

Summary

Nutrition during childhood can have immediate and long-term effects on growth and development. Important lifelong habits and preferences are developed during this time. These can have a long-term impact on the child's life, even after he or she attains adulthood. Many families are misinformed and confused about what is correct and appropriate for their children relating to nutrition. The goal of health care providers should be to guide children and families to follow healthy dietary guidelines.

For a list of references for this chapter, please visit the University of Pennsylvania School of Medicine's Nutrition Education and Prevention Program web site: *http://www.med.upenn.edu/nutrimed/articles.html*

Case 1

Overweight Child with Insulin Resistance

Andrew M. Tershakovec and Lisa Hark

Objectives

- Take an appropriate dietary and medical history, including family history of overweight or obesity, and social history regarding physical activity, sedentary activity, and other lifestyle issues.
- Perform an appropriate physical examination for an overweight or obese child or adolescent, and evaluate the patient for other signs and symptoms of chronic diseases related to obesity (i.e., hypertension, insulin resistance, dyslipidemia, sleep apnea, orthopedic problems, etc.).
- Identify factors responsible for increasing weight in order to recommend suitable dietary or lifestyle changes.
- Recognize the importance of the patient's and patient's family's involvement in making changes and the social, emotional, and psychological factors that may support the development of obesity and may influence the response to intervention.

TR is an 11-year-old boy who comes to see his physician for a health maintenance visit. His parents note that he has gained a lot of weight since last year but feel that he "does not eat that much" and is an active boy. They are at a loss to explain his weight gain.

Past Medical History

TR was a full-term infant (birth weight 3950 g). His mother notes that he has always had a good appetite and grew rapidly as a young child (she says he is "big boned"). In kindergarten, he was a head taller than most of the other children. TR's mother notes that his weight gain had been relatively stable until he reached the age of 7, when his rate of weight gain increased steadily over the next 4 years.

TR had recurrent ear infections and was a loud snorer as a toddler. A tonsillectomy and adenoidectomy (T&A) was performed when TR was 2 years old. TR was diagnosed with asthma at the age of 9. He currently uses an albuterol inhaler on a daily basis for preventive care. He has never been admitted to the hospital for an asthma attack, but his mother says she does not want him running too much, as he easily gets short of breath.

Family History

TR's family history is remarkable for type 2 diabetes, obesity, and heart disease. His mother (age 35) is obese and has type 2 diabetes (BMI 35 kg/m^2). His father (age 36) is overweight (BMI 28 kg/m^2). His maternal grandmother (age 65) is obese and has type 2 diabetes; his maternal grandfather (age 67) had a myocardial infarction (MI) at age 53.

Social/Development/Puberty

TR's development is described as normal. He walked at age 15 months and was toilet trained at 2^1/$_2$ years. He is described as an average student who keeps mostly to himself. He admits that the kids at school have been teasing him about his weight for several years and call him "fatty boy." He has few friends and spends most of his free time alone. TR denies smoking, alcohol, drugs, or sexual activity.

Social History

TR's mother works from 9:00 a.m. to 5:00 p.m. daily in food services. TR's father works the night shift in maintenance at a local refinery (10:00 p.m. to 6:00 a.m.). TR goes to his grandmother's house directly after school. He is an only child.

Diet/Physical Activity History

TR's parents state that he "does not eat that much." When asked what he eats during the day (24-hour recall), the parents reveal that he enjoys eating breakfast with his father when he arrives home at 7:00 a.m. (usually scrambled eggs, toast, and juice), a sandwich for lunch at school (peanut butter and jelly with 2 cookies and juice or chocolate milk), and a healthy dinner (baked chicken, potatoes, green beans, and milk), which they all eat together when mom arrives home from work. TR's parents state that he is active with soccer (goalie position) and baseball during the year. TR is described as a restless sleeper. He reports feeling tired during the day and frequently falls asleep while watching TV.

Review of Systems

Skin: No history of rashes

Neurologic: No headaches, tremors, seizures

Endocrine: No polyphagia, polydipsia, or polyuria

Pulmonary: Snoring remitted after the T&A but has recurred over the last few months

Joints: No swelling; complains that his legs hurt if has to walk for a long distance

Physical Examination

Vital Signs

Temperature: 99°F (37°C)

Heart rate: 95 beats per minute (BPM)

Respiratory rate: 26 BPM

Blood pressure: 130/75 mm Hg

Current weight: 82 kg (180 lb) (>ninety-fifth percentile for age)

Current height: 162 cm (63.8 in.) (>ninety-fifth percentile for age)

BMI: 31.2 kg/m^2 (>eighty-fifth percentile for age)

Weight history

    8 years old: 40 kg (>ninety-fifth percentile)

    9 years old: 55 kg (>ninety-fifth percentile)

    10 years old: 70 kg (>ninety-fifth percentile)

General: Overweight boy in no acute distress, no hirsutism or striae, no edema, no cushingoid features

Head, ears, eyes, nose, throat (HEENT): Increased pigmentation and wrinkled, hypertrophied skin at base of neck (acanthosis nigricans), nonpalpable thyroid

Eyes: Extraocular movements intact (EOMI), pupils equally round and reactive to light (PERRL), normal disc margins

Abdomen: Bowel sounds (BS) (+), soft, no masses or organomegaly palpable, liver span by percussion 8 cm, stretch marks noted

Cardiac: Regular rate and rhythm (RRR) S$_1$, S$_2$, no murmurs

Chest: Clear

Genitalia: Tanner I boy, phallus largely obscured by fat pad, testes normal

Neurologic: Alert, strength 5/5, deep tendon reflex (DTR) +2 upper and lower extremities, normal tone

Orthopedic: Wide-based gait, mild bowing of lower aspect of legs bilaterally

Laboratory Data

Patient's Fasting Values	Normal Values
Glucose: 87 mg/dL	70–100 mg/dL
Insulin: 28 μU/mL	<20 μU/mL
Hemoglobin (Hgb) A1C: 4.3 mg/dL	<4.5 mg/dL
Cholesterol: 212 mg/dL	<200 mg/dL
Triglycerides: 145 mg/dL	<120 mg/dL
Low-density lipoprotein cholesterol (LDL-C): 105 mg/dL	<130 mg/dL
High-density lipoprotein cholesterol (HDL-C): 38 mg/dL	≥40 mg/dL

Alanine aminotransferase (ALT): 37 units per liter	10–30 units per liter
Aspartate aminotransferase (AST): 55 units per liter	10–30 units per liter
Thyroid-stimulating hormone (TSH): 2.3 μU per liter	0.5–5.0 μU per liter

Case Questions

1. Describe methods that can be used to assess TR's weight.
2. Describe the risk factors and health consequences associated with being an overweight child or adolescent.
3. What additional information should be asked regarding TR's increasing weight over the past 4 years?
4. Before treatment is recommended, how can TR and his family's readiness to change be assessed and how should this treatment process be explained?
5. What are the appropriate medical nutrition therapy and physical activity recommendations for TR and his family?
6. What type of behavior modification techniques can be used to help TR and his family implement these dietary and lifestyle suggestions?

Case Answers

Part 1: Diagnosis

1. **Describe methods that can be used to assess TR's weight.**

   Using the current Centers for Disease Control (CDC) growth charts that include BMI growth curves for children and adolescents, *at-risk for overweight* is defined as a BMI between the eighty-fifth and ninety-fifth percentile, and *overweight* is defined as BMI greater than the ninety-fifth percentile. However, BMI is only a screening tool and the patient's degree of overweight can be confirmed on physical examination. Such screening is necessary to identify those who require intervention. The goal of intervention may be weight loss or weight stabilization depending on the specific circumstances. Decreasing the rate of weight gain while a child is growing will help decrease ultimate gain in relative weight.

   It is apparent from his weight history that TR was always a large child but began to gain weight rapidly over the last few years. It is common that overweight prepubertal children are taller than their normal-weight counterparts. These overweight children tend to enter puberty earlier, have their growth spurt earlier, and then attain a normal adult height.

2. **Describe the risk factors and health consequences associated with being an overweight child or adolescent.**

   Overweight children and adolescents are at risk for similar health problems as adults who are overweight or obese, including type 2 diabetes, hypertension, dyslipidemia, sleep apnea, asthma, gallbladder disease, orthopedic problems, and nonalcoholic steatohepatitis. TR was diagnosed with asthma at age 9. It is not known if the asthma limits his activity and thus contributes to his weight gain or if the asthma itself somehow contributes to the development of obesity. It is not clear if TR's dyspnea on exertion is due to asthma or his poor cardiovascular fitness. Appropriate treatment should allow TR to participate in normal physical activity without restriction.

Sleep Apnea

On further questioning about his sleep patterns, TR and his parents indicate that he is a restless sleeper, has daytime sleepiness, and snores loudly. These symptoms may be consistent with sleep apnea. TR should be referred to a pulmonary specialist for further evaluation and possibly a formal sleep study.

Diabetes

Recently, there has been a dramatic increase in the prevalence of type 2 diabetes in children and adolescents, especially in African-American and Hispanic populations. This may be explained, in part, by the parallel increase in the prevalence of overweight among children and teenagers. A positive family history of type 2 diabetes is associated with an increased risk of insulin resistance (insulin resistance is thought to be part of the etiology of type 2 diabetes). The increased skin pigmentation that TR demonstrates could be acanthosis nigricans, which can be associated with insulin resistance. Thus, a fasting serum glucose, insulin, and HgbA1c were obtained. The normal glucose (87 mg/dL) and HgbA1c (4.3 mg/dL), with an elevated insulin level (28 mIU/mL), is consistent with insulin resistance.

Heart Disease/Hypertension

Because of TR's family history of heart disease, as well as the fact that his blood pressure is elevated using the age/height–specific blood pressure criteria, a fasting lipid panel was ordered. These results, when compared to the age-appropriate percentiles, indicate that TR has elevated cholesterol and triglyceride and a reduced HDL level. Hypertriglyceridemia and low HDL-C are the most common lipid abnormalities associated with insulin resistance.

Nonalcoholic Steatohepatitis

Overweight children may present with increased liver enzymes ALT and AST, which may be indicative of fatty infiltration into the liver. Abnormal liver function tests have been described in 6% to 10% of obese adolescents. This condition, know as *nonalcoholic steatohepatitis*, has been described to progress to cirrhosis and liver failure in adults. Obesity-associated nonalcoholic steatohepatitis may be associated with low antioxidant levels and may respond to vitamin E therapy and weight loss.

Part 2: Nutrition Assessment

3. **What additional information should be asked regarding TR's increasing weight over the past 4 years?**

    TR's 24-hour recall looks "healthy" on first glance. Although TR's parents feel that he is "not a big eater," it is important to probe for excess calories, such as sodas and juices, as well as high-fat foods. Dietary information provided for obese individuals tends to be grossly underreported. Studies suggest that obese adolescents underreport their caloric intake by as much as 40% to 60% and that obese individuals underreport to a greater degree than nonobese individuals.

    Further questioning reveals that TR eats breakfast with his father at 7:00 a.m. and then again with his mother at 8:00 a.m. [bowl of Cocoa Puffs cereal with whole milk and a 16-oz (480-mL) glass of orange juice]. He eats his lunch from home but also has access to the soda machine, where he buys a 20-oz (600-mL) bottle of soda every day with lunch. After school he spends most days with his grandmother, who serves him a hamburger, fries, and a 16-oz soda or another sandwich with chocolate milk at 3:30 p.m for a snack. He eats dinner at 6:00 p.m. when he arrives home. TR also enjoys either ice cream and a few chocolate chip cookies or an 8-oz (240-mL) glass of whole milk with peanut butter crackers before bed.

    TR's parents stated that he is active with soccer in the fall and baseball in the spring. He usually has one game each week and plays goalie or a defensive position that involves very little running. As both teams have many players, TR never plays more than half a game or approximately 25 minutes. After the game TR's family often goes to a fast food restaurant to celebrate. TR is sedentary during the winter months.

    Further questioning about TR's television, video, and computer game usage reveals that on weekdays, on average, he watches 3 hours of television per day. On weekends TR watches television, plays video or computer games, or "surfs the web" for up to 6 hours per day.

4. **Before treatment is recommended, how can TR and his family's readiness to change be assessed and how should this treatment process be explained?**

    Before recommending any dietary or lifestyle suggestions, it is very important to assess both TR and his family's interest in making changes. It is best to directly address the motivation and willingness to change with TR and his parents. Some families may express significant interest in changing behaviors yet will be unable to identify concrete changes that they are willing to undertake. It is also important to assess other potential environmental obstacles (e.g., other uncooperative family members).

TR's parents stated in the initial workup that he has gained a lot of weight since last year; they seem to realize that there may be a problem with his weight. However, the fact that they do not recognize his sedentary lifestyle and increased caloric intake as a problem suggests some denial or lack of willingness to change. Because TR says he dislikes the teasing, he may have some interest in changing. However, the fact that he is becoming more and more withdrawn may suggest depression or other psychosocial issues that may be necessary to address before weight management interventions can be successful.

When explaining the process of weight management and the implications of excessive weight gain, it is useful to show the family the child's growth curve. The specific medical issues affecting the child should also be discussed. In TR's case, his asthma, insulin resistance, sleep apnea, hypertension, and dyslipidemia are likely related to his obesity.

In general, the initial goals of a pediatric weight management program are to decrease the rate of weight gain. Keeping weight stable while a child grows decreases relative weight. With significant obesity, actual weight loss may be appropriate.

Part 3: Medical Nutrition Therapy

5. **What are the appropriate medical nutrition therapy and physical activity recommendations for TR and his family?**

The most important dietary change that should be recommended for TR is to establish a regular eating pattern. Most days, TR is eating two breakfasts, two dinners, and an evening snack. The first step would be to eliminate one of his breakfast meals and to reduce the amount of juice he is drinking at breakfast to approximately 6 oz (180 mL) per day. He could also try a low-sugar cereal, such as Cheerios, Life, or Rice Krispies, and change to 2%, reduced-fat milk to be later changed to 1% low-fat or fat-free milk, all of which will considerably reduce his carbohydrate, saturated fat, and caloric intake. Lunch could remain the same, with the addition of a fresh fruit and carrot sticks. Purchasing soda with lunch should be discouraged, and eliminating all soda and sugar-containing drinks should be considered. Maybe he could bring a bottle of water or purchase one from the vending machine, which is now available in most schools.

TR's grandmother should be included in any discussions since she is his afterschool caregiver. Because she has type 2 diabetes, she may be receptive to the idea of prevention in her grandson. Healthy afterschool snack suggestions for TR include fruit, low-fat yogurt, low-fat granola bar, bowl of cereal with low-fat milk, microwave "lite" popcorn, or a frozen fruit bar. Snacks are a normal and important part of a child's diet; however, choices should not be high in calories.

Beverage choices are another common problem with overweight children. Efforts should be made to limit the intake of all sugar-containing beverages including juices. Many families seem to feel that since juices are "natural" their intake should not be limited. It is not unusual to see a child ingest 500 to 1000 calories a day in juice, soda, and other sugar-sweetened beverages. Just eliminating this will likely stop excessive weight gain.

Dinner meals seem to be the healthiest and could remain the same, although TR should be served low-fat or skim milk at home to reduce his fat intake. In addition to a healthy diet, families should be instructed on proper serving sizes for children.

Parents and families should assess and plan opportunities for increased physical activity. One should find activities that the child enjoys (i.e., one should not expect a child to use a treadmill regularly). Parents need to provide an environment in which being active several times a week is normal and expected. Parents should be role models and participate in activities with their children. They should not assume that children are active during school recess, as physical education has been consistently decreased and often eliminated from the school curriculum. Parents should also monitor and set daily limits for sedentary activities, such as watching TV and playing computer and video games, as less than 2 hours per day is suggested by the AAP. According to the CDC, children and adolescents should engage in at least 1 hour of physical activity every day.

6. **What type of behavior modification techniques can be used to help TR and his family implement these dietary and lifestyle suggestions?**

It is important to assess the child and family's psychosocial well-being before initiating a behavior modification program. For example, if the child is depressed, the depression will probably make the weight management more difficult. In some cases, it may be best to defer the weight management program until the psychological issues are addressed. Similarly, significant family difficulties, such as a family member with anorexia or a substance abuse problem, should be identified.

The issues surrounding eating and weight are complex and frequently emotionally charged. As few families have the insight to address these issues as part of a "self-help" program without outside assistance, it is important to institute a behavior modification program with the guidance of a behavior specialist. Little research has directly assessed the efficacy of different behavioral components of a weight management program. However, several factors are commonly included in most weight management programs. Some of these include the following.

Motivation

It is important to assess the child's and family's motivation to participate in the weight management program. Experience suggests that in addition to being interested and motivated participants, children do better in the program when a parent is also an active and supportive participant.

Stimulus Control and Environmental Modification

One should provide an environment that only includes healthy choices. However, trying to restrict a child from eating certain foods in the home (e.g., chips, soda) may be counterproductive.

Role Modeling

It is important to have as many people as possible and, it is hoped, the whole family, act as role models in all aspects of the behavior modification program.

Positive Reinforcement

Parents should be instructed in methods of positive reinforcement.

Self-Monitoring

Parents and children should be instructed in methods of self-monitoring (keeping a diet diary and activity log), generally focusing on dietary intake and physical activity. Experience suggests that persons who self-monitor significantly decrease caloric intake and generally do much better in weight management programs.

Case 2

Malnutrition and Refeeding Syndrome in Children

John A. Kerner and Jo Ann T. Hattner

Objectives

- Describe the physiologic and metabolic adaptations that occur during starvation.
- Describe the physiologic processes that occur when refeeding an undernourished patient.
- Identify potential clinical manifestations of the refeeding syndrome and explain the most common laboratory abnormalities that may occur during refeeding.
- Summarize the clinical recommendations for minimizing or avoiding the complications associated with refeeding.

RD is an 8-year-old boy of Liberian descent who lives in the United States with his parents. In October, RD and his family flew to Liberia to spend a few months with their extended family. Several weeks after his arrival, political unrest erupted. RD and his family were forced from their homes at gunpoint, taken to a university, and held against their will in overcrowded, unsanitary conditions. Medical and food supplies were scarce. Food was provided by soldiers outside the camp who lowered buckets of rice and occasionally fish over the barbed-wire fences. Daily tea was also provided. Many of the hostages died from starvation. RD and his family escaped after 3 months of captivity and sought refuge in the American Embassy. From there, they were airlifted to a neighboring country. Shortly thereafter, RD returned to the United States. At the US Embassy, RD's vital signs were as follows:

Temperature: 97°F (36°C)
Heart rate: 45 beats per minute (BPM)
Respiratory rate: 18 BPM
Blood pressure: 100/80 mm Hg

After 3 months of virtual starvation, the family reported that RD ate "everything he could get his hands on." On follow-up with his local physician in the United States, RD was immediately referred to the local emergency room for evaluation of undernutrition.

Past Medical History

RD tested positive for malaria in the past; no other problems were noted. On admission, he was not taking any medications or vitamins. RD has no known food allergies. He was having four to five loose stools per day.

Social/Diet History

By report, before his imprisonment in the refugee camp, RD's food supply met 100% of his needs. While in the refugee camp, his estimated intake amounted to only 250 to 300 kcal per day, with 30 g protein per week. Four days after he escaped, his intake had risen to an estimated 2500 to 3000 kcal per day, with 80 to 90 g protein per day. Further evaluation in the hospital produced the following clinical picture.

Physical Examination

Vital Signs

Temperature: 101.8°F (38°C)
Heart rate: 120 beats per minute (BPM)
Respiratory rate: 30 BPM
Blood pressure: 80/50 mm Hg
General: Eight-year-old boy who appears apathetic and emaciated
Skin: Dry, scaly dermatitis
Head: Alopecia, thinning hair lacking in luster
Abdomen: Mildly distended
Extremities: Bipedal edema; temporal and interosseous muscle wasting

Physical Exam Data

See Table 5-6.

Laboratory Data

See Table 5-7.

Case Questions

1. What nutrition-related changes in body function probably occurred during the past 3-month period of starvation?
2. Based on the physical examination and laboratory data, what clinical and biochemical manifestations of undernutrition does RD exhibit?
3. What metabolic and physiologic changes occur as RD begins to eat again? Why are his electrolyte abnormalities of primary concern?

Table 5-6   Physical exam data.

DATE	Cm (in.)	PERCENTILE	kg (lb)	PERCENTILE, g/m^2	BMI	BMI PERCENTILE
	HEIGHT		**WEIGHT**			
1/7*	127 (50")	50th	19 (42)	<5	11.8	<5th
1/10	127 (50")	50th	22 (48)	10-25	13.6	<5th

* At initial presentation to the emergency room.

Table 5-7   Laboratory data.

DATE	Ca (mg/dL)	PO$_4$ (mg/dL)	Mg (mg/dL)	K (mEq/L)	ALBUMIN (g/dL)
1/7*	8.0	3.0	1.8	3.6	2.7
1/10	6.3	1.0	0.9	2.0	2.4
Normal	(9–11)	(2.5–4.6)	(1.8–2.9)	(3.5–5.3)	(3.5–5.8)

* At initial presentation to the emergency room.

4. Based on RD's physical examination and laboratory data, what complications of refeeding does he exhibit?

5. How could the complications of refeeding that RD experienced have been minimized or avoided?

Case Answers

Part 1: Physiology

1. **What nutrition-related changes in body function probably occurred during the past 3-month period of starvation?**

The body's systems adapt to calorie and protein deficits in a complex manner. Chronic nutritional deprivation results in a mildly catabolic state. The body's compensatory mechanisms involve changes in energy metabolism and hormone regulation. Fat from adipose tissue and protein from muscle mass are mobilized and converted to energy via glucose and ketones. The catabolism of fat and protein results in a loss of lean body mass, electrolytes, and water. The basal metabolic rate (BMR) decreases to conserve energy; the body becomes hypothermic, hypotensive, and bradycardic, and physical activity decreases. Growth hormone and thyroid hormone regulation decrease or stop growth, which helps to lower the BMR. Production of insulin, which promotes anabolism of catecholamines, cortisol, and glucagon, also decreases. The net effect facilitates survival by decreasing the BMR and promoting conservation of protein and organ function.

Overall decreases in cellular mass may eventually result in functional loss in vital organs. Respiratory muscle loss may lessen respiratory efficiency. Myocardial atrophy may reduce cardiac output. Decreased intravascular fluid volume results in decreased cardiac output.

GI atrophy slows motility and gastric acid secretion and causes thinning of the mucosa, villous atrophy, and decreased production of digestive enzymes. These effects reduce GI function and can result in malabsorption and diarrhea, further exacerbating the malnutrition and possibly increasing susceptibility to infection. Liver wasting also causes altered metabolism and decreased protein synthesis. Lastly, the kidney's ability to concentrate urine decreases, causing diuresis.

2. **Based on the physical examination and laboratory data, what clinical and biochemical manifestations of undernutrition does RD exhibit?**

   Specific manifestations include wasting and apparent emaciation (depleted somatic protein and subcutaneous fat stores) due to protein-energy undernutrition. Although protein status may be depleted at initial presentation, serum albumin and protein values are commonly normal due to the decreased blood volume (hemoconcentration). However, as the child is refed, the total blood volume increases, and albumin and protein concentrations may decrease (hemodilution). The changes in calcium, phosphate, magnesium, and potassium levels may be associated with his undernutrition as well as his rapid refeeding. Bradycardia, hypothermia, and a decreased respiratory rate are common bodily defense mechanisms in undernutrition that result in decreased energy needs. In addition, RD exhibited signs and symptoms of vitamin and mineral deficiencies as listed, such as dry scaly dermatitis (essential fatty acids, vitamin A, niacin), alopecia (protein, biotin), and thinning hair, lacking luster (essential fatty acids, zinc, protein). Nonspecific manifestations include decreased growth rate and physical activity. The child generally appears apathetic with a flat affect.

   RD presents with severe wasting demonstrated by his low BMI and weight change, suggesting acute undernutrition. If RD's starvation had continued, he would have manifested stunting or slowed height growth. His low serum albumin level suggests depleted visceral protein status as well, although most children with marasmus have normal albumin levels.

Part 2: Initiating Refeeding

3. **What metabolic and physiologic changes occur as RD begins to eat again? Why are his electrolyte abnormalities of primary concern?**

   Refeeding syndrome is defined as the broad range of metabolic abnormalities and physiologic consequences that can occur as a result of rapid reinstitution of feeding in a person with nutritional deprivation. These changes can lead to significant pathologic consequences, including death. Awareness of the physiologic adaptation and metabolic changes with fluid and electrolyte shifts with refeeding is of primary concern. It is important to note that these changes occur, to a greater or lesser degree, in every

Table 5-8   Diagnoses or conditions of patients at risk for refeeding syndrome.

Anorexia nervosa
Chronic undernutrition (e.g., from neglect)
Crohn's disease
Cystic fibrosis
Chronic infections
Diabetic ketoacidosis
Dysphagia caused by neuromuscular diseases
Human immunodeficiency virus (HIV)+/acquired immunodeficiency syndrome (AIDS)
Malignancies
Burns
Protein calorie undernutrition (e.g., refugees or famine victims)
Any conditions associated with wasting or acute or
    chronic weight loss

pediatric or adult patient who has been deprived of adequate nutrients. Pediatric patients with the diagnoses listed in Table 5-8 are at particular risk for refeeding syndrome.

When refeeding is initiated in the undernourished patient, anabolism begins almost immediately. A rapid alteration in hormonal levels, primarily an increase in insulin production, occurs as the shift from fat to carbohydrate metabolism occurs and glucose becomes the predominant fuel. The glucose load with corresponding insulin release results in cellular uptake of glucose, phosphate, potassium, magnesium, and water, as well as protein synthesis. At this time the basal metabolic rate increases. Anabolism requires energy, nutrients, and enzymes as intermediate compounds to act as building blocks for regrowth. Increased requirements for anabolism may cause or unmask deficiencies, including life-threatening imbalances, thus inhibiting anabolism.

The cardiovascular adaptations of undernutrition, including myocardial atrophy and volume contraction, must also be considered when refeeding an undernourished patient. A rapid alteration in calories, fluid, and particularly sodium intake may produce fluid shifts and intravascular volume overload, causing the patient to go into congestive heart failure.

The most common laboratory abnormalities encountered when refeeding undernourished patients involve potassium, phosphate, magnesium, and calcium. The etiology of each of these abnormalities includes the following.

Potassium

Insulin, secreted in response to the increased glucose load during refeeding, causes glucose and potassium to enter the intracellular space. This may result in a rapid fall in serum potassium. Hypokalemia may alter nerve and muscle function, resulting in cardiac arrhythmias, hypotension, and cardiac arrest. A potassium concentration of less than 3.0 mEq per liter is considered severe hypokalemia.

Phosphate

Hypophosphatemia is one of the predominant features of the refeeding syndrome. As anabolism increases, the need for phosphorylated intermediates also increases. Phosphate bound to these compounds is, in effect, "trapped" intracellularly. The resulting imbalance may cause severe hypophosphatemia, which may lead to cell damage and dysfunction resulting in organ failure.

Magnesium

The refeeding syndrome is associated with hypomagnesemia. The mechanism is probably multifactorial. Intracellular movement of magnesium into cells with carbohydrate feeding and preexisting magnesium status are two of the possible factors. Magnesium is also a cofactor for the enzyme adenosine triphosphatase (ATPase). As the metabolic rate increases, magnesium requirements rise. Magnesium is also required for normal parathyroid function. Thus, hypomagnesemia may cause dysmetabolism by altering ATPase function and calcium and phosphate homeostasis.

Calcium

As growth is initiated, calcium requirements increase. Maintenance of calcium levels may be affected if hypomagnesemia is present. Serum levels of calcium are maintained in such cases at the expense of bone deposits. Thus, chronic undernutrition alters bone mineralization. Hypocalcemia may alter muscle and myocardial function, causing tetany and cardiac arrhythmias.

4. **Based on RD's physical examination and laboratory data, what complications of refeeding does he exhibit?**

RD exhibits fluid overload, as evidenced by the edema. This condition could be exacerbated by his low albumin level as fluid leaks from the capillaries because of decreased oncotic pressure. In addition, he may be in congestive heart failure because of his decreased cardiac output secondary to loss of heart muscle function from protein catabolism. The stress of a restored blood volume on a depleted cardiac muscle could result in cardiac decompensation. Furthermore, his myocardial function may be altered by electrolyte imbalances, putting him at greater risk for cardiac arrhythmia.

RD demonstrated dangerously low serum calcium, phosphate, magnesium, and potassium levels after refeeding because of rapid utilization of depleted mineral stores to initiate anabolism.

5. **How could the complications of refeeding that RD experienced have been minimized or avoided?**

    The following treatment recommendations will help to avoid or minimize the complications of refeeding in children and adults.

    • Refeed slowly, with gradual increases in fluid, salt, and calories. Begin with 50% to 75% of basal caloric needs.

    • Provide multivitamin and mineral supplements.

    • Correct electrolyte abnormalities before initiation of enteral or parenteral nutrition support and monitor serum levels.

    • Increase calories by 10% each day while closely monitoring laboratory values, specifically calcium, phosphate, sodium, glucose, potassium, and magnesium and the patient's overall clinical state. Consider stopping or slowing the advancement of calories if fluid overload, congestive heart failure, or electrolyte imbalance develops.

    • Monitor vital signs closely during this process to detect changes in cardiorespiratory function early. Continuous electrocardiographic monitoring may be appropriate.

    • Monitor fluid intake and output carefully to avoid stressing the undernourished cardiorespiratory system and to avoid potential fluid overload.

    • Monitor daily weight gain. Excessive weight gain suggests fluid retention.

Case 3

Eating Disorders in Adolescent Athletes

Diane Barsky and Marion Fitzgibbon

Objectives

- Recognize how rapid growth during puberty alters adolescents' nutritional requirements.
- Identify teenagers at risk for eating disorders and determine appropriate interventions.
- Assess the nutrient intake of adolescent athletes and their risk of developing nutritional deficiencies.
- Outline the time sequence of the adolescent growth spurt and the stages of pubertal development described by Tanner.

AB is a 15-year-old girl who has been a member of her school's cross-country running team for the past 2 years. She presents to her physician after an episode of fainting while she was competing in a 5-km race. Before fainting she felt dizzy, but she has denied heart pounding, shortness of breath, or visual changes. She reports drinking water before starting the race. AB has experienced episodes of muscle cramping and headaches over the past 2 weeks.

History of Present Illness

Six months ago AB reported abdominal pain and a burning sensation in her chest. Her symptoms subsequently improved with the use of antacids and a change in her eating pattern by consuming small, more frequent meals. According to her medical records, AB was at the fiftieth percentile for her weight-for-age on the growth charts until last year. She has lost 15 lb (6.8 kg) during the past year and is currently at the fifth percentile for weight-for-age.

Past Medical History

AB's history appears negative for heart disease, asthma, epilepsy, or diabetes. She has no previous history of fainting. AB takes antacids occasionally, but she is not taking any over-the-counter supplements, medications, vitamins, or minerals. She has no known allergies.

Social/Development

AB is a high-achieving student. Her current circle of friends includes mostly school athletes. On further questioning, AB expresses concern over recent changes in her body, such as breast development and widening hips. She wants to maintain a trim, muscular physique and fears that excessive weight gain will affect her speed and athletic agility. She denies smoking, alcohol, drugs, or sexual activity.

Diet History

To prepare herself for the race, AB had been consuming a high-protein (80 to 100 g per day), low-fat, and low-carbohydrate diet for the past few weeks. Twenty-four hours before the race, she consumed two high-carbohydrate meals.

AB states that she enjoys eating but follows a low-fat regimen to minimize weight gain. On occasion, she indulges in high-fat or high-sugar foods. She admits to small weight fluctuations during the past year, but she increases the intensity of her exercise routine to keep her weight at 90 lb (41 kg). She denies vomiting or abuse of laxatives, enemas, or diuretics. AB frequently skips meals and compensates by snacking. During the interview, she frequently expresses concern that she is overweight and not muscular enough for long-distance running. Based on a 24-hour dietary recall, AB consumes approximately 900 to 1000 kcal per day.

Menstrual History

Menses started when AB was 12 years of age. She reports a normal cycle every 30 days until 8 months ago, when menses abruptly ceased.

Physical Examination

Vital Signs

Temperature: 96°F (35.6°C)

Heart rate: 68 beats per minute (BPM)

Respiratory rate: 14 BPM

Blood pressure: 90/62 mm Hg

Height: 162 cm (64 in.; fiftieth percentile for age)

Current weight: 41 kg (90 lb; fifth percentile for age)

Ideal weight: 53 kg (117 lb; fiftieth percentile for age)

BMI: 15.6 kg/m^2

General: Thin, muscular female appearing sad, anxious, and younger than her age

HEENT: Pale face, pale conjunctiva; no palpable goiter, dental erosions; gag reflex somewhat diminished; enlarged salivary glands

Cardiac: Normal rate and rhythm

Breasts: Elevation of breast mound with areola, Tanner 3

Genitalia: Coarse pubic hair with sparse distribution, Tanner 3
Neurologic: Reflexes slightly decreased in upper and lower extremities
Extremities: Dry, coarse skin at dorsum of hand

Laboratory Data

Patient's Laboratory Values	Normal Values
Sodium: 142 mEq per liter	133–143 mEq per liter
Potassium: 2.5 mEq per liter	3.5–5.3 mEq per liter
CO_2: 32 mmol per liter	24–32 mmol per liter
Calcium: 8.2 mg/dL	9–11 mg/dL
Phosphate: 4.2 mg/dL	2.5–4.6 mg/dL
Albumin: 3.5 g/dL	3.5–5.8 g/dL
Hgb: 11.2 g/dL	11.8–15.5 g/dL

Case Questions

1. What clues in AB's medical history indicate that she may have an eating disorder?
2. Based on AB's laboratory values, what are the possible causes of her fainting spell, muscle cramps, and headaches?
3. Is AB's Tanner staging appropriate for her age?
4. Is AB's current diet appropriate for her age and physical activity level?
5. What nutrient deficiencies is AB at risk for developing?
6. What treatment recommendations are appropriate for AB at this time?

Case Answers

Part 1: Diagnosis

1. **What clues in AB's medical history indicate that she may have an eating disorder?**

   Several clues in AB's past medical history may lead the clinician to suspect that she has an eating disorder. The history of a burning sensation in her chest and abdominal pain that responded to antacids signal possible esophagitis, which may be secondary to self-induced vomiting, or purging. Purging behavior may be associated with both anorexia nervosa and bulimia nervosa. Bulimia nervosa is a disorder characterized by frequent episodes of binge eating followed by purging (self-induced vomiting or ingestion of laxatives or cathartics to induce vomiting). Patients with bulimia nervosa tend to be of normal or increased weight. The hallmark of anorexia nervosa is an altered perception of body image, with resulting

Table 5-9   Diagnostic criteria for bulimia nervosa.

Recurrent episodes of binge eating. An episode of binge eating is characterized by both of the following:

1. Eating, in a discrete period of time (e.g., within any 2-hr period), an amount of food that is definitely larger than most people would eat during a similar period of time in similar circumstances; and

2. A sense of lack of control over eating during the episode (e.g., a feeling that one cannot stop eating or control what or how much one is eating).

Recurrent inappropriate compensatory behavior in order to prevent weight gain, such as self-induced vomiting; misuse of laxatives, diuretics, or other medications; fasting; or excessive exercise.

The binge eating and inappropriate compensatory behaviors occur, on average, at least twice a week for 3 mo.

Self-evaluation is unduly influenced by body shape and weight.

The disturbance does not occur exclusively during episodes of anorexia nervosa.

SPECIFY TYPE

Purging type: The person regularly engages in self-induced vomiting or the misuse of laxatives or diuretics.

Nonpurging type: The person uses other inappropriate compensatory behaviors, such as fasting or excessive exercise, but does not regularly engage in self-induced vomiting or the misuse of laxatives or diuretics.

SOURCE: Reprinted with permission from American Psychiatric Association. Diagnostic and Statistical Manual of Mental Disorders. 4th ed. Washington, DC: American Psychiatric Association, 1994. Copyright 1994 American Psychiatric Association.

Table 5-10   Diagnostic criteria for anorexia nervosa.

Refusal to maintain body weight over a minimal normal weight for age and height (e.g., weight loss leading to maintenance of body weight 15% below that expected; or failure to make expected weight gain during period of growth, leading to body weight 15% below that expected).

Intense fear of gaining weight or becoming fat, even though underweight.

Disturbance in the way in which one's body weight or shape is experienced, undue influence of body shape and weight on self-evaluation, or denial of the seriousness of current low body weight.

In females, absence of at least three consecutive menstrual cycles when otherwise expected to occur (primary or secondary amenorrhea). (A woman is considered to have amenorrhea if her periods occur only following hormone, e.g., estrogen, administration.)

SPECIFY TYPE

Restricting type: During the episode of anorexia nervosa, the person does not regularly engage in binge eating or purging behavior (i.e., self-induced vomiting or the misuse of laxatives or diuretics).

Binge eating/purging type: During the episode of anorexia nervosa, the person regularly engages in binge eating or purging behavior (i.e., self-induced vomiting or the misuse of laxatives or diuretics).

SOURCE: Reprinted with permission from American Psychiatric Association. Diagnostic and Statistical Manual of Mental Disorders. 4th ed. Washington, DC: American Psychiatric Association, 1994. Copyright 1994 American Psychiatric Association.

restriction of calories and body weight maintained significantly below normal weight for age and height (<85% expected weight) (Tables 5-9 and 5-10).

AB's presentation is consistent with anorexia nervosa, purging type. She is preoccupied with her body image, expressing an intense fear of gaining weight, and exercises vigorously to maintain herself at a low weight. Despite her degree of undernutrition, AB views herself as overweight, unable to acknowledge the seriousness of her condition. These symptoms are typical of the anorexia nervosa diagnosis.

AB's medical problems could be explained by her eating disorder. Although she denied vomiting, her possible esophagitis and electrolyte abnormalities (hypokalemia and alkalosis) suggest vomiting in an effort to keep her weight down. It is not unusual for patients who purge food to deny vomiting or laxative abuse.

AB's low body weight, and therefore low body fat, cannot support normal menstrual cycles, resulting in secondary amenorrhea, defined as an absence of menses for 6 months or for three usual cycle intervals following previous normal menstruation. Amenorrhea is more common among female athletes than in the general population; however, unless women with amenorrhea meet the other diagnostic criteria for eating disorders as shown in Table 5-11, amenorrhea does not confirm an eating disorder.

Eating disorders primarily occur in adolescents and college-aged women. They are more often found in industrialized cultures and occur in all socioeconomic levels and across all major ethnic groups. Given the emphasis on weight, certain athletes are at higher risk for the development of eating disorders. Those especially at risk include dancers, long-distance runners, figure skaters, actors, models, wrestlers, gymnasts, and jockeys.

2. **Based on AB's laboratory values, what are the possible causes of her fainting spell, muscle cramps, and headaches?**

    Electrolyte abnormalities are probable causes of AB's fainting spells, dizziness, and muscle cramps. Her low potassium level and metabolic alkalosis, indicated by an elevated carbon dioxide level (characteristic of base excess), are probably due to losses of potassium and hydrogen ions during self-induced vomiting. Low serum potassium or low serum calcium levels, or both can lead to muscle cramps, headaches, dizziness, and abnormal heart rhythms. Her low serum calcium level may be secondary to insufficient intake of calcium or vitamin D deficiency.

    AB is at risk for dehydration if she has been inducing vomiting without orally replacing her fluid loss. During a race, she will lose additional free water sodium and potassium from sweating. Dehydration can cause headaches and weakness. Also, depletion of glycogen reserves, due to inadequate consumption of energy and carbohydrates, may result in poor muscle endurance and cramping. AB's low Hgb level, which may be indicative of iron-deficiency anemia, may also contribute to her early fatigue and muscle weakness because of her diminished capacity to transport oxygen (see Table 5-11).

3. **Is AB's Tanner staging appropriate for her age?**

    AB demonstrates an arrest of her pubertal development. Puberty starts in girls at an earlier age than in boys. Girls usually demonstrate acceleration

Table 5-11   Medical complications of anorexia nervosa and bulimia nervosa.

ANOREXIA NERVOSA	BULIMIA NERVOSA
Physical signs and symptoms	
Cachexia, body fat depletion	Ulceration or scarring of knuckles (due to abrasions received while inducing vomiting)
Bradycardia, hypotension, hypothermia	
Salivary gland hypertrophy	Salivary gland hypertrophy
Lanugo hair	Dental enamel erosion, tooth decay
Amenorrhea	Oligomenorrhea or amenorrhea
Edema	Enlarged parotids
Constipation	Loss of gag reflex
Polyuria	Esophagitis
	Constipation/diarrhea
	Peripheral edema
	Irregular menses
Laboratory findings	
Anemia, leukopenia	Electrolyte abnormalities (hypokalemic alkalosis)
Elevated liver enzymes	Elevated serum amylase
Hypoglycemia	Metabolic alkalosis/acidosis
Increased serum cholesterol	Hypoglycemia
Hypothalamic/pituitary/endocrine gland abnormalities	Hypocalcemia
	Dehydration
Delayed gastric emptying	
Cortical atrophy on computed tomography	
Complications	
Sudden death possibly related to the presence of prolonged QT interval	Pancreatitis
Acute gastric dilatation	Ipecac-induced cardiomyopathy
Osteoporosis	Esophageal or gastric rupture
	Pneumomediastinum
	"Cathartic colon"

SOURCE: Reprinted with permission from Devlin MJ, Walsh T. Anorexia nervosa and bulimia nervosa. In Bjorntorp P, Brodoff BN, eds. Obesity. Philadelphia: Lippincott, 1992:137.

of linear growth at the onset of puberty and reach peak growth velocity early, at Tanner stage two or three, whereas boys reach peak growth velocity when genital and pubic hair are at Tanner stage four or five. In healthy females, menarche usually occurs 1 year after their growth peak and after the rise in estrogen-stimulated closure of their growth plates. Females typically reach their maximal growth velocity (a rate of 9.0 cm per year) at a mean age of 12.5 years. AB's height is already at the ninetieth percentile for her age, and she has experienced menarche. Therefore, her Tanner stage should be more advanced, but being undernourished and having a reduced amount of body fat prevents an appropriate hormonal milieu to support the progression of puberty.

Part 2: Nutrition Assessment

4. **Is AB's current diet appropriate for her age and physical activity level?**

    No. AB's diet is inadequate to meet her needs, as she is consuming fewer than 1000 kcal per day and frequently skips meals. A sufficient diet would not normally maintain an adolescent at only 90 lb (41 kg). Growing adolescents have increased energy requirements to support their rapid growth (calories per kilogram). In addition, vigorous exercise, such as running, further increases energy requirements 30% to 50% above basal metabolic needs. Her restriction of the variety and quantity of food she consumes places her at risk for several vitamin and mineral deficiencies as described below.

5. **What nutrient deficiencies is AB at risk for developing?**

    AB is at risk for developing a calcium deficiency. The highest requirements for calcium are during infancy and adolescence. An adolescent's high calcium requirements are due to increased bone modeling with calcium deposition, promoted by the hormonal changes associated with puberty and the associated growth peak (1300 mg per day). Maximal bone mass during skeletal maturation is achieved by adolescence or early adulthood and provides the best protection against bone loss after menopause (osteoporosis). However, according to the NHANES III, only 20% of teenage girls meet the dietary reference intake (DRI) for calcium. AB intentionally avoids dairy products such as cheese and ice cream because they are high in fat, but she could eat low-fat or fat-free sources and calcium-fortified foods or drinks.

    As previously stated, AB most likely has iron-deficiency anemia. Adolescents also require increased dietary iron to support growth. Foods rich in iron, which include liver, red meat, legumes, dried fruits, and green vegetables, are often lacking in an adolescent's diet.

6. **What treatment recommendations are appropriate for AB at this time?**

    A team approach that combines medical management, cognitive-behavioral interventions, and nutritional counseling is important in the treatment of patients with eating disorders. Eating disorders are viewed as psychiatric conditions, but these patients must be observed medically since significant morbidity and mortality are associated with these conditions. The many potential medical complications include delayed gastric emptying, heart failure, pancreatitis, diarrhea, osteopenia, and life-threatening electrolyte disturbances. Patients with anorexia may also experience cognitive deficits secondary to undernutrition or the subsequent refeeding process.

    Psychotherapeutic assessment and intervention are crucial in establishing a diagnosis, evaluating the risk of suicide, and assessing the severity of the psychological symptoms as well as other comorbid conditions, such as depression, anxiety, substance abuse, or personality disorders. If AB's prognosis is to improve, she needs to recognize her problem, improve her perceived body image, and set and reinforce nutritional and weight goals. In addition to psychiatric/psychological and medical intervention, a dietitian should provide guidance for nutritional rehabilitation and education.

The initial goals of medical nutrition therapy for AB should be to gain control over her purging behavior, stop her caloric restriction, and support steady weight gain. Increases in caloric intake should be gradual to avoid refeeding syndrome. Efforts to help AB accept a healthier weight goal would be undertaken. If purging continues despite psychological intervention, medication may reduce her binging and purging. However, psychopharmacologic interventions (antidepressants and neuroleptics) have been less successful with anorexia nervosa than with bulimia nervosa.

Treatment for eating disorders can usually be initiated as outpatient therapy as long as the patient is medically and psychiatrically stable. Those who are 25% to 30% below their ideal weight are often hospitalized because the severity of their undernutrition is life-threatening. Because AB is only 90 lb (41 kg), she will require close monitoring by her physician and may need to be hospitalized if her weight does not increase in the next few weeks.

See Chapter Review Questions, pages A-17 to A-20.

6

Older Adults

Jane V. White and Richard J. Ham

Objectives*

- Describe the physiologic changes associated with aging and their impact on nutrient requirements, absorption, and metabolism.
- List common risk factors associated with poor nutritional status in older Americans.
- Identify the tools used to assess nutritional, functional, cognitive, and emotional status in older adults and the impact that alterations in any one or more of these parameters have on health and quality of life.
- Identify common drug-nutrient interactions in older adults and recognize why this population is at risk for such interactions.

The older adult population in the United States and in most Western nations is rapidly expanding. By the year 2030, an estimated 70 million Americans will be 65 years of age or older. Of these, approximately 18 million Americans will be 85 years of age or older. Minority populations (Hispanics, Asians/Pacific Islanders, Native Americans, and African-Americans) are projected to represent more than 25% of the elderly population by 2030. Women continue to significantly outnumber men as age increases.

Information on the health and nutritional status of older Americans from the third National Health and Nutrition Examination Survey (NHANES III) suggests that diet plays a major role in the health and disease of adults aged 65 years and older. For many low-income and minority older adults, it may be the most important factor. Only 21% of older Americans had diets that were rated "good" according to the Healthy Eating Index when compared to younger adults; 13% reported diets rated "poor," and 67% consumed diets that

* SOURCE: Objectives for chapter and cases adapted from the *NIH Nutrition Curriculum Guide for Training Physicians* (*http://www.nhlbi.nih.gov/funding/training/naa*).

"need improvement." Inadequate physical activity is a health risk in older people, with one-third of older adults reporting no leisure time activity in a 2-week period.

Older adults are at increased risk of consuming an inadequate diet due to the presence of disease, physical disability, inability to chew food adequately, polypharmacy, social isolation, and poverty. Among older adults, nutrient intake tends to decline as age increases and regulation of energy intake in response to over- or underfeeding is less precise. Total calories and intakes of calcium, vitamin B_{12}, and folate fall well below those suggested by the recommended dietary allowances (RDAs) and the dietary reference intakes (DRIs) (see Table 2-2).

Physiologic Changes Associated with Aging

Recognition of the physiologic changes that usually occur with the aging process is essential to evaluating diet and health. Physiologic decline escalates in the fifth decade, with some functional measures changing very little (i.e., conduction velocity of cardiac myocytes) and others undergoing substantial alteration (i.e., renal plasma flow). Not all organs age in the same manner or at the same rate. Total body water decreases by approximately 20%, and body fat increases with age. Basal metabolic rate (BMR) decreases with age as a result of reductions in lean body mass and increased adipose tissue.

Moderate exercise helps to preserve lean body mass, thereby slowing the rate at which this process occurs. Among individuals of the same age and gender, however, body fat content is much more variable than is lean body mass. Digestion and absorption of macronutrients appear to be well preserved as aging occurs. Reduction in gastric acid secretion and gastric motility, however, may contribute to decreased absorption of critical nutrients such as folate, vitamin B_{12}, vitamin D, and calcium.

Although an independent effect of age on taste and smell has been demonstrated, it is highly variable among individuals and its impact on food intake and diet quality is uncertain. Chronic disease, medication use, poor oral hygiene, dentures, smoking, and poor nutritional status itself are significant contributors to age-related changes in taste and smell. Changes in the sleep cycle often lead to poor sleep quality, insomnia, daytime drowsiness, reduced participation in activities, and depression; ability to access and to prepare a healthy diet may therefore be impaired. Table 6-1 highlights age-related physiologic changes and their potential consequences.

Risk Factors for Poor Nutritional Status in Older Adults

Acute and Chronic Diseases or Disorders

Most older adults have at least one chronic disease or condition, and many have several. The prevalence of chronic disease increases with advancing age and varies according to gender and race. The most common are cardiovascular

Table 6-1 Age-related physiologic changes with potential nutrition-related outcomes.

ORGAN SYSTEM	CHANGE	POTENTIAL OUTCOME
Body composition	↑ Fat	↓ Basal metabolic rate
		↑ Fat-soluble drug storage, with prolonged half-life
	↓ Body water	↑ Concentration of water-soluble drugs
Gastrointestinal	↓ Gastric acid secretion	↓ Absorption of folate, protein-bound vitamin B_{12}
	↓ Gastric motility	↓ Bioavailability of minerals, vitamins, protein
	↓ Lactase activity	Avoidance of milk products, with reduced intake vitamin D and calcium
Hepatic	↓ Size and blood flow	↓ Albumin synthesis rate
	↓ Activity drug-metabolizing enzymes	Poor or delayed metabolism of certain drugs
Immune	↓ T-cell function	Anergy
		↓ Resistance to infection
Neurologic	Brain atrophy	↓ Cognitive function
Renal	↓ Glomerular filtration rate	Reduced renal excretion of metabolites, drugs
Sensory-perceptual	↓ Taste buds, papilla on tongue	Altered taste threshold, reduced ability to detect sweet/salt, increased use of salt/sugar
	↓ Olfactory nerve endings	Altered smell threshold, reduced palatability causing poor food intake
Skeletal	↓ Bone density	↓ Fractures

SOURCE: Nutrition Screening Initiative. 2626 Pennsylvania Ave NW, Suite 301, Washington, DC 20037.

disease (65%), arthritis (49%), hypertension (36%), hearing impairment (30%), orthopedic impairment (18%), cataracts (17%), sinusitis (12%), and diabetes (10%). These data underestimate the prevalence of the dementias, a group of illnesses dominated by Alzheimer's disease (AD). Leading causes of death in this age group include heart disease, cancer, and stroke, respectively.

The presence of a chronic disease or condition often results in a prescribed or self-imposed modification in food intake. Such modifications frequently limit variety and result in decreased total nutrient intake.

AD is the main cause of progressive dementia in old age. The characteristic, extremely slow onset of AD makes its early recognition difficult for family and clinician alike, and authorities encourage earlier diagnosis. This would lead to earlier medical treatment and earlier training of family caregivers, who have essential roles, including ensuring nutrition and hydration. A meta-analysis of reported early symptoms of AD confirms that apathy is the most frequent early behavioral manifestation, with indecisiveness, impaired abstract thinking, and reduced ability in complex instrumental activities of daily living (IADLs; i.e., planning and conceptualizing shopping and food preparation) also very characteristic. This one illness even before the patient has enough impairment to be described as suffering from "dementia" is an often unrecognized contributor to overt undernutrition. In summary, patients who present with unintentional weight loss or signs/symptoms of undernutrition in conjunction with acute or chronic illness should be monitored closely.

Oral Health Problems

Approximately 23% of the older US population is edentulous, with the prevalence by state ranging from 14% in Hawaii to 48% in West Virginia. Edentulism is higher among minorities and among those who smoke, are uninsured, have less formal education, and reside in a nursing home. Nearly one-third of older Americans with natural teeth had untreated root or crown cavities, and 41% had periodontal disease. Incidence of periodontal disease is higher in those with cardiovascular disease or diabetes. Patients who have loose, decaying, or missing teeth; difficulty chewing; or ill-fitting dentures or who fail to wear their dentures are at increased risk for poor nutritional status due to a decreased or modified food intake.

Cognitive and Emotional Impairment

Changes in the level of cognitive function that are associated with normal aging are difficult to quantify. The limited data from longitudinal sources suggest that short-term memory (20 seconds or less) declines with age. Progressive dementia is characterized by a gradual decline in multiple cognitive functions that causes loss of the ability to make choices, to initiate activities (such as shopping and food preparation), and to simply remember to eat appropriately. Clearly, dementia is a major risk factor for undernutrition. Extensive evidence has shown that patients with dementia often become undernourished.

Grief or mourning is viewed as a normal part of life, yet the elderly are forced to suffer its effects more often because they are more likely to experience loss—death of friends, spouses, or loved ones; retirement; decline in personal income; and decline in general health. In individuals of all ages, grief may dramatically disrupt memory and can result in a general sense of confusion and disorganization. Disease processes for which mourners may be at increased risk include myocardial infarction, gastrointestinal cancer, hypertension, neurodermatitis, rheumatoid arthritis, diabetes, thyrotoxicosis (women in particular), depression, alcohol/drug abuse, undernutrition, headaches, low back pain, colds/flu, excessive fatigue, impotence, and sleep disorders. Although the symptoms of grief, such as insomnia, changes in appetite, difficulty in decision-making, and problems in cognition, can mimic those of a depressive disorder, it is important to distinguish between these conditions. Older adults may need more frequent contact with their physician during the first 2 years following a grief-inducing incident.

In older people, depression can present as cognitive impairment, with memory and concentration being particularly affected. However, change in appetite (usually a reduction but sometimes a pathologic increase) is a defining feature of "major depression," that is, a depression that will likely respond to treatment with antidepressant drugs. The depressed individual will become undernourished with decreased food intake as a result of feelings of poor self-esteem, lack of motivation, and negativity. New onset of reduced food intake should always lead to consideration of depression as a cause.

Isolation

Seventeen percent of men and 40% of women aged 65 years and older live alone. The likelihood of living alone increases as age advances. Loneliness is greater among divorced, widowed, or childless men; older women who have outlived spouse and friends; older adults who live alone; those with few contacts; those more physically disabled; those who subjectively feel that their health is poorer or that their economic condition is inadequate; and those with hearing or visual impairments.

Elderly people who have limited social interaction or infrequent contact with family, friends, or neighbors on an individual level, and who are unable or unwilling to access social support systems on a broader level, may experience decreased food intake, lack of appetite, and limited motivation to shop and prepare meals as a result. Eating is a social event that is often enhanced by the presence of others. Loneliness, and in particular the lack of a companion at mealtimes, tends to have a negative impact on food intake.

Alcohol/Drug Use

The potential benefits of moderate alcohol use (1 to 2 drinks per day) described in the literature for older individuals include mood enhancement, stress reduction, sociability, social integration, maintenance of long-term cognitive functioning, improved cardiovascular health, and enhanced bone mineral density. However, 6% to 11% of elderly patients admitted to hospitals and 14% of those in emergency rooms exhibit symptoms of alcoholism. In nursing homes, the percentage may be as high as 49%. Studies of elderly living in the community suggest that although 62% report alcohol consumption, approximately 13% of men and 2% of women drink heavily. Generally, about 6% of US elderly are considered heavy alcohol users (>2 drinks per day). Early-onset alcoholics frequently have a family history of alcoholism and higher prevalence of antisocial behavior. Poverty and family estrangement are common in this group. Late-onset drinkers usually have higher education and income levels. They are more likely to have greater resources, family support, and better treatment outcomes. Depression, loneliness, and lack of social support are the most frequent reasons given for late-onset drinking by the elderly.

The type of alcohol/drug consumed and the duration and frequency of alcohol/drug consumption should be ascertained using a simple questionnaire (CAGE; see Chapter 8, Case 1). Interviewing family members may also be helpful. Remember that denial or understatement of amount or frequency of alcohol consumption is common. Ascertain the presence of anxiety, depression, or other psychiatric/personality disorders and look for isolation, falls, accidents, or other clues for intoxication. Remind patients that use of pre-scription or over-the-counter medications may be a contraindication to alcohol consumption.

Socioeconomic Status

Approximately 17% of the older US population were poor and near poor in 2000. Women, minorities, and elders living in central cities, rural areas, and the South had higher than average poverty rates. Elders living alone or with nonrelatives were more likely to be poor than those living in families. Highest poverty rates were experienced by older Hispanic women (38.3%) living alone or with nonrelatives.

Many older individuals are reluctant to use food stamps or similar feeding programs because of "welfare stigma" and their pride. Many do not know how to access federal programs, are uncomfortable going to a congregate dining site, do not qualify for home-delivered meals, or are placed on a long waiting list. Food/meals provision activities sponsored by churches or other nongovernmental agencies are often the type of help that most elders find acceptable. Consideration of the older person's socioeconomic status and knowledge of available social service options are essential to reducing nutritional risk in elders.

Functional Status

More than half of older Americans report some degree of disability, and over one-third report severe disability. Approximately 14% report limitation in the activities of daily living (ADLs), which reflect an individual's capacity for self-care, and 21% report limitation in the IADLs, which reflect more complex tasks that enable a person to live independently in the community (Table 6-2). The percent with disability increases with increased age.

Even after controlling for demographic, socioeconomic, gender, and racial factors, level of disability predicts increased mortality risk. It is imperative that,

Table 6-2   Commonly used measures of functional capacity.

ACTIVITIES OF DAILY LIVING (ADLs) (REFLECT CAPACITY FOR SELF-CARE)	INSTRUMENTAL ACTIVITIES OF DAILY LIVING (IADLs) (REFLECT CAPACITY FOR INDEPENDENT LIVING)
Bathing	Telephone use
Dressing	Walking
Toileting	Shopping: groceries/clothes
Transferring	Meal preparation
Continence	Housework/laundry
Feeding	Home maintenance/repair
	Taking medicines
	Managing money

SOURCE: Nutrition Screening Initiative. 2626 Pennsylvania Ave NW, Suite 301, Washington, DC 20037.

when taking a medical history in older individuals, questions regarding functional capacity be included.

Polypharmacy

A recent survey of adult Americans showed that in those aged 65 and older, 91% of men used at least 1 drug, 44% used 5 or more drugs, and 12% used 10 or more drugs during the preceding week. For older women, the figures were 94%, 57%, and 12%, respectively. The most common reasons for taking drugs were hypertension and headache. However, several concurrent medications are the standard of care for an increasing number of conditions (e.g., chronic obstructive pulmonary disease, cardiovascular illnesses), and other medications are widely regarded as underprescribed (e.g., cholinesterase inhibitors that postpone the progression of AD, antidepressants, analgesics—including narcotics—for relief of chronic severe pain). Thus, multiple medications are often necessary in elders; unfortunately, the prescriber rarely considers the potential detriment to nutritional health of each and every prescription. Elderly people in poor health and on multiple medications are at highest risk for undernutrition.

Vitamin/mineral supplement use was reported by 47% and 59% of older men and women, respectively, and the use of herbal supplements was reported by 11% and 14%. Vitamins/minerals and herbs were taken because they "promote health/are good for you." Foods/nutrients have the potential to alter the effects of drugs by affecting their pharmacokinetics (absorption, distribution, metabolism, or excretion) and influencing their pharmacologic actions or effects. Drug categories and specific examples of drugs within these categories that may be affected by food are listed in Table 6-3. It is increasingly clear that some complementary/alternative medicines are pharmacologically active substances and should be regarded as "real" medicines, although unregulated and freely available (i.e., St. John's wort, ginkgo biloba) (Chapter 3).

Nutrition Screening and Assessment Tools

No single physical or biochemical parameter accurately measures nutritional status. Thus, a number of tools have been developed in an attempt to provide relevant information that clinicians can use in the identification of poor nutritional status in the elderly. The Nutrition Screening Initiative's (NSI) Determine Your Nutritional Health Checklist and Level 2 Screen, Subjective Global Assessment, the Meals on Wheels mnemonic and Mini Nutritional Assessment, the NSI Care Alerts, and the Health Care Financing Administration (Centers for Medicare and Medicaid Services) Nutrition and Hydration Care are examples of structured approaches to nutrition screening and assessment in the elderly. All tools are available online and are listed in the reference section. Each has benefits and limitations. Regardless of the tool used, a structured approach to nutrition screening and assessment must become an integral component of your care of each older person, either free living or institutionalized.

Table 6-3   Common medications and nutrition-related side effects.

Antimicrobial agents

- Absorption of tetracyclines and certain fluoroquinolones may be decreased by chelation with dietary cations such as calcium and magnesium in milk products.
- Absorption of macrolide agents (i.e., azithromycin, erythromycin) may be reduced by food/meals.
- A disulfiram-like reaction is produced by the ingestion of metronidazole or cephalosporins and alcohol.
- Vitamin B_6 metabolism is impaired by isoniazid; the effect is dose related and can lead to the development of peripheral neuropathy.
- Absorption of didanosine is decreased by food.
- Absorption of griseofulvin is increased by food.

Cardiovascular and cholesterol-lowering drugs

- Concentrations of digoxin may be reduced by food/fiber intake.
- Hyperkalemia and/or changes in taste may be caused by angiotensin-converting enzyme (ACE) inhibitors.
- Flavonoid compounds in grapefruit increase serum felodipine concentrations.
- Foods high in soluble fiber decrease absorption of 3-hydroxy-3-methyl-glutaryl-coenzyme A (HMG-CoA) reductase inhibitors.
- Bile acid sequestrants decrease absorption of the fat-soluble vitamins (A, D, E, K).

Oral anticoagulants

- Foods high in vitamin K (including enteral formulations) may counteract the effects of oral anticoagulants.
- Ginkgo biloba and allium sativum (garlic) augment the anticoagulant effect of oral anticoagulants.

Bronchodilators

- Protein and carbohydrate alter hepatic clearance of theophylline.
- Food may induce dose-dumping of sustained-release theophylline preparations.
- Caffeine increases serum theophylline concentrations and enhances its pharmacologic effects.

Anticonvulsants

- Enteral formulations reduce serum phenytoin levels.
- Applesauce increases serum phenytoin levels.
- Reductions in serum folate levels caused by valproic acid may result in neural tube defects in the infants of women taking this drug. Carbamazepine, phenobarbital, and primidone produce a similar effect.
- Folic acid may reduce serum phenytoin levels and decrease seizure control.
- Vitamin D metabolism is altered by phenytoin and phenobarbital and may result in osteoporosis.

Anti-Parkinson drugs

- Protein may delay absorption of levodopa.
- Tyramine-containing foods may interact with selegiline hydrochloride.

Antidepressants

- Tyramine-containing foods interact with monoamine oxidase (MAO) inhibitors, which may produce a hypertensive crisis and chest pain.
- High- and low-sodium diets may increase and decrease renal lithium excretion, respectively; decreased lithium excretion may result in lithium toxicity.
- Appetite is temporarily suppressed by fluoxetine hydrochloride and similar serotonin reuptake inhibitors (SSRIs), although anorexia from the depression itself may respond to SSRIs.
- Ginkgo biloba may increase digoxin toxicity.

Table 6-3 (continued)

Laxatives

- Stimulant or saline laxatives decrease absorption of electrolytes.
- Stimulant laxatives, if taken with milk, may dissolve in the stomach rather than the small intestine, causing gastric irritation and abdominal cramps.
- Mineral oil decreases absorption of the fat-soluble vitamins (A, D, E, K).

Antacids

- Aluminum-containing antacids may decrease the absorption of phosphate.

Antineoplastic drugs

- Numerous antineoplastic drugs may suppress appetite, resulting in weight loss.

Nutritional Needs of Older Adults

The nutritional needs of older adults are difficult to quantify due to "physiologic diversity and heterogeneity" and the prevalence of chronic diseases. Deficiency signs and symptoms are uncommon in elderly individuals who live in the community but are occasionally seen in people who are frail, homebound, and must rely on others to meet basic needs. In general, nutrient needs in older adults appear to be similar to those for middle-aged adult populations. However, for some nutrients, clear evidence of increased need exists.

The recently revised DRIs (see Table 2-2) represent quantitative estimates that are useful in planning and assessing diets for healthy people. To date, DRIs have been established for the vitamins/minerals essential for maintenance of bone health and for the B-complex vitamins and choline. Those nutrients for which clear evidence of increased need in older adults has been established are discussed below.

Calcium

Osteoporosis is a major health risk for older women and men. Calcium recommendations were set at levels associated with maximum retention of body calcium since bones that are calcium rich are known to be less susceptible to fracture. For men and women aged 51 years and older including those over age 70, the DRI value for calcium is 1200 mg per day, and the tolerable upper intake level (UL) for calcium is 2500 mg per day. Supplements should be considered for those whose dietary intake of calcium is poor.

Vitamin D

For vitamin D, the DRI value for men and women aged 51 to 70 years is 10 μg per day (400 IU), and for those over age 70, it is 15 μg per day (600 IU). The tolerable UL for vitamin D for adults is 50 μg per day (2000 IU). Supplements should be considered for frail homebound or institutionalized elderly patients whose exposure to sunlight is limited or those in whom evidence of osteomalacia or osteoporosis is documented.

Folate

The DRI value for folate for adults aged 51 years and older is set at 400 μg per day. Because folate fortification of grain products is now widespread in the United

States, it is believed that most older people can obtain an adequate folate intake from their diet. The upper intake limit for folate has been set at 1000 μg per day (1 mg per day). Excessive consumption of folic acid may mask a vitamin B_{12} deficiency, allowing the neurologic sequelae to progress even though the anemia associated with this deficiency resolves.

The Warning Signs of poor nutritional health are often overlooked. Use this Checklist to find out if you or someone you know is at nutritional risk.

DETERMINE YOUR NUTRITIONAL HEALTH

Read the statements below. Circle the number in the "yes" column for those that apply to you or someone you know. For each "yes" answer, score the number in the box. Total your nutritional score.

	YES
I have an illness or condition that made me change the kind and/or amount of food I eat.	2
I eat fewer than 2 meals per day.	3
I eat few fruits or vegetables or milk products.	2
I have 3 or more drinks of beer, liquor or wine almost every day.	2
I have tooth or mouth problems that make it hard for me to eat.	2
I don't always have enough money to buy the food I need.	4
I eat alone most of the time.	1
I take 3 or more different prescribed or over-the-counter drugs a day.	1
Without wanting to, I have lost or gained 10 pounds in the last 6 months.	2
I am not always physically able to shop, cook and/or feed myself.	2
TOTAL	

Total Your Nutritional Score. If it's –

0-2   Good! Recheck your nutritional score in 6 months.

3-5   You are at moderate nutritional risk. See what can be done to improve your eating habits and lifestyle. Your office on aging, senior nutrition program, senior citizens center or health department can help. Recheck your nutritional score in 3 months.

6 or more   You are at high nutritional risk. Bring this Checklist the next time you see your doctor, dietitian or other qualified health or social service professional. Talk with them about any problems you may have. Ask for help to improve your nutritional health.

Remember that Warning Signs suggest risk, but do not represent a diagnosis of any condition. Turn the page to learn more about the Warning Signs of poor nutritional health.

These materials are developed and distributed by the Nutrition Screening Initiative, a project of:

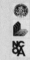

AMERICAN ACADEMY OF FAMILY PHYSICIANS

THE AMERICAN DIETETIC ASSOCIATION

THE NATIONAL COUNCIL ON THE AGING, INC.

The Nutrition Screening Initiative • 1010 Wisconsin Avenue, NW • Suite 800 • Washington, DC 20007
The Nutrition Screening Initiative is funded in part by a grant from Ross Products Division of Abbott Laboratories, Inc.

Figure 6-1   **Determine your nutritional health.**

SOURCE: The Nutritional Screening Initiative

The Nutrition Checklist is based on the Warning Signs described below. Use the word <u>DETERMINE</u> to remind you of the Warning Signs.

DISEASE

Any disease, illness or chronic condition which causes you to change the way you eat, or makes it hard for you to eat, puts your nutritional health at risk. Four out of five adults have chronic diseases that are affected by diet. Confusion or memory loss that keeps getting worse is estimated to affect one out of five or more of older adults. This can make it hard to remember what, when or if you've eaten. Feeling sad or depressed, which happens to about one in eight older adults, can cause big changes in appetite, digestion, energy level, weight and well-being.

EATING POORLY

Eating too little and eating too much both lead to poor health. Eating the same foods day after day or not eating fruit, vegetables, and milk products daily will also cause poor nutritional health. One in five adults skip meals daily. Only 13% of adults eat the minimum amount of fruit and vegetables needed. One in four older adults drink too much alcohol. Many health problems become worse if you drink more than one or two alcoholic beverages per day.

TOOTH LOSS / MOUTH PAIN

A healthy mouth, teeth and gums are needed to eat. Missing, loose or rotten teeth or dentures which don't fit well, or cause mouth sores, make it hard to eat.

ECONOMIC HARDSHIP

As many as 40% of older Americans have incomes of less than $6,000 per year. Having less -- or choosing to spend less -- than $25-30 per week for food makes it very hard to get the foods you need to stay healthy.

REDUCED SOCIAL CONTACT

One-third of all older people live alone. Being with people daily has a positive effect on morale, well-being and eating.

MULTIPLE MEDICINES

Many older Americans must take medicines for health problems. Almost half of older Americans take multiple medicines daily. Growing old may change the way we respond to drugs. The more medicines you take, the greater the chance for side effects such as increased or decreased appetite, change in taste, constipation, weakness, drowsiness, diarrhea, nausea, and others. Vitamins or minerals, when taken in large doses, act like drugs and can cause harm. Alert your doctor to everything you take.

INVOLUNTARY WEIGHT LOSS / GAIN

Losing or gaining a lot of weight when you are not trying to do so is an important warning sign that must not be ignored. Being overweight or underweight also increases your chance of poor health.

NEEDS ASSISTANCE IN SELF CARE

Although most older people are able to eat, one of every five have trouble walking, shopping, buying and cooking food, especially as they get older.

ELDER YEARS ABOVE AGE 80

Most older people lead full and productive lives. But as age increases, risk of frailty and health problems increase. Checking your nutritional health regularly makes good sense.

The Nutrition Screening Initiative • 1010 Wisconsin Avenue, NW • Suite 800 • Washington, DC 20007
The Nutrition Screening Initiative is funded in part by a grant from Ross Products Division of Abbott Laboratories, Inc.

Figure 6-1 (continued)

Level II Screen

Complete the following screen by interviewing the patient directly and/or by referring to the patient chart. If you do not routinely perform all of the described tests or ask all of the listed questions, please consider including them but do not be concerned if the entire screen is not completed. Please try to conduct a minimal screen on as many older patients as possible, and please try to collect serial measurements, which are extremely valuable in monitoring nutritional status. Please refer to the manual for additional information.

Anthropometrics

Measure height to the nearest inch and weight to the nearest pound. Record the values below and mark them on the Body Mass Index (BMI) scale to the right. Then use a straight edge (paper, ruler) to connect the two points and circle the spot where this straight line crosses the center line (body mass index). Record the number below; healthy older adults should have a BMI between 24 and 27; check the appropriate box to flag an abnormally high or low value.

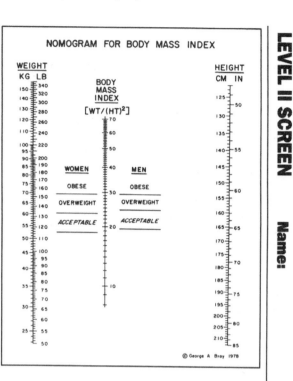

Height (in):_____
Weight (lbs):_____
Body Mass Index
(weight/height²):_____

Please place a check by any statement regarding BMI and recent weight loss that is true for the patient.

☐ Body mass index <24

☐ Body mass index >27

☐ Has lost or gained 10 pounds (or more) of body weight in the past 6 months

Record the measurement of mid-arm circumference to the nearest 0.1 centimeter and of triceps skinfold to the nearest 2 millimeters.

Mid-Arm Circumference (cm):_____
Triceps Skinfold (mm):_____
Mid-Arm Muscle Circumference (cm):_____

Refer to the table and check any abnormal values:

☐ Mid-arm muscle circumference <10th percentile

☐ Triceps skinfold <10th percentile

☐ Triceps skinfold >95th percentile

Note: mid-arm circumference (cm) - {0.314 x triceps skinfold (mm)}= mid-arm *muscle* circumference (cm)

For the remaining sections, please place a check by any statements that are true for the patient.

Laboratory Data

☐ Serum albumin below 3.5 g/dl

☐ Serum cholesterol below 160 mg/dl

☐ Serum cholesterol above 240 mg/dl

Drug Use

☐ Three or more prescription drugs, OTC medications, and/or vitamin/mineral supplements daily

Figure 6-2   Determine your nutritional health level II screen.

SOURCE: The Nutritional Screening Institute

Clinical Features

Presence of (check each that apply):

❑ Problems with mouth, teeth, or gums

❑ Difficulty chewing

❑ Difficulty swallowing

❑ Angular stomatitis

❑ Glossitis

❑ History of bone pain

❑ History of bone fractures

❑ Skin changes (dry, loose, nonspecific lesions, edema)

	Men		Women	
Percentile	55-65 y	65-75 y	55-65 y	65-75 y
Arm circumference (cm)				
10th	27.3	26.3	25.7	25.2
50th	31.7	30.7	30.3	29.9
95th	36.9	35.5	38.5	37.3
Arm muscle circumference (cm)				
10th	24.5	23.5	19.6	19.5
50th	27.8	26.8	22.5	22.5
95th	32.0	30.6	28.0	27.9
Triceps skinfold (mm)				
10th	6	6	16	14
50th	11	11	25	24
95th	22	22	38	36

From: Frisancho AR. New norms of upper limb fat and muscle areas for assessment of nutritional status. Am J Clin Nutr 1981; 34:2540-2545. © 1981 American Society for Clinical Nutrition.

Eating Habits

❑ Does not have enough food to eat each day

❑ Usually eats alone

❑ Does not eat anything on one or more days each month

❑ Has poor appetite

❑ Is on a special diet

❑ Eats vegetables two or fewer times daily

❑ Eats milk or milk products once or not at all daily

❑ Eats fruit or drinks fruit juice once or not at all daily

❑ Eats breads, cereals, pasta, rice, or other grains five or fewer times daily

❑ Has more than one alcoholic drink per day (if woman); more than two drinks per day (if man)

Living Environment

❑ Lives on an income of less than $6000 per year (per individual in the household)

❑ Lives alone

❑ Is housebound

❑ Is concerned about home security

❑ Lives in a home with inadequate heating or cooling

❑ Does not have a stove and/or refrigerator

❑ Is unable or prefers not to spend money on food (<$25-30 per person spent on food each week)

Functional Status

Usually or always needs assistance with (check each that apply):

❑ Bathing

❑ Dressing

❑ Grooming

❑ Toileting

❑ Eating

❑ Walking or moving about

❑ Traveling (outside the home)

❑ Preparing food

❑ Shopping for food or other necessities

Mental/Cognitive Status

❑ Clinical evidence of impairment, e.g. Folstein<26

❑ Clinical evidence of depressive illness, e.g. Beck Depression Inventory>15, Geriatric Depression Scale>5

Patients in whom you have identified one or more major indicator (see pg 2) of poor nutritional status require immediate medical attention; if minor indicators are found, ensure that they are known to a health professional or to the patient's own physician. Patients who display risk factors (see pg 2) of poor nutritional status should be referred to the appropriate health care or social service professional (dietitian, nurse, dentist, case manager, etc.).

These materials developed by the Nutrition Screening Initiative.

Figure 6-2   (continued)

Table 6-4   Nutrition-related questions for the history and physical examination of older adults.

Medical history

Chief complaint (especially if nutrition problem suspected).

History of chronic disease [allergy, anemia, anorexia/cachexia, arthritis, cancer, cardiovascular disease (CVD), diabetes, hypertension, hepatic disease, malabsorption, obesity, psychiatric disorder, chronic obstructive pulmonary disease (COPD), pneumonia, renal disease].

History of recent surgery/illness.

Current or past use of enteral or parenteral nutrition therapies.

Medications

Medications, including over-the-counter products and alternative/complementary therapies.

Vitamin, mineral, herbal, or dietary fiber supplements; use or abuse.

Addicting substances use (type, frequency, amount; alcohol, cigarettes, drugs).

Family history

Pertinent family history.

Review of systems

Changes in appetite, weight, nausea, vomiting, diarrhea.

Handicaps to feeding (change in appetite; biting, chewing, swallowing problems; ill-fitting dentures or rotten, missing, or decayed teeth; persistent nausea, vomiting, constipation, diarrhea, heartburn).

Psychosocial history

Occupation.

Living arrangements (family members in the home, food preparation/storage facilities, transportation).

Income level (food budget, reliance on medical/food assistance programs).

Cognitive/emotional status (including grief).

Functional status [activities of daily living (ADLs) and instrumental activities of daily living (IADLs)].

Cultural, ethnic, religious factors that affect food intake.

Education level (literacy, learning style, motivation/receptiveness).

Diet history

Current eating pattern (meals/snacks, type/amounts of food consumed).

Prescribed/self-imposed dietary modifications.

Food aversions/restrictions.

Activity level/sleep patterns.

Physical examination

Vital signs, including height, weight, body mass index (BMI), waist circumference, weight loss.

Signs of passive or self-neglect or even physical abuse (poor hygiene, bruising).

Mobility/balance difficulty.

Poor oral health (dry mouth, caries, periodontal disease, ill-fitting dentures).

Signs of loss of skin strength or actual skin breakdown, e.g., healed or unhealed areas.

Laboratory data (as indicated by history/physical)

Albumin, prealbumin, transferrin, complete blood count (CBC) with hematocrit/hemoglobin (ferritin, vitamin B_{12}, folate), glucose, cholesterol, triglycerides, low-density lipoprotein (LDL), high-density lipoprotein (HDL), blood urea nitrogen (BUN), and electrolytes (potassium, sodium, magnesium).

SOURCE: Lisa Hark, Ph D, RD, University of Pennsylvania School of Medicine. Used with permission.

Vitamin B₁₂

The DRI for vitamin B_{12} for people over age 50 has been set at 2.4 μg per day. Although most Americans who consume animal products can get sufficient vitamin B_{12} from food, it is estimated that between 10% and 30% of older people have lost the ability to absorb protein-bound vitamin B_{12} adequately. Thus, the Food and Nutrition Board recommends that people over age 50 meet most of their dietary requirement for vitamin B_{12} with synthetic B_{12} (free vs. protein-bound) from fortified foods or supplements. Most oral supplements currently on the market contain free versus protein-bound B_{12}. Intrinsic factor and hydrochloric acid (needed to cleave B_{12} from its protein carrier) are not required for the digestion/absorption of this form of B_{12} versus the food form of B_{12}; thus, widespread use of vitamin B_{12} injections is no longer necessary if the free form of B_{12} is given as an oral supplement.

Vitamin B₆

The DRI for vitamin B_6 in adults over age 50 is 1.5 mg per day, which can be met through dietary means. It has been suggested that adequate intakes of this vitamin also help to reduce homocysteine levels and thus the risk of cardiovascular disease. The upper intake for vitamin B_6 has been set at 100 mg per day. Adults who take doses of vitamin B_6 above this level are at increased risk of developing progressive, crippling neurologic damage.

Summary

In summary, poor nutritional status is a common yet frequently overlooked problem in old age. It is a potential sign of treatable illness, which must be sought. It has medical consequences, both short- and long-term, including being a major factor in the prevention, treatment, and ability to recover from acute/chronic illness. It is a contributor to morbidity in the majority of frail, dependent elders. By considering nutrition in all aspects of medical decision-making (e.g., diagnosis, medication prescription, surgery, rehabilitation, referral, placement), quality of life can be improved and successful aging can be the outcome for a higher proportion of our nation's adults.

For a list of references for this chapter, please visit the University of Pennsylvania School of Medicine's Nutrition Education and Prevention Program web site: *http://www.med.upenn.edu/nutrimed/articles.html*

Case 1

Malnutrition and Depression

Katherine Galluzzi and Larry Finkelstein

Objectives

- Identify common risk factors for poor nutritional status in older adults.
- Describe the effects of undernutrition on physiologic function in geriatric patients.
- Develop a nutritional care plan for an older adult with poor nutritional status and weight loss secondary to altered living situation.
- Provide nutritional counseling appropriate to the physiologic, emotional, social, and financial changes that occur with aging.
- Recognize the unique contribution of different members of a health care team, including social workers, home health aides, and community volunteers, in the effort to improve the nutritional status of older people.

ML is a 75-year-old widow who was brought to her primary care physician's office by the local Older Americans Transportation Service. She had missed her two prior scheduled office visits because of the recent death of her husband and a subsequent fall, which resulted in an intertrochanteric fracture of her right hip.

On presentation, ML appeared withdrawn and much more frail than on previous visits. She answered in a monotone with terse, nonspontaneous speech, and she lacked expression. When asked about how she has been coping after the loss of her husband, she became tearful. She admitted that in addition to the loss of companionship, the loss of his pension has caused tremendous financial hardship.

Past Medical History

ML tripped on the steps in her house 2 months ago and fractured her hip. She underwent an open reduction/internal fixation surgery to repair the fracture, and the operation went well. She had no serious operative complications, but she lost approximately 350 cm^3 blood during the procedure (1 unit = 500 cm^3). ML underwent inpatient rehabilitation for 10 days after discharge from the surgical service and then returned home, where she lives alone. She ambulates slowly with a cane and can climb stairs only with difficulty.

During her inpatient rehabilitation stay, she was diagnosed with depression and she was started on an antidepressant. She has no major chronic diseases except for osteoporosis, discovered at the time of her hip fractures 2 month ago. ML had an appendectomy at age 46 and bilateral cataract surgeries 10 years ago. She has no previous history of pneumonia, tuberculosis, hepatitis, or urinary tract infection.

Medications

ML currently takes fluoxetine (Prozac), 20 mg daily, for depression and an iron supplement for anemia three times per day. She also self-medicates with over-the-counter preparations of ibuprofen (200 to 400 mg three times a day) and frequently uses over-the-counter laxatives and glycerin suppositories for her constipation, which she attributes to her iron tablets. She does not take a multiple vitamin, calcium, or vitamin D. She has no known food allergies.

Social History

ML lives alone in the four-bedroom, two-story home she has occupied since she married 55 years ago. Her son and daughter both live out of state. Although they call her every few weeks, they have not visited since her husband's death. ML also explains that she used to attend church and visit the local senior center regularly with her husband but has not been to either lately. ML explains that she has no energy to "get up and go" anymore and she falls asleep in front of the television. She also reports being constipated and that her food does not have much taste. She avoids alcohol and tobacco and drinks one cup of coffee and two cups of tea daily.

Review of Systems

General: Weakness, fatigue, weight loss, and depression.

Mouth: Food lacks taste (hypogeusia); dry, "thick-feeling" tongue; sores in corners of mouth.

Gastrointestinal (GI): Poor appetite, constipation.

Extremities: Hip pain when climbing stairs, some tenderness at old incision site, and chronic low back pain.

Physical Examination

Vital Signs

Temperature: 97.0°F (36°C)

Heart rate: 88 beats per minute (BPM)

Respiration: 18 BPM

Blood pressure: 130/80 mm Hg

Height: 5'6" (168 cm)
Current weight: 110 lb (50 kg)
Usual weight: 140 lb (64 kg)
BMI: 18 kg/m^2
Weight 6 months ago to surgery: 125 lb (57 kg)
Percent weight change: 12% (125 to 110/125 × 100)

General: Thin, elderly woman who is appropriately conversant but withdrawn. She is well groomed, but her clothes are loose fitting, suggesting weight loss.

Skin: Warm to touch, patches of dryness and flaking to elbows and lower extremities

Head, ears, eyes, nose, throat (HEENT): Temporal muscle wasting, no enlargement of thyroid

Mouth: Ill-fitting dentures, sore beneath bottom plate; cracks/fissures at corners of mouth (angular chelitis)

Cardiac: Regular rate at 88 BPM, soft systolic murmur

Abdomen: Well-healed appendectomy site scar, no enlargement of liver or spleen, diffusely diminished bowel sounds

Extremities: Well-healed hip surgery incision with slight surrounding erythema, no sores on feet, trace pretibial edema to both lower extremities

Rectal: Hard stool in vault, stool test for occult blood negative

Neurologic: Alert, good memory, no evidence of sensory loss

Gait: Slightly wide-based with decreased arm swing, antalgic and tentative but with safe, appropriate use of cane

Laboratory Data

Patient's Laboratory Values	Normal Values
Albumin: 2.5 g/dL	3.5–5.8 g/dL
Hemoglobin: 11.0 g/dL	11.8–15.5 g/dL
Hematocrit: 33.0%	36%–46%

ML's 24-Hour Dietary Recall

At her physician's request, ML provided the following 24-hour dietary recall, stating that this represents her usual daily intake:

Breakfast (home)	Jelly doughnut	1 whole
	White toast	1 slice
	Jelly	2 Tbsp.
	Coffee	1 cup
Lunch (home)	Butter cookies	2
	Chicken and rice soup	1 cup
	Saltine crackers	6
	Tea	2 cups

Dinner (home)	White bread	1 slice
	Jelly	2 Tbsp.
	Peanut butter	2 Tbsp.
	Butter cookies	2

Total calories: 1270 kcal
Protein: 25 g per day (8% of calories)
Fat: 42 g (30% of calories)
Carbohydrate: 201 g (63% of calories)
Calcium: 153 mg
Iron: 6 mg

Case Questions

1. What information from the case history would cause you concern over ML's functional status?
2. Based on that information, what medical, environmental, and social factors could lead to nutritional problems in this patient?
3. What do ML's BMI and percent weight change indicate about her nutritional status?
4. What are ML's calorie and protein requirements for repletion? What general conclusions can you draw regarding ML's diet?
5. How can ML's diet be improved to meet her increased requirements, achieve weight gain, and relieve her constipation?
6. What specific recommendations would you offer to improve ML's nutritional status?

Case Answers

Part 1: Assessing Activities of Daily Living

1. What information from the case history would cause you concern over ML's functional status?

Activities of Daily Living

Although ML can feed herself, she has trouble chewing because of her loose dentures and a sore in her mouth. She has insufficient money for a visit to the dentist. ML also exhibits poor mobility; she walks with a cane, has difficulty with stairs, and fears falling since her hip fracture. Although she is mobile, she reports pain with movement and moves slowly about the house. Finally, ML dislikes eating alone, which may have a negative impact on her food intake.

Instrumental Activities of Daily Living

Since her injury, ML has been afraid to go outside, which may be secondary to fear of falling or lack of energy from exertion. Because she does not drive and is unaccustomed to using public transportation, she has difficulty shopping for food and other necessities. ML reports a very limited social life; since her husband's death she has avoided church, community programs, and the senior center. Her reported dislike of cooking for one person most likely has a negative effect on the quality and quantity of her food intake. She denies difficulty with dressing, grooming, or toileting, however, and feels that if her husband were alive she would still be doing cooking duties.

2. **Based on that information, what medical, environmental, and social factors could lead to nutritional problems in this patient?**

ML's ill-fitting dentures and hypogeusia may lead to decreased intake and undernutrition. Depression over the loss of her husband may decrease her appetite. Also, ML lives alone in a large house and may be unable to clean and cook for herself because of her poor mobility, and she lacks money for assistance with household tasks. Because she is homebound, her exposure to sunlight is limited, which may result in vitamin D deficiency. Furthermore, she no longer participates in community activities that could provide support, meals, and social interaction. Her children have not visited recently or provided any assistance. Finally, the loss of her husband's pension has significantly reduced her income.

Part 2: Nutrition Assessment

3. **What do ML's BMI and percent weight change indicate about her nutritional status?**

It should be noted that in this case the value used for ML's usual weight is 125 lb (57 kg), her weight 6 months earlier (rather than her usual weight of 140 lb). Her percent weight change is greater than 10% in a period of 6 months, which represents a clinical indicator of the risk for undernutrition. ML's BMI of 18 kg/m^2 also indicates that she is underweight and may be at risk for undernutrition; normal BMI values fall in the range of 18.5 to 24.9 kg/m^2.

4. **What are ML's calorie and protein requirements for repletion? What general conclusions can you draw regarding ML's diet?**

ML's total estimated daily calorie requirements, based on the RDA, are 25 to 30 kcal/kg body weight for weight maintenance and an additional 250 to 500 calories per day to gain $1/2$ to 1 lb (0.22 to 0.45 kg) per week.

$$(50 \text{ kg}) \times (25 \text{ to } 30 \text{ kcal/kg}) = 1250 \text{ to } 1500 \text{ kcal/day} + 250$$
$$\text{to } 500 \text{ additional calories} = 1500 \text{ to } 2000 \text{ kcal/day}$$

The estimated total daily protein requirements are 1.5 g/kg weight.

$$(50 \text{ kg}) \times (1.5 \text{ g/kg}) = 75 \text{ g per day}$$

ML's usual daily intake provides 1270 calories and 25 g protein. Her diet is low in calories due to her lack of appetite and poor selection of foods. ML's limited consumption of meats and poultry products, resulting in a poor overall protein and iron intake, probably is due to her limited income and poor dentition. Because ML stopped drinking milk many years ago and does not shop for dairy products regularly, her diet is deficient in calcium and vitamin D. The fissures at the corners of her mouth most likely indicate a riboflavin deficiency. Riboflavin is also found in dairy products. Fruits, vegetables, and fluids also appear to be below acceptable limits in ML's diet.

Part 3: Medical Nutrition Therapy

5. **How can ML's diet be improved to meet her increased requirements, achieve weight gain, and relieve her constipation?**

    Constipation, very common in older adults, can often be corrected by increasing fiber and fluid intake; physical activity should also be encouraged. Examples of high-fiber foods include fresh fruits, vegetables, bran cereals, and whole-grain products such as whole-wheat bread and brown rice. One bowl of raisin bran cereal or oatmeal every day would most likely be sufficient to achieve bowel regularity. If these measures are not sufficient, fiber supplements can be recommended. She should be advised to drink at least one liter of water daily and preferably more if tolerated. Increasing fluid intake will also help alleviate constipation. The elderly, however, are prone to hypodypsia (blunted thirst response), which leads to inadequate fluid intake. Older adults may require prompting or frequent reminders to ensure adequate fluid intake. In light of her weight loss and inadequate dietary intake, ML's diet clearly needs to be higher in calories, protein, and calcium to fulfill her current requirements. She should also be asked whether she is taking her iron supplements, as older adults tend to discontinue these minerals if constipation occurs.

High-Calorie, High-Protein Dietary Recommendations

Breakfast (home)	Coffee	1 cup
	Instant oatmeal	1 package
	Lactose-free 2% milk	6 oz (180 mL)
	Orange juice	4 oz (120 mL)
Lunch (senior center)	Chicken drumstick	3 oz (85 g)
	Baked potato	1 medium

	Margarine	2 Tbsp.
	Green beans	4 Tbsp.
Snack (senior center)	Lactose-free 2% milk or yogurt	8 oz (240 mL)
	Canned peaches	$^{1}/_{2}$ cup
Dinner (home)	Tuna salad	4 oz (113 g)
	Saltine crackers	6
	Tomatoes	3 slices
	Vanilla pudding	5 oz (142 g)
Snack (home)	Applesauce	$^{1}/_{2}$ cup

Total calories: 1540 kcal
Protein: 72 g (19% of calories)
Fat: 57 g (33% of calories)
Carbohydrate: 190 g (49% of calories)
Calcium: 974 mg
Iron 15 mg

6. **What specific recommendations would you offer to improve ML's nutritional status?**

   In addition to the recommended dietary modifications, ML or her primary care physician, or both, should take the following steps to ensure her continued well-being.

   - Contact her other health care providers, specifically her psychiatrist or psychologist, regarding recommended changes in medications and make arrangements to have her dentures properly adjusted.
   - Drink high-calorie, high-protein liquid supplements or suggest adding nonfat powdered milk to puddings to increase her intake of calories, protein, vitamins, and minerals.
   - Prescribe a multivitamin and mineral supplement with 100% of the RDA for older adults and calcium (600 mg twice a day) with vitamin D.
   - Use a microwave oven to prepare convenience foods and decrease cooking time.
   - Contact a social worker to help ML get in touch with the area council on aging, Meals on Wheels, and other community resources.
   - Consider a home health aide to monitor ML's weekly weight and food intake and assess whether her ambulatory status is improving or whether she is at increased risk of falling again.
   - Use community volunteers to shop for food or contact a grocery store that delivers.

- Contact her children and other family members for support and to help her arrange to move to an apartment or a smaller, single-story home.
- Undergo further rehabilitation and exercise therapy to increase her diminished mobility.
- Contact a neighbor with whom ML could share meals or travel to the senior center daily for a hot lunch.

See Chapter Review Questions, pages A-20 to A-22.

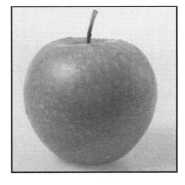

PART III

Integrative Systems and Disease

7

Cardiovascular Disease

Jo Ann S. Carson and Scott M. Grundy

Objectives*

- Identify patients at risk for coronary heart disease, including identification of risk factors, assessment of abdominal obesity by waist circumference, and use of a nutrition history that targets dietary components relevant to atherosclerosis, hypertension, and/or heart failure.
- Given a patient's medical history and laboratory data, propose an optimal set of goals for nutritional risk factor reduction using the National Cholesterol Education Program (NCEP) and American Heart Association (AHA) guidelines for nutrition and exercise.
- Describe the parameters of the NCEP's Therapeutic Lifestyle Changes (TLC) diet.
- Discuss potential benefits of vitamin supplementation for prevention or treatment of cardiovascular disease.
- Summarize the dietary parameters of the Dietary Approaches to Stop Hypertension (DASH) diet for the hypertensive patient.
- Prioritize nutritional goals for the patient with heart failure.

According to the National Center for Health Statistics and the AHA, cardiovascular disease (CVD) ranks as the number one killer in the United States, accounting for 40.1% of all deaths. Nutrition plays a key role in the prevention and treatment of various types of cardiovascular disease, particularly the most common forms in the American population: coronary heart disease (CHD) and hypertension.

* SOURCE: Objectives for chapter and cases adapted from the *NIH Nutrition Curriculum Guide for Training Physicians* (*http://www.nhlbi.nih.gov/funding/training/naa*).

The importance of nutrition in CHD has heightened with the growing aware-ness of metabolic syndrome, in which altered serum lipid levels, insulin resistance, and hypertension interplay with abdominal obesity to increase the potential for morbidity and mortality from heart disease. The positive association between di-etary fat, particularly saturated fat intake, and the risk for development of CHD is irrefutable. This association is presumed to reflect the increased serum choles-terol and low-density lipoprotein (LDL) levels that result from a high intake of saturated fat. The association of obesity with the development of hypertension, type 2 diabetes, and consequent CVD further heightens the need for all health care workers to be educated in the role of nutrition in health promotion and disease prevention.

Evidence Base for Diet and Heart Disease

The evidence base that diet, through its effect on serum lipids, influences the incidence of heart disease is perhaps greater than that for any other diet and disease connection. Intake of saturated fat increases LDL cholesterol (LDL-C) level, thereby increasing the risk of CHD. In the last decade, several large-scale clinical trials have shown conclusively that reducing serum LDL levels reduces the number of acute cardiac events and deaths from CHD both in patients with existing disease and those at risk due to elevated lipids. Angiographic studies have demonstrated that LDL reduction slows the progression of atherosclerosis in patients with known disease.

Dietary Lipids

An understanding of the basic biochemistry of fat and fatty acids is needed to address the role of dietary fat in the prevention and treatment of heart disease. Di-etary fats are composed chiefly of three fatty acids attached to a glycerol molecule. All fats are a combination of saturated, monounsaturated, and polyunsaturated fatty acids. Fat is the most calorically dense nutrient, supplying 9 calories per gram. Therefore, a diet high in fat is generally high in calories. Reducing total fat intake and adhering to an exercise program can help an individual lose weight. The effects of different types of fats on serum lipids are discussed below and summarized in Table 7-1.

Saturated Fat

Saturated fats are fatty acids with no double bonds. With the exception of palm and coconut oil, foods high in saturated fat are solid at room temperature and are primarily from animal sources. Major contributors of saturated fat include fatty meats, such as cold cuts, sausage, and bacon, and regular-fat dairy products, including whole or 2% milk, cheese, and ice cream. According to the National Health and Nutrition Examination Survey (NHANES) III data (1988 to 1994), approximately 11% of the calories in the American diet come from saturated fat. Saturated fatty acids, when contrasted with unsaturated fatty acids, decrease

Table 7-1   Summary of dietary changes to impact serum lipids.

LIPID GOAL	DIETARY MANIPULATION	DIETARY ADVICE
To lower LDL	• Decrease saturated fat	Limit portion size of meats; use lean meats and fat-free dairy products
	• Replace saturated fat with MUFA and/or PUFA	Use canola or olive oil for MUFA; can use safflower or corn oil for PUFA
	• Limit trans-fatty acids	Use soft, trans-free margarine; limit baked goods with partially hydrogenated oils
	• Limit cholesterol	Limit egg yolks, organ meats, butterfat, and high-fat meats
To lower triglycerides	• Include MUFA	Use olive or canola oil, peanuts, pecans
	• Include omega-3	Have cold-water fish weekly
	• Eliminate alcohol	
	• Lose weight if overweight	
To raise HDL	• Use MUFA in place of PUFA	Use canola or olive oil
	• Lose weight if overweight	
	• Limit trans-fatty acid intake	
	• Avoid high-carbohydrate diets	

LDL, low-density lipoprotein; MUFA, monounsaturated fat; PUFA, polyunsaturated fat; HDL, high-density lipoprotein.

synthesis and activity of LDL receptors, promoting an increase in serum LDL-C, thereby contributing to atherogenesis. An increase of 1 mg/dL in serum LDL increases CHD risk by 1%. A meta-analysis of dietary studies concludes that for every 1% increase in calories from saturated fat, serum LDL-C increases approximately 2%.

Polyunsaturated Fats

Two major categories of polyunsaturated fats (PUFA) are omega-3 and omega-6 fatty acids. Vegetable oils such as corn, sunflower, safflower, and soybean contain omega-6 fatty acids. The essential omega-6 fatty acid is linoleic acid, which cannot be synthesized by the body and is required in the diet. Arachidonic acid, which is synthesized from linoleic acid, is the major omega-6 fatty acid found in cell membranes and the precursor of prostaglandins. The dietary requirement for linoleic acid is 2% to 3% of total calories or approximately 5 g (1 tsp.) per day. Substitution of PUFA for saturated fat in the diet lowers LDL and high-density lipoprotein cholesterol (HDL-C) and reduces risk for CHD; however, long-term high intakes of PUFA have not been proven safe in large populations.

Omega-3 fatty acids include the very-long-chain eicosapentanoic acid (EPA) and docosahexanoic acid (DHA), as well as the 18-carbon linolenic acid, another essential fatty acid. Linolenic acid is present in flaxseed oil and to some extent in soybean oil. EPA and DHA are fish oils found in cold-water fish, including tuna, swordfish, salmon, mackerel, sardines, and herring. Very-long omega-3 fatty acids (EPA/DHA) decrease serum triglyceride and platelet aggregation. A lower incidence of acute myocardial infarction has been reported in patients who consumed at least one meal per week of fish rich in omega-3 fatty acids. Whether this benefit is due to the omega-3 fatty acid content of fish is uncertain. The AHA advises consumption of fish at least twice a week.

Monounsaturated Fats

Monounsaturated fats (MUFA) contain one double bond; oleic acid is the most common dietary form. Oils high in oleic acid include canola and olive oil. Other dietary sources of MUFA include avocados, peanuts, and pecans. Epidemiologic evidence from the Mediterranean region, where diets are rich in MUFA, have demonstrated a lower incidence of CHD. This finding has recently been corroborated by a clinical trial, the Lyon Diet Heart Study. Substitution of oleic acid for saturated fatty acids reduces LDL-C levels. A diet high in MUFA lowers LDL-C and serum triglycerides without lowering HDL-C. Thus, providing some calories from MUFA, which might otherwise be provided from PUFA or carbohydrate, can lower LDL without lowering HDL or raising triglyceride levels.

Trans-Fatty Acids

Hydrogenation, the addition of hydrogen atoms to an unsaturated fat, can change a fatty acid double bond from a cis to trans configuration. The major source of trans-fatty acids are partially hydrogenated vegetable oils. Food manufacturers use this process to prolong the shelf life of foods such as crackers, cookies, potato chips, and puddings. Randomized clinical trials indicate that trans-fatty acids raise LDL-C levels when compared with naturally occurring cis-fatty acids (but less so than do saturated fatty acids). Although margarines contain trans-fatty acids, use of a soft or liquid margarine (preferably trans-free) maintains a lower LDL-C than does a comparable diet containing butter (a source of saturated fat and cholesterol). The Food and Drug Administration (FDA) is currently considering a regulation change to add trans-fatty acid information to food labels (proposed regulation is at *http://frwebgate5.access.gpo.gov*).

Dietary Cholesterol

Although saturated fat is perhaps the major dietary factor responsible for raising serum LDL-C levels, a high intake of cholesterol in the diet can also increase serum LDL-C. Animal foods are sources of cholesterol, with the highest being egg yolk and organ meats. Meat and dairy sources of saturated fat, such as cheese, cream, and fatty meats, also contain substantial amounts of cholesterol.

Hyperlipidemia

Hyperlipidemia, the clinical term used to describe elevated cholesterol, LDL, or triglyceride levels, increases the risk of atherosclerosis. When atherosclerosis proceeds to occlusion or rupture of a blood vessel, myocardial infarction, stroke, or peripheral vascular disease results (depending on the affected site). Various lipoproteins transport cholesterol and triglyceride in the blood. The majority of

Table 7-2 Major risk factors (exclusive of low-density lipoprotein cholesterol) that modify low-density lipoprotein goals.*

- Cigarette smoking
- Hypertension (blood pressure ≥140/90 mm Hg or on antihypertensive medication)
- Low high-density lipoprotein (HDL) cholesterol (<40 mg/dL)†
- Family history of premature coronary heart disease (CHD; CHD in male first-degree relative <55 yr; CHD in female first-degree relative <65 yr)
- Age (men ≥45 yr; women ≥55 yr)

* Diabetes is regarded as a CHD risk equivalent.
† HDL cholesterol ≥60 mg/dL counts as a "negative" risk factor; its presence removes one risk factor from the total count.
SOURCE: From the Executive Summary of the Third Report of the National Cholesterol Education Program (NCEP), Expert Panel on Detection, Education, and Treatment of High Blood Cholesterol in Adults (Adult Treatment Panel III or ATP III).

cholesterol is carried in the blood by LDL and transported to the cells via LDL receptors. LDLs are the major atherogenic lipoproteins. In contrast, cholesterol carried by HDL represents cholesterol being released by the cells. The majority of serum triglyceride is present in very-low-density lipoproteins (VLDL). Rather than an earlier clinical approach of assessing total cholesterol, a fasting lipid profile of the patient's LDL, HDL, and triglyceride levels is now recommended by the National Cholesterol Education Program, Third Adult Treatment Panel (NCEP ATP III).

Assessment of the Hyperlipidemic Patient (Framingham Data)

The clinical approach to the hyperlipidemic patient is well outlined in the NCEP ATP III guidelines. Key steps include the assessment of risk factors, which allows determination of lipoprotein goals and delineation of the need for lifestyle change and, if needed, the addition of pharmacologic treatment. Individuals with existing evidence of CHD or diabetes, which is a CHD equivalent, should aim for a goal LDL of 100 g/dL or less. Individuals without either diagnosis, but with two or more risk factors (Table 7-2), are further stratified as to their risk of a coronary event within the next 10 years based on Framingham data. This estimate of risk takes into account age, gender, total cholesterol, smoking, HDL, and blood pressure.

Metabolic Syndrome

Recent attention regarding risk for CHD has focused on a constellation of characteristics termed *metabolic syndrome*. Metabolic syndrome includes 1) insulin resistance; 2) hypertension; 3) dyslipidemia that can include elevated serum triglycerides, low HDL-C, and small, dense LDL-C; 4) a prothrombotic state; and 5) a proinflammatory state. Although sophisticated laboratory analyses, such as determination of C-reactive protein or measurement of insulin resistance, can strengthen the diagnosis of metabolic syndrome, a series of simple measurements shown in Table 7-3 provide a reliable means of clinical identification of

Table 7-3   Clinical identification of metabolic syndrome.

RISK FACTOR	DEFINING LEVEL
Abdominal obesity	Waist circumference
Men	>40 in.
Women	>35 in.
Triglycerides	≥150 mg/dL
HDL cholesterol	
Men	<40 mg/dL
Women	<50 mg/dL
Blood pressure	≥130/≥85 mm Hg
Fasting glucose	≥110 mg/dL

HDL, high-density lipoprotein.
SOURCE: From the Executive Summary of the Third Report of the National Cholesterol Education Program (NCEP), Expert Panel on Detection, Education, and Treatment of High Blood Cholesterol in Adults (Adult Treatment Panel III or ATP III).

individuals at risk for metabolic syndrome. The presence of abdominal obesity is a valuable clue to metabolic syndrome. It can easily be assessed via the patient's waist circumference, which is described in detail in Chapter 1.

Medical Nutrition Therapy for Hyperlipidemia and Metabolic Syndrome

Table 7-4 delineates LDL goals and indications for diet and drug treatment for hyperlipidemia. Diet and exercise are cornerstones of the effective treatment of hyperlipidemia. The NCEP ATP III Guidelines enumerated four essential components of the TLC for achievement of LDL goals. They encompass the following:

- LDL-raising nutrients should be minimized.
  - Keep dietary intake of saturated fat to less than 7% of total calories.
  - Keep dietary cholesterol intake to less than 200 mg per day.
  - Total fat is allowed within the range of 25% to 35% of calories.
- Therapeutic options can be added for further LDL lowering.
  - Include 2 g plant stanol/sterol esters per day.
  - Increase viscous fiber intake to 10 to 25 g per day.
- Total calories should be adjusted to maintain desirable body weight and prevent weight gain.
- Physical activity should include enough moderate exercise to expend at least 200 calories per day.

Table 7-4   Low-density lipoprotein cholesterol goals and cutpoints for therapeutic lifestyle changes and drug therapy in different risk categories.

RISK CATEGORY	LDL-C GOAL	LDL LEVEL AT WHICH TO INITIATE TLC	LDL LEVEL AT WHICH TO CONSIDER DRUG THERAPY
CHD or CHD risk equivalents (10-yr risk >20%)	<100 mg/dL	≥100 mg/dL	≥130 mg/dL (100–129 mg/dL: drug optional)[a]
2+ Risk factors (10-yr risk ≤20%)	<130 mg/dL	≥130 mg/dL	10-yr risk 10%–20%: ≥130 mg/dL 10-yr risk <10%: ≥160 mg/dL
0–1 Risk factor[b]	<160 mg/dL	≥160 mg/dL	≥190 mg/dL (169–189 mg/dL: LDL–lowering drug optional)

LDL, low-density lipoprotein; TLC, therapeutic lifestyle changes; CHD, coronary heart disease.
[a] Some authorities recommend use of LDL-lowering drugs in this category if an LDL cholesterol <100 mg/dL cannot be achieved by TLC. Others prefer use of drugs that primarily modify triglycerides and high-density lipoprotein, e.g., nicotinic acid or fibrate.
[b] Almost all people with 0–1 risk factors have a 10-year risk <10%; thus, 10-year risk assessment in people with 0–1 risk factor is not necessary.
SOURCE: From the Executive Summary of the Third Report of the National Cholesterol Education Program (NCEP), Expert Panel on Detection, Education, and Treatment of High Blood Cholesterol in Adults (Adult Treatment Panel III or ATP III).

The ATP III–recommended distribution for macronutrients is shown in Table 7-5, and specific food-based guidance is provided in Table 7-6. Adopting lifestyle changes that incorporate new long-term dietary habits demands an investment of time and family support. Referral to a registered dietitian for medical nutrition therapy provides a comprehensive assessment of nutritional status, development of negotiated tailored behavior change goals, and strategies to achieve these goals. The dietitian can assist patients with problem areas, such as portion size, eating out, and tips for food purchasing and preparation. Continued reinforcement and monitoring of behavior change by health care professionals is important for achieving and maintaining lifestyle changes. Many Lipid Centers have full-time or part-time dietitians on staff who routinely counsel patients and work closely with the health care team.

Homocysteine, Folic Acid, and Cardiovascular Risk

In addition to the major risk factors listed in ATP III, current evidence points to several emerging risk factors, including various abnormalities of lipoproteins and elevation of plasma homocysteine level. Hyperhomocysteinemia is now identified as an independent risk factor for CHD. Although it is not as common as the major risk factors, evidence suggests that a 10% increase in homocysteine results in a 10% increase in a patient's CHD risk. Genetic polymorphisms resulting in decreased enzyme activities in metabolic pathways for homocysteine can be overcome with an adequate supply of B-complex vitamins: folate, B_6, and

Table 7-5   Macronutrient recommendations for the therapeutic lifestyle changes diet.

COMPONENT	RECOMMENDATION
Saturated fat	<7% of total calories
Polyunsaturated fat	Up to 10% of total calories
Monounsaturated fat	Up to 20% of total calories
Total fat	25%–35% of total calories[a]
Carbohydrate[b]	50%–60% of total calories[a]
Dietary fiber	20–30 g/d
Protein	~ 15% of total calories

[a]The Adult Treatment Panel III allows an increase of total fat to 35% of total calories and a reduction in carbohydrate to 50% for persons with the metabolic syndrome. Any increase in fat intake should be in the form of either polyunsaturated or monounsaturated fat.
[b]Carbohydrate should derive predominantly from foods rich in complex carbohydrates, including grain—especially whole grains—fruits, and vegetables.
SOURCE: From the Executive Summary of the Third Report of the National Cholesterol Education Program (NCEP), Expert Panel on Detection, Education, and Treatment of High Blood Cholesterol in Adults (Adult Treatment Panel III or ATP III).

B_{12} (Figure 7-1). Folate is most likely to be deficient in the diet since 70% of Americans do not consume five vegetables and fruits every day. A diet adequate in folic acid (via fortified grains as well) and vitamins B_6 and B_{12} can help ensure adequate homocysteine metabolism. Folate is present primarily in dark-green leafy vegetables, whole-grain cereals, beans, and oranges.

Other Nutritional Components

Stanol/Sterol Esters

Plant sterols and their chemically modified counterpart, plant stanols, have been esterified and incorporated into some brands of margarine. Consuming 2 Tbsp. per day provides 2 to 3 g sterol/stanol esters per day, which has been shown to lower LDL levels by 6% to 15%. In the gastrointestinal tract, sterol/stanol esters compete with cholesterol for incorporation into micelles and thus absorption. Two possible concerns regarding use of plant sterol/stanol fortified margarines are 1) if margarine use is increased, some means of caloric adjustment is needed to maintain energy balance, and 2) concurrent reduced absorption of dietary carotenoids suggests the need for attention to consume an adequate intake of fruits and vegetables.

Table 7-6   Food-based advice for therapeutic lifestyle changes diet.

FOOD ITEMS TO CHOOSE MORE OFTEN	FOOD ITEMS TO CHOOSE LESS OFTEN
Breads and cereals	
≥6 servings per day, adjusted to caloric needs	Many bakery products, including doughnuts, biscuits, butter croissants, Danish, pies, cookies
Breads, cereals, especially whole grain; pasta; rice; potatoes; dry beans and peas; low-fat crackers and cookies	Many grain-based snacks, including chips, cheese puffs, snack mix, regular crackers, buttered popcorn
Vegetables and fruits	
3–5 servings vegetables per day fresh, frozen, or canned, without added fat, sauce, or salt	Vegetables fried or prepared with butter, cheese, or cream sauce
2–4 servings fruits per day fresh, frozen, canned, dried	Fruits fried or served with butter or cream
Dairy products	
2–3 servings per day fat-free, 1/2%, 1% milk; buttermilk; yogurt; cottage cheese; fat-free and low-fat cheese	Whole milk/2% milk, whole-milk yogurt, ice cream, cream, cheese
Eggs	
≤ 2 egg yolks per week Egg whites or egg substitute	Egg yolks, whole eggs
Meat, fish, and poultry	
≤ 5 oz/d Lean cuts loin, leg, round; extra-lean hamburger; cold cuts made with lean meat or soy protein; skinless poultry; fish	Higher-fat meat cuts: ribs, t-bone steak, regular hamburger, bacon, sausage; cold cuts: salami, bologna, hot dogs; organ meats: liver, brains, sweetbreads; poultry with skin; fried meat; fried poultry; fried fish
Fats and oils	
Amount adjusted to caloric level: unsaturated oils; soft or liquid margarines and vegetable oil spreads, salad dressings, seeds, and nuts	Butter, shortening, stick margarine, chocolate, coconut

SOURCE: From the Executive Summary of the Third Report of the National Cholesterol Education Program (NCEP), Expert Panel on Detection, Education, and Treatment of High Blood Cholesterol in Adults (Adult Treatment Panel III or ATP III).

Dietary Fiber

Inclusion of viscous or soluble fiber in the diet can decrease LDL levels. Based on evidence from a meta-analysis of over 50 clinical trials, ATP III recommends inclusion of at least 5 to 10 g viscous fiber daily, with the option of greater intakes in the range of 10 to 25 g daily. The 5- to 10-g level has been shown to reduce LDL by approximately 5%. The hypocholesterolemic effect of soluble fiber results from its ability to form a gel-like substance in the gut, which binds and removes bile acids from the body through the stool before they are reabsorbed. Hepatic conversion of cholesterol into new bile acids reduces serum cholesterol. Some of

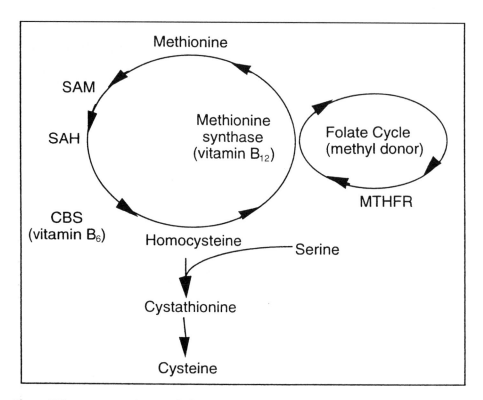

Figure 7-1   Homocysteine metabolism. SAM, *S*-adenosyl methionine; SAH, *S*-adenosyl homocysteine; MS, methionine synthase; MTHFR, methylenetetrahydrofolate reductase; CBS, cystathionine β-synthase.

SOURCE: Fallest-Strobl PC, Koch DD, Stein JH, et al. Homocysteine: a new risk factor for atherosclerosis. Am Fam Physician 1997;56:1607–1612. Used with permission from the October 15, 1997 issue of American Family Physician. Copyright American Academy of Family Physicians. All Rights Reserved.

the best dietary sources that provide 2 to 4 g viscous fiber per serving include dried beans (lima, pinto, kidney), oatmeal, oat bran, citrus fruits, pears, and brussels sprouts.

Soy

The benefit of soy in lowering cholesterol is less well substantiated than the nutritional approaches discussed above. Based on current evidence, the FDA has approved a health claim for soy foods that 25 g soy protein per day, as part of a diet low in saturated fat and cholesterol, may reduce the risk of heart disease. Studies have shown that this level of soy protein lowers LDL levels by approximately 5%. The number of Americans consuming 25 g soy protein per day and its associated isoflavones from natural foods is small. Part of the observed benefits of soy may result from the substitution of vegetable protein for animal protein and fat. Currently, neither the AHA nor NCEP includes a specific recommendation to incorporate soy to reduce the risk of CHD.

Supplemental Vitamins

Two sets of supplemental vitamins have drawn attention for prevention and treatment of CHD. Intake of folate, B_6, and B_{12} can lower homocysteine levels. Although elevated homocysteine levels are associated with increased CHD, there is not yet direct evidence that nutritional manipulations to lower homocysteine lower CHD risk. Recent data suggest that folic acid improves endothelial function independent of homocysteine levels. Daily supplementation with 1 mg folic acid, 400 mcg B_{12}, and 10 mg B_6 decreased serum homocysteine levels and the rate of restenosis after angioplasty. The recommended dietary allowance (RDA) for folate is 400 mcg daily, with an upper limit for safety set at 1000 mcg daily.

Other supplemental vitamins of interest in heart disease are the antioxidants. Although there is evidence that supplementation with alpha tocopherol (vitamin E) reduces LDL oxidation, results from recent trials are contradictory regarding its benefit in reducing CHD. This may be partly due to the amounts and form of supplementation. The Heart Outcomes Prevention Evaluation (HOPE; 400 IU daily) and Gruppo Italiano per lo Studio della Streptochinasi nell'Infarto Miocardico (GISSI; 300 mg daily) trials did not demonstrate a protective effect. The Cambridge Heart Antioxidant Study (CHAOS) did report significant reduction in risk of recurrent myocardial infarction among CHD patients receiving 400 to 800 IU vitamin E daily. Other antioxidants that continue to be studied for benefit in heart disease include vitamin C, beta-carotene, coenzyme Q10, and selenium (see Chapter 2).

Medical Nutrition Therapy for Coronary Heart Disease

Nutrition issues should be addressed with patients who have hyperlipidemia, CHD, or a family history of heart disease during most routine primary care visits. One quick reminder of nutrition issues to consider is the use of WAVE, an acronym suggesting consideration of the patient's *weight*, *activity*, and diet in terms of *variety* and *excess*. (See *http://www.utsouthwestern.edu/naa/wave/ wave_info.htm*.) Specific to hyperlipidemia, it is valuable to address the excesses in the diet that would contribute saturated fat and cholesterol.

Weight Control

Attention to calorie balance is important for most patients. Fostering control of caloric intake and encouraging increased physical activity are key to weight maintenance and weight reduction. Weight reduction in overweight patients improves parameters associated with metabolic syndrome, including reducing LDL-C and triglycerides, increasing HDL-C, reducing blood pressure, and normalizing elevated serum glucose levels. In many cases, as little as 7% to 10% weight reduction alone can eliminate the need for drug therapy in these clinical syndromes. Furthermore, this concept, when explained to the patient, can result in increased patient motivation and improved dietary adherence.

On the other hand, sometimes patients begun on lipid-lowering medication feel that attention to diet is no longer needed. Failure to follow an appropriate diet with use of drugs can necessitate higher doses of drugs, increasing any potential for side effects. Therefore, physicians should continue to emphasize the underlying benefit of a calorically balanced, low-saturated-fat diet when lipid-lowering drugs are used.

Alcohol

In addition to the general lifestyle issues of diet and exercise, a specific issue often raised in patient conversations regarding heart disease is consumption of alcohol. Alcohol, in relation to heart disease, has both positive and negative effects. A first step in advising patients regarding alcohol is to obtain an adequate alcohol intake history.

Although light to moderate intake of alcohol may reduce the risk of CHD, intake over 30 g per day (more than 2 drinks) is associated with an increased mortality due to hypertension, pancreatitis, hypertriglyceridemia, gastrointestinal malignancies, stroke, cardiomyopathy, cirrhosis, accidents, and breast cancer. Moderate alcohol intake is defined as no more than two drinks per day for men and one drink per day for women. A drink is defined as 6 oz wine, $1^1/_2$ oz 80-proof liquor, or 12 oz beer.

On the positive side, alcohol, specifically red wine, may have cardioprotective effects by increasing HDL levels and reducing LDL oxidation via the antioxidant polyphenols (catechin, quercetin, resveratrol). A CHD patient can continue to drink alcohol in moderation if free of other medical, psychiatric, or social problems. However, it is *not* appropriate to recommend alcohol intake to a non-drinker or an at-risk drinker for its cardioprotective effect, as there are many other effective nonpharmacologic therapies.

Hypertension

Hypertension affects over 50 million people in the United States and is a major risk factor for the development of CHD, cardiomyopathy, and stroke. Diet and other lifestyle factors have enormous potential for the prevention and treatment of hypertension and in some cases can obviate the need for drug therapy or lower the dose required. This is particularly evident in patients with high normal blood pressure (130/85 to 139/89 mm Hg).

Nutritional factors that may contribute to the development of essential hypertension include obesity, high sodium intake, low potassium and calcium intake, and excessive alcohol consumption. Although earlier studies have pointed to a number of dietary components in addition to sodium, the DASH trial and the later DASH-sodium trials have substantiated the benefit of a comprehensive dietary approach in prevention and treatment of hypertension.

Table 7-7 DASH diet.

This Dietary Approaches to Stop Hypertension (DASH) eating plan is based on 2000 calories a day. The number of servings may vary from those listed depending on caloric needs.

FOOD GROUP	DAILY SERVINGS	SERVING SIZES
Grains and grain products	7–8	1 slice bread
		1 cup dry cereal[a]
		$1/2$ cup cooked rice, pasta, or cereal
Vegetables	4–5	1 cup raw leafy vegetable
		$1/2$ cup cooked vegetable
		6 oz vegetable juice
Fruits	4–5	6 oz fruit juice
		1 medium fruit
		$1/4$ cup dried fruit
		$1/2$ cup fresh, frozen, or canned fruit
Low-fat or fat-free dairy foods	2–3	8 oz milk
		1 cup yogurt
		$1 1/2$ oz cheese
Meats, poultry, and fish	2 or less	3 oz cooked meats, poultry, or fish
Nuts, seeds, and dry beans	4–5 per week	1/3 cup or $1 1/2$ oz nuts
		2 Tbsp. or $1/2$ oz seeds
		$1/2$ cup cooked dry beans
Fats and oils[b]	2–3	1 tsp. soft margarine
		1 Tbsp. low-fat mayonnaise
		2 Tbsp. light salad dressing
		1 tsp. vegetable oil
Sweets	5 per week	1 Tbsp. sugar
		1 Tbsp. jelly or jam
		$1/2$ oz jelly beans
		8 oz lemonade

[a] Serving sizes may vary between $1/2$ and $1 1/4$ cups. Check the product's nutrition label.
[b] Fat content changes serving counts for fats and oils: For example, 1 Tbsp. regular salad dressing equals $1/2$ serving; 1 Tbsp. of fat-free dressing equals 0 servings.
SOURCE: From NHLBI's Facts about DASH Diet.

The DASH diet, outlined in Table 7-7, provides for a substantial intake of potassium and calcium through the inclusion of fruits and vegetables and low-fat dairy products. In addition, meat portions are limited and nuts are used to provide magnesium and additional fiber. The diet limits saturated fat and cholesterol comparable to the dietary parameters of the TLC diet of ATP III. Results from the clinical trial of the DASH diet indicated reduction of diastolic blood pressure by as much as 5 mm Hg, regardless of age, gender, ethnicity, or preexisting hypertension. The diet was more effective among African-American and hypertensive individuals. For patients with stage 1 hypertension (blood pressure 140/90 to 159/99 mm Hg), the diet's effectiveness in lowering blood pressure was similar to that of a single-agent antihypertensive therapy.

After the original trial, the DASH-sodium trial investigated the effect of the DASH diet combined with three different levels of sodium (3300 mg, 2400 mg, and 1500 mg). Reductions in blood pressure were proportional to the level of sodium restriction. Thus, optimum medical nutrition therapy for hypertension provides a diet that includes:

- Reduced sodium level
- Generous amounts of potassium and calcium
- Abstinence or moderation of alcohol intake
- Continued weight control

Obesity and Hypertension

Obesity is a major risk factor in the development of hypertension. It has been estimated that 60% of the hypertensive population are more than 20% overweight. A linear relationship exits between the degree of obesity and the severity of hypertension. The beneficial effect of weight reduction in hypertensive individuals has been clearly documented. Controlled dietary intervention trials estimate that a mean reduction in body weight of 20 lb (9.2 kg) is associated with a 6.3 mm Hg reduction in systolic blood pressure and a 3.1 mm Hg reduction in diastolic blood pressure. The exact mechanism of obesity-induced hypertension is unclear, but increased cardiac output, sodium retention, and increased sympathetic activity in response to elevated insulin levels are all thought to be significant contributors. Weight reduction should be the primary goal for the overweight hypertensive patient, since 10% change in body weight is sufficient to reduce blood pressure (see Chapter 1, Case 1).

Dietary Sodium Intake

Population studies have repeatedly demonstrated a relationship of hypertension to higher sodium intakes. However, not all individuals respond the same way to dietary sodium. Depletion and loading studies indicate that up to 50% of hypertensive patients are salt-sensitive. Salt sensitivity appears to be associated with several demographic variables, such as obesity, African-American race, and older age. Unfortunately, there is no simple way to determine salt sensitivity in the clinical setting.

The Joint National Committee on Prevention, Detection, Evaluation and Treatment of High Blood Pressure (JNC VI) recommends limiting sodium to 2400 mg daily for patients with hypertension. The typical American diet contains approximately 4 to 8 g sodium per day. Table salt and foods high in sodium, such as salted, smoked, canned, and highly processed foods, should be limited. The use of convenience foods, fast foods, and eating out frequently all contribute to higher sodium intakes among Americans today. Key questions for patients with hypertension are the following:

- Do you use a salt shaker at the table or in cooking?
- Do you read labels for sodium content? (Recommend <400 mg per serving.)
- How often do you eat canned, smoked, frozen, and processed foods?

Dietary Potassium Intake

Epidemiologic and observational studies have reported an inverse correlation between potassium intake and blood pressure, especially among African-Americans and individuals who consume a high-sodium diet. More recently, several small intervention studies have shown that potassium supplementation results in a modest hypotensive effect. Although the exact mechanism remains unclear, effects of potassium supplementation include naturesis, inhibition of renin release, and decreased thromboxane production. For practical purposes, increasing dietary intake of potassium may have a beneficial effect on blood pressure. Foods high in potassium include oranges, orange juice, potatoes (especially with the skins), and bananas. To maintain a high potassium intake, the DASH diet includes 8 to 10 servings of fruits and vegetables daily. Diuretic therapy, a first-line modality for treating hypertension, frequently induces potassium wasting. Increasing dietary intake in these patients may obviate the need for synthetic potassium supplements, which require close monitoring.

Dietary Calcium Intake

Calcium intake may be lower among hypertensive patients than among normotensive individuals. Increased dietary intake may reduce the incidence of hypertension, and calcium supplements may produce a hypotensive effect in some patients. Although it appears that calcium supplements have no role in the treatment of hypertension, an adequate dietary intake is essential. Dietary calcium has been correlated with blood pressure, but calcium supplementation has not been shown to lower blood pressure significantly. On the other hand, the inclusion of low-fat dairy products within the framework of the DASH diet did provide additional blood pressure lowering, as outlined in Table 7-7, which advises two to three servings per day of low-fat dairy products.

Alcohol Intake

Alcohol consumption in amounts of three or more drinks per day is estimated to account for 5% to 7% of the diagnosed cases of hypertension. Although alcohol, when ingested, acts as a vasodilator, chronic alcohol ingestion is associated with increased formation of the vasoconstrictor thromboxane. Chronically increased levels of this prostaglandin metabolite may be partially responsible for the hypertensive effect of chronic alcohol ingestion. In controlled studies, reducing alcohol consumption in this population has been associated with a modest reduction in blood pressure.

Heart Failure

Heart failure (HF), which affects nearly 5 million adults in the United States, is characterized by decreased cardiac output, venous stasis, sodium and fluid retention, multiple organ failure (kidney, liver, heart, brain), and undernutrition. A triad of classic symptoms includes shortness of breath, fatigue, and congestion.

The absence of clinical trials regarding medical nutrition therapy for HF provides a much weaker evidence base than the basis for nutritional intervention for hyperlipidemia or hypertension. Nevertheless, attention to medical nutrition therapy in the management of patients with HF is critical.

Causes of Undernutrition in Heart Failure

Cardiac cachexia is the term used to describe the wasting and undernutrition seen in patients with long-standing HF. As myocardial function progressively deteriorates, patients present with loss of adipose tissue and lean body mass secondary to poor nutritional intake and decreased activity. Upper-body and temporal wasting with lower-extremity edema are the hallmark features of this condition. The proposed mechanisms to explain cardiac cachexia include:

- Impaired cellular oxygen supply
- Increased nutrient losses
- Increased nutritional requirements
- Decreased nutritional intake

Impaired Cellular Oxygen Supply

Decreased cardiac output reduces oxygen delivery to cells, resulting in inefficient substrate oxidation and inadequate synthesis of high-energy intermediary metabolites.

Increased Nutrient Losses

Hypoxemia and increased venous pressure may cause bowel edema, with subsequent fat and protein malabsorption. Decreased synthesis of hepatic bile salts and pancreatic enzymes caused by oxygen deprivation to the liver and pancreas may further contribute to this. Proteinuria is also a feature of HF secondary to the reduced renal blood flow characteristic of this disorder.

Increased Nutritional Requirements

Patients with HF can be hypermetabolic and therefore have increased nutritional requirements. This hypermetabolic state is caused by the increased work required for breathing, the mechanical work of the heart, and oxygen consumption related to alterations in neuroendocrine activity. If additional calories are not ingested to meet these increased demands, weight loss ensues.

Decreased Nutritional Intake

Factors that may result in an inadequate food intake in patients with HF include one or all of the following:

- Hepatomegaly and ascites reduce functional gastric volume causing early satiety.
- Dyspnea and fatigue induced by eating.
- Unpalatable low-sodium diets.
- Anorexia, nausea, or vomiting from medications used to treat congestive heart failure (CHF).

Medical Nutrition Therapy for Heart Failure

Medical nutrition therapy for patients with HF should be aimed at controlling sodium and fluid retention; restoring and maintaining body weight; providing adequate energy, protein, vitamins, and minerals; and repleting protein stores in patients who have lost lean body mass.

Dietary Sodium Intake

Patients with HF retain sodium and fluid, and, therefore, dietary sodium restriction is a necessary adjunct to diuretic therapy. The level of sodium restriction should be individualized according to the severity of the HF. It is recommended that patients with symptomatic chronic HF reduce dietary sodium intake to 2 to 3 g (2000 to 3000 mg) per day. Restricting sodium intake supports the effectiveness of diuretic agents in achieving negative sodium balance. Failure to adhere to dietary sodium advice has been attributed to one-fifth of hospital readmissions for patients with HF. Patients need more than to be told "stay away from salt." They need to be able to state their recommended level of dietary sodium, use values on the nutrition label to guide their intake, and distinguish between very high and very low sources of sodium.

A recent study in an urban teaching hospital reported that only 14% of patients seen in a chronic HF clinic could accurately identify their recommended level of sodium intake. Whether patients are seen in the acute care or ambulatory care setting, referral to the registered dietitian for assessment of their nutritional status and assistance in achieving the skills needed to manage a sodium-restricted diet at home are appropriate for cost-effective management of HF. Salt substitutes are available to flavor foods, but many of them substitute potassium for sodium. Patients with renal failure or those taking potassium-sparing diuretics should avoid these products.

Fluid

Heart failure associated with dilutional hyponatremia may require restricting fluid intake to 1500 to 2000 mL per day. The fluid may be restricted slightly more in the hospital setting. Some suggest limiting daily fluid intake to an amount equal to the 24-hour urine output volume plus 500 mL. Traditional nutrition assessment parameters such as actual body weight or weight change may not accurately reflect nutritional status in patients with CHF. For example, cardiac cachexia may go undetected if body weight is normal or elevated because of sodium and water retention, with resultant enlargement of the extracellular fluid compartment. In addition, serum protein levels, such as albumin, may be decreased secondary to either undernutrition or artifactually as a result of fluid overload.

Calories and Protein

The daily caloric intake should be adequate to promote weight gain (if needed) in patients with HF. Therefore, to support anabolism, current recommendations are to estimate dietary calories at 1.5 times the basal energy expenditure. The amount of protein necessary to promote anabolism and achieve positive nitrogen balance in a patient with cardiac cachexia is thought to be 1.5 to 2.0 g/kg per day. High-protein, high-calorie supplements are often necessary to achieve this calorie requirement, especially when the patient has a poor appetite. Nutritional supplements, both liquid and pudding forms, are available and provide a high concentration of calories and protein in a relatively small volume. The sodium and fluid content of HF supplements must be considered in the total daily sodium and fluid allowance. Small, frequent meals also may help HF patients achieve an adequate dietary intake. Patients who cannot meet their caloric and protein requirements orally may require enteral tube feeding (see Chapter 12). Enteral feeding in an HF patient can be precarious, as it can result in overfeeding, which will aggravate the primary condition.

For some patients, obesity places additional strain on an already compromised heart. Thus, careful assessment of nutritional status and monitoring of dietary intake are valuable in providing for optimum nutritional support.

For a list of references for this chapter, please visit the University of Pennsylvania School of Medicine's Nutrition Education and Prevention Program web site: *http://www.med.upenn.edu/nutrimed/articles.html*

Case 1

Adult Hyperlipidemia

Wahida Karmally and Henry Ginsberg

Objectives

- Identify cardiac risk factors for coronary artery disease in obese patients without known disease.
- Describe the scientific basis for nutritional and lifestyle recommendations for patients with hyperlipidemia.
- Provide a nutritional care plan including physical activity and alcohol consumption for patients with hyperlipidemia.
- Apply the current NCEP guidelines for screening, evaluation, and treatment of hyperlipidemia in patient care.
- Recognize the importance of medical nutrition therapy and lifestyle recommendations for treatment and prevention of cardiovascular disease.

HC is a 52-year-old man who consults a new physician for a routine physical examination since his employer has recently changed their health insurance plan. He has not seen a physician for the past 3 years.

Past Medical History

HC has no prior history of hospitalizations or chronic illnesses. He is not taking any medications or over-the-counter dietary or herbal supplements, and he has no known food allergies.

Family History

HC's family history is positive for heart disease. His father had a fatal heart attack at age 54, and his father's brother had a heart attack at age 55. HC's uncle is currently being treated for hypercholesterolemia. He has no family history of hypertension, diabetes, or obesity.

Social History

HC works as an accountant and reports a high stress level both at work and at home. Because his work commitments do not allow him much free time, he frequently orders lunch in and eats at his desk. After a long day at work and his 45-minute commute home, HC feels too tired to exercise. Over the past 3 years he has experienced a 12-lb weight gain. HC attributes this to his sedentary, high-stress lifestyle, in addition to dining out with clients on average 2 to 3 nights per week. HC is a nonsmoker. He drinks a 20 oz (600-mL) cup of coffee every morning and two alcoholic beverages every evening. HC is married and has one daughter who is currently in her junior year in college.

Dietary Intake

Using the 24-hour recall method, HC's physician obtained the following information about his typical diet.

Breakfast (office)

Bagel	1 large (4 oz/113 g)
Cream cheese	2 Tbsp.
Coffee	20 oz (600 mL)
Half-and-half	2 oz (60 mL)

Lunch (restaurant)

Pizza with cheese	2 slices
Soda (cola)	12 oz (360 mL)

Snack (office)

Jelly beans	1 oz (28 g)

Evening (restaurant)

Beer	24 oz (720 mL)
Hamburger	6 oz (170 g)
Bun	1 large
French fries	1 cup
Vanilla ice cream	1 cup

Total calories: 2718 kcal
Protein: 106 g (16% of total calories)
Fat: 101 g (33% of total calories)
Saturated fat: 46 g (15% of total calories)
Monounsaturated fat: 26 g (9% of total calories)
Polyunsaturated fat: 4 g (1% of total calories)
Trans-fat: 2.75 g
Carbohydrate: 311 g (45% of total calories)
Alcohol: 26 g (7% of total calories)
Cholesterol: 309 mg
Sodium: 2680 mg
Dietary fiber: 14 g
Folic acid: 215 mcg

Review of Systems

Noncontributory.

Physical Examination

Vital Signs

Temperature: 98°F (37°C)

Heart rate: 76 beats per minute (BPM)

Respiration: 20 BPM

Blood pressure: 139/88 mm Hg (high normal 130–139/85–89)

Height: 5'10" (178 cm)

Current weight: 212 lb (96 kg)

Body mass index (BMI): 30.4 kg/m^2

Weight 2 years ago: 200 lb (91 kg)

Waist circumference: 42 in. (107 cm)

General: Obese male in no acute distress

The remainder of the physical examination was normal and unremarkable.

Laboratory Data

HC's lipid profile, after a 12-hour overnight fast, produced the following laboratory values:

Patient's Laboratory Values	Normal Values
Total cholesterol: 260 mg/dL	Desirable <200 mg/dL
HDL-C: 32 mg/dL	≥40 mg/dL
LDL-C: 158 mg/dL	<130 mg/dL
Triglycerides: 350 mg/dL	<150 mg/dL
Homocysteine: 8 mol per liter	<12 mol per liter
Lipoprotein (a): 11 mg/dL	<20 mg/dL
Plasma glucose: 95 mg/dL	70 to 110 mg/dL

Framingham Point Score: 10-year risk for CHD is 12%

Case Questions

1. What additional questions should be asked of all patients during the general health maintenance screening?

2. What physical examination findings should one look for in a patient suspected of having hyperlipidemia?

3. What additional screening and laboratory data should be performed on patients suspected of having hyperlipidemia?

4. Based on HC's medical history, physical examination, and laboratory data, how would you classify and diagnose his lipid disorder?

5. Is HC's current nutrient intake within the recommended guidelines of the Adult Treatment Panel (ATP) III TLC diet?

6. What are the best dietary approaches for this patient?

7. How can HC translate the recommended dietary guidelines into food choices?

8. Should HC receive a lipid-lowering medication at this time?

Case Answers

Part 1: Screening, Risk Assessment, and Diagnosis

1. **What additional questions should be asked of all patients during general health maintenance screening?**

   During the general health maintenance screen, a thorough history should include questions related to cardiac risk factors. Traditional risk factors for coronary artery disease in this patient include elevated total, LDL-C and triglyceride levels, age (men older than 45), family history of heart disease, low HDL, borderline hypertension, and obesity (BMI ≥ 30). Nutrient intake, average weekly alcohol consumption, alternative medicine use, exercise habits, and stress levels are also important areas to explore. In addition the physician should consider in the past medical history any diseases that directly increase cardiovascular risk (i.e., diabetes) or any secondary medical disorder that could be contributing or causing the hyperlipidemia (Table 7-8).

2. **What physical examination findings should one look for in a patient suspected of having hyperlipidemia?**

   In addition to general health screening, patients suspected of having hyperlipidemia should undergo an examination of pulses (palpation of all pulses and auscultation for bruits in the carotids and femoral arteries), thyroid palpation (hypothyroidism is a possible secondary cause of

Table 7-8   Causes of secondary hyperlipidemia.

ENDOCRINE/METABOLIC	DRUGS
Diabetes mellitus	Alcohol
Obesity	Cyclosporine
Hypothyroidism	Androgens
Hypogonadism	Estrogens
Hypercortisolism	Progestins

hypercholesterolemia), an eye examination for corneal arcus senilis, and a tendon and skin examination for xanthelasmas or xanthomas.

3. **What additional screening and laboratory data should be performed on patients suspected of having hyperlipidemia?**

The current NCEP ATP III guidelines recommend a complete lipoprotein profile (total cholesterol, LDL-C, HDL-C, and triglycerides) as the preferred initial laboratory test, rather than screening for total cholesterol and HDL alone. In addition, ATP III's major new focus is on primary prevention of CHD in persons with multiple risk factors. Primary prevention is the treatment of high-risk individuals without established cardiovascular disease.

LDL-C can be calculated using the following equation, but techniques for its direct measurement also are available.

$$\text{Total cholesterol} = \text{HDL-C} + \text{LDL-C} + \text{VLDL-C or}$$
$$\text{LDL-C} = \text{total cholesterol} - (\text{HDL-C} + \text{VLDL-C})$$
$$\text{VLDL-C} = \frac{\text{triglyceride level}}{5}$$

In hyperlipidemic states, a triglyceride level greater than 400 mg/dL invalidates the results of this equation.

In addition to the screening tests described above, a plasma homocysteine and Lp(a) level were considered because of HC's family history of premature heart disease. Preliminary data suggest that treating high levels of homocysteine may offer protection. Two recent studies have shown a reduction in the restenosis rate following coronary angioplasty in patients receiving a supplement containing folate, vitamin B_{12}, and vitamin B_6.

To rule out secondary or contributory causes of hyperlipidemia, fasting serum glucose to diagnose glucose intolerance or diabetes mellitus and thyroid-stimulating hormone to diagnose hypothyroidism should also be measured. If lipid-lowering drug therapy is required, baseline liver transaminases [alanine aminotransferase (ALT) and aspartate aminotransferase (AST)] and uric acid levels may be helpful in choosing the appropriate type of drug therapy.

Patients with abdominal obesity should be evaluated for metabolic syndrome. Each of the five clinical criteria for metabolic syndrome can be obtained via a focused medical history, brief physical examination, and fasting laboratory data (see Table 7-3). HC has four of the five criteria for metabolic syndrome, including abdominal obesity, elevated triglycerides, low HDL-C, and borderline high blood pressure. Recent estimates suggest that 24% of the US population meets the current NCEP criteria for metabolic syndrome. NCEP has identified metabolic syndrome as a secondary target of therapy in hypercholesterolemic patients.

4. **Based on HC's medical history, physical examination, and laboratory data, how would you classify and diagnose his lipid disorder?**

This type of lipid disorder is called *combined hyperlipidemia*, since HC's total plasma triglycerides and LDL-C concentrations are both elevated compared with those of age-matched control subjects. Although it is likely that a variety of combinations of regulatory defects in lipid metabolism account for a significant number of individuals with this phenotype, familial forms of combined hyperlipidemia (FCHL) have been identified in which members of the same family may have combined hyperlipidemia, only hypertriglyceridemia, or only elevated LDL-C concentrations. In the familial disorder, which appears to be transmitted as an autosomal dominant gene, the diagnosis must rest on the presentation of combined hyperlipidemia or the presence of various phenotypes in first-degree family members along with either isolated hypertriglyceridemia or isolated LDL-C elevation in the patient. FCHL is estimated to occur in 1 out of 100 Americans and is the most common familial lipid disorder found in survivors of myocardial infarction.

FCHL appears to be associated with the secretion of increased numbers of VLDL particles. Once individuals with FCHL assemble and secrete increased numbers of large, triglyceride-rich VLDLs, their plasma triglyceride concentrations depend on their ability to hydrolyze VLDL triglycerides with lipoprotein lipase and, to a lesser degree, with hepatic lipase.

The ability to hydrolyze VLDL triglycerides also regulates the generation of LDLs in the plasma. Thus, subjects with FCHL who have very-high VLDL triglyceride concentrations (and are not able to efficiently catabolize VLDLs) might have normal or reduced numbers of LDL particles in the circulation and thus a normal LDL-C concentration. If these same individuals were able to efficiently catabolize the increased numbers of VLDL particles that were entering the plasma, they would generate increased numbers of LDL particles and have both hypertriglyceridemia and a high LDL-C level. Patients with FCHL who synthesize only normal quantities of triglycerides and secrete increased numbers of VLDLs carrying normal triglyceride loads would generate increased numbers of LDL particles and have elevated plasma LDL-C concentrations only.

Part 2: Medical Nutrition Therapy

5. **Is HC's current nutrient intake within the recommended guidelines of the ATP III TLC diet?**

HC's current diet is not within the recommended guidelines of the TLC diet. According to the nutritional analysis of his current intake, HC's fat intake is 33% of his total caloric intake. His saturated fat intake is

15% of his caloric intake (recommended is <7%), and cholesterol intake is 309 mg (recommended <200 mg per day). Significant sources of saturated fat in HC's diet come from high-fat dairy foods, including half-and-half, cream cheese, mozzarella cheese, and ice cream as well as ground red meat. His caloric intake is approximately 2700 calories per day. This excessive calorie intake combined with his sedentary lifestyle will continue to promote weight gain unless he reduces total calories and routinely participates in some physical activity. In order to lose 1 to 2 lb body weight per week (which is the recommended rate of weight loss), HC must reduce his weight maintenance caloric needs by at least 500 calories and increase activity by 250 calories daily. Alternatively, he may choose to exercise more rather than eat less to achieve the targeted weight loss.

HC's typical diet is deficient in fruit and vegetables, which are generally low in calories and nutrient dense. HC's diet contains only 14 g dietary fiber, compared to the TLC diet, which recommends 20 to 30 g fiber per day as adjunctive therapy to reduce LDL-C. HC's folate intake is below the updated dietary reference intake for folate, which is now set at 400 mcg per day for adults. Sources of folate in HC's diet are the bread products (bagel and hamburger roll), which are fortified with folic acid.

6. **What are the best lifestyle approaches for this patient?**

HC's modifiable risk factors include obesity, high-saturated-fat diet, sedentary lifestyle, and excessive alcohol consumption. Implementing a number of lifestyle and behavioral changes should improve HC's risk profile significantly.

The first line of therapy for all lipid and nonlipid factors associated with the metabolic syndrome are weight reduction and increased physical activity. The ATP III guidelines recognize overweight and obesity as major underlying risk factors for CHD. Regular physical activity is a component in the management of hyperlipidemia.

In order to make dietary recommendations, it is necessary to first define the desired endpoint or goal for each individual. Is the goal to reduce triglycerides and LDL-C with/without weight reduction? For HC the goal is to lower total cholesterol, LDL-C, and triglycerides; raise HDL-C levels; and reduce weight. He can achieve this by adhering to the TLC diet and reducing his total caloric intake. MUFA and omega-3 fatty acids should be favored in place of both saturated and omega-6 fatty acids, while keeping total fat to a maximum of 35% of total calories.

The specific dietary recommendations include reducing total calories and saturated fat intake (<7%), having a moderate carbohydrate intake (<50%), increasing MUFA (up to 20%), and reducing alcohol intake. For patients who have a low HDL-C or high triglycerides, or both, a very-low-fat eating plan can aggravate their metabolic abnormalities unless they lose weight.

7. **How can HC translate the recommended dietary guidelines into food choices?**

A hypocaloric diet that favors MUFA (see recommended meal plan) is recommended for HC. Sources of MUFAs are canola oil, olive oil, olives, hazelnuts, almonds, cashews, peanuts, peanut butter, pecans, pistachios, avocado, and high oleic acid safflower oil and sunflower oil. The main sources of omega-3 fatty acids are fatty fish, such as salmon, mackerel, and sardines, and plant foods, such as flaxseeds and walnuts. HC should eat plenty of fruits and vegetables (5 to 8 servings per day), whole grains, beans and legumes (7 to 8 servings per day), only nonfat or very-low-fat dairy products, and chicken without skin, fish, or lean meats limited to 5 to 6 oz per day. If he enjoys eggs, he can include two large eggs per week.

His fiber intake would be significantly increased with the recommended servings of fresh fruits, vegetables, and whole grains. Therapeutic options for enhancing LDL reduction include increased intake of viscous (soluble) fiber (10 to 25 g per day) from oats, psyllium, dried beans, and fruits. Margarine containing plant stanol/sterols (2 g per day) could be included to further lower LDL-C in place of other spreads that the patient is currently using. Plant stanols/sterols can be obtained from Benecol and Take Control and smaller amounts from soy, flaxseeds, beans, corn, wheat, and rice. HC may benefit from a reduction in alcohol and sodium intake. Alcohol adds calories to HC's diet but has been shown to have some cardioprotective benefit.

HC's Recommended Sample Low-Fat Diet

Breakfast	Oat cereal	2 cups
	Skim milk	1 cup
	Orange, navel	1
Lunch	Tuna, canned, water pack	0.5 cup
	Whole-wheat bread	2 slices
	Tomato	$^{1}/_{2}$ medium
	Mayonnaise	1.5 Tbsp.
	Nonfat flavored yogurt	1 cup
Dinner	Chicken breast, baked	3 oz (85 g)
	Noodles, cooked	1 cup
	Broccoli	1 cup
	Romaine lettuce	2 cups
	Olive oil	1 Tbsp.
	Vinegar	1 Tbsp.
	Banana	1 small

Snack	Apple	1 small
	Peanut butter	2 Tbsp.
	Skim milk	6 oz (180 mL)

Total calories: 1916 kcal

Protein: 117 g (24% protein calories)

Carbohydrate: 239 g (49% carbohydrate calories)

Total fat: 63 g (29% fat calories)

Saturated fat: 12 g (6% saturated fat calories)

Polyunsaturated fat: 19 g (9% calories)

Monounsaturated fat: 27 g (13% calories)

Cholesterol: 184 mg

Fiber: 30 g

Soluble fiber: 10 g

Sodium: 2223 mg

Potassium: 3754 mg

Folic acid: 920 μg

Part 3: Lipid-Lowering Medication

8. **Should HC receive a lipid-lowering medication at this time?**

    HC may require drug therapy at some point in the future, but only after an adequate trial of lifestyle modification has been undertaken; therefore, the answer is no. It should be emphasized, however, that if pharmacologic intervention becomes necessary it should be thought of as an adjunct and not as a substitute to lifestyle modifications as a way to reduce his lipid levels.

    The physician needs to set the stage for dietary treatment and increasing physical activity. The physician's positive attitude toward lifestyle changes can influence the patient's attitude and success toward making these changes. An explanation of the effects that lifestyle modification can have on HC's prognosis should be highlighted. These benefits include lower LDL-C and triglyceride levels, increased HDL-C levels (usually only modestly), decreased blood pressure, increased cardiac output, increased collateral blood supply, and stress relief. Regardless of age, patients should begin any exercise program gradually and include 5 to 10 minutes of warming up at the beginning of exercise and cooling down at the end. The ultimate goal is to increase the total workout to 30 minutes daily. HC would need a stress test (>40 years of age) before he starts an exercise program.

    Referring the patient to a registered dietitian helps facilitate diet modification. The patient's readiness to make behavioral changes needs to be assessed. Most patients are not ready to make dramatic changes in lifestyle habits during the first meeting. In addition, assessment of the patient's compliance is essential to determine if the diet changes are optimal to maximize their effects on lipid metabolism. Diet instruction may require several follow-up visits. Early initial follow-up (every 4 to 6 weeks) is important because it affords opportunities to verify adherence to and provide support for diet and exercise changes. Later, the patient can be monitored at intervals deemed appropriate to reinforce the *TLC* treatment plan and to check lipid levels. In a patient such as HC, lifestyle changes should be attempted for 4 to 6 months before drug therapy is considered, because they may bring about a significant decrease in lipid parameters, thereby obviating the need for drug therapy.

Drug Treatment

If HC's lipid profile does not respond to diet and exercise, drug treatment should be initiated. The primary goal is lowering LDL-C, and secondary goals are to lower triglycerides (TG) and raise HDL-C. The following drugs can be considered:

- Nicotinic acid (niacin):
  Lowers LDL-C and TG levels and raises HDL-C. It can also increase insulin resistance, as this would be less of a risk if HC loses weight concomitantly.
- Statin: Lowers LDL-C and can lower TG at higher doses.
- Fibric acid derivatives: Lowers TG and raises HDL-C.

See Chapter Review Questions, pages A-22 to A-25.

8

Gastrointestinal Disease

Charlene Compher and Gary R. Lichtenstein

Objectives*

- Demonstrate how to incorporate nutrition into the medical history, review of systems, and physical examination of patients with gastrointestinal (GI) diseases.
- Discuss the process of nutrient digestion and absorption and how it is impaired in specific GI diseases.
- Describe the causes of undernutrition in inflammatory bowel disease, short bowel syndrome, liver disease, pancreatitis, and malabsorption syndromes.
- Identify the association between diet and lower esophageal sphincter pressure in gastroesophageal reflux disease.
- Recognize why sodium and fluid restriction may be necessary for patients with liver disease.

Normal Digestion and Absorption

The digestion of nutrients from dietary food sources requires a coordinated process of mechanical and chemical processes, including enzymatic, secretory, and absorptive responses. Defects in any of these phases of digestion or absorption can lead to maldigestion or malabsorption of nutrients, with subsequent undernutrition. The products of the digestive processes have an impact on intestinal function.

* SOURCE: Objectives for chapter and cases adapted from the *NIH Nutrition Curriculum Guide for Training Physicians* (*http://www.nhlbi.nih.gov/funding/training/naa*).

Dietary Carbohydrates

For the digestion of carbohydrates, adequate amylase activity is needed to break down food starches to disaccharides, and then specific intestinal enzymes are required to hydrolyze each of the disaccharides to their constituent monosaccharides. For the absorption of monosaccharides, diffusion or active transport is employed.

Dietary Fiber

Fibers are structural parts of plants, found in fruits, grains, legumes, and vegetables, which can have an impact on intestinal function. In general, soluble fibers (such as pectin from fruits and hemicellulose from oats, barley, and legumes) delay intestinal transit time, delay glucose absorption and limit cholesterol absorption, and provide a feeling of satiety from the meal. Soluble fibers have shown promise in improving glucose and cholesterol control and are encouraged in weight-loss regimens. By contrast, insoluble fibers (such as cellulose and lignins from whole grains, some vegetables) speed intestinal transit, increase fecal bulk, and slow starch hydrolysis and glucose absorption. Insoluble fibers are effective at preventing constipation and are believed to be important for prevention of diverticulosis.

Dietary Fat

Lipids and sterols include compounds with very different chemical and physical properties: triglycerides, diglycerides, monoglycerides, fatty acids, phospholipids, cholesterol, cholesterol esters, and bile acids. Lipids require the most complicated sequence of digestive and absorptive processes; fat-soluble vitamins are absorbed similarly. The digestion of dietary fats requires the action of lingual, gastric, pancreatic, and intestinal lipases to hydrolyze fatty acids from the glycerol backbone of triglycerides. The absorption of monoglycerides, glycerol, fatty acids, and fat-soluble vitamins requires emulsification by bile acids to carry these water-insoluble nutrients through the watery intestinal juices in order to allow them to diffuse across the cell membrane of enterocytes.

Dietary Protein

The digestion of proteins requires adequate gastric acidity to uncoil proteins and activate pepsin and intestinal and pancreatic proteases to complete the breakdown of proteins into their constituent amino acid components. Absorption occurs by a carrier-mediated process.

Malabsorption

Malabsorption involves defective digestion and absorption of carbohydrates, proteins, fats, vitamins, and minerals, either in combination or independently.

From a clinical standpoint malabsorption should be differentiated from maldigestion. A thorough history and a detailed physical examination are essential to detect the signs and symptoms of malabsorption. Successful management of malabsorption hinges on identifying the underlying defect and implementing specific therapy to correct it.

Defects Associated with Malabsorption

Four categories of defects have been identified as the major causes of malabsorption:

- Impairment of mechanical digestion
- Impairment of chemical digestion
- Impairment of solubilization
- Anatomic or pathologic impairment of absorption

Malabsorption of Specific Nutrients

Carbohydrate Malabsorption

Malabsorption of carbohydrates can cause osmotic diarrhea and other symptoms. The most common carbohydrate malabsorption syndrome is lactose intolerance. Lactose is a disaccharide found in milk and dairy products. Normally, lactose is hydrolyzed to glucose and galactose by an enzyme called *lactase*. Approximately 15% of whites; more than 80% of African-Americans, Asian-Americans, and Native Americans; and 50% of Hispanics are lactase deficient. The development of clinical symptoms, usually in late childhood to adulthood, of lactose intolerance—bloating, abdominal cramps, and diarrhea—depends on whether the level of lactase activity is adequate to hydrolyze the lactose load delivered to the intestine.

Medical nutrition therapy for lactose intolerance or lactase deficiency involves the following measures, individually or in combination, based on the severity of the patient's intolerance:

- Reducing or avoiding lactose intake (milk and dairy products)
- Pretreating milk with lactase derived from bacteria
- Ingesting only lactase-treated dairy products (such as Lactaid or Dairy Ease)

Individuals who avoid all products containing lactose will have difficulty meeting their daily calcium requirement. Calcium supplementation with 800 to 1200 mg per day calcium carbonate is advisable for these patients.

Fat Malabsorption

More than 99% of all ingested triglyceride is normally absorbed. A number of problems can arise in individuals whose intake of these substances exceeds their capacity to break them down.

Clinical Manifestations of Fat Malabsorption Malabsorption of fat can cause steatorrhea, the result of impairment of either the digestive or the absorptive process. Steatorrhea is described by patients as a frothy stool that floats in the toilet. They may also describe seeing oil droplets in the toilet bowl. If left untreated, clinical signs and symptoms of undernutrition, which can be secondary to fat malabsorption, include

- Weight loss, muscle wasting
- Failure to thrive, growth retardation, and fatigue, especially in infants, children, and adolescents
- Tetany, osteomalacia, bone pain, compression fracture of vertebral bodies due to hypocalcemia secondary to calcium and vitamin D malabsorption
- Infertility, dysmenorrhea, amenorrhea

In addition, fat malabsorption is often responsible for a number of fat-soluble vitamin deficiencies. Clinical signs vary as follows according to the vitamin deficiency involved:

Vitamin A: Night blindness, hyperkeratosis, skin changes
Vitamin D: Hypocalcemia, osteomalacia, rickets, hypophosphatemia
Vitamin K: Prolongation of prothrombin time, easy bruisability, osteopenia
Vitamin E: Neuropathy, hemolytic anemia

Renal Manifestations of Fat Malabsorption Oxalate stones, the primary renal manifestation of fat malabsorption, are generally caused by bile salt malabsorption resulting from a pathologic disease process in the intestinal lumen. Most dietary oxalic acid is normally precipitated in the lumen as calcium oxalate and excreted in the feces without being absorbed. However, in the presence of certain pathologic processes, such as ileal Crohn's disease or surgical resection of the ileum, the small bowel is unable to reabsorb bile salts. As a result, excess bile salts are lost in the stool and fatty acids are not emulsified adequately for absorption. Fatty acids in the bowel lumen bind calcium to form a calcium soap and are unavailable to bind with oxalate. Consequently, dietary oxalic acid in these patients binds with sodium to form sodium oxalate, which becomes available for colonic absorption.

After oxalate is absorbed in the colon, the kidney excretes it, which contributes secondarily to the formation of oxalate stones. In addition, these patients tend to be volume depleted secondary to diarrhea and may have concentrated urine, another factor contributing to increased precipitation of oxalate stones. To avoid the formation of stones, patients with bile salt malabsorption should avoid foods high in oxalate, such as spinach, rhubarb, cocoa, chocolate, tea, green beans, collards, kale, peanut butter, and beer. They should also drink adequate volumes of liquid to help dilute and flush through oxalate salts in the kidney. The use of bile acid resins to bind bile acids in the intestinal tract may also be helpful (see Chapter 11). Additionally, use of oral supplementation of calcium might bind the oxalate in the bowel and not permit its uptake in the colon.

Protein Malabsorption

Celiac disease, due to a sensitivity to the gliadin fraction of wheat or other similar proteins in rye and barley, may affect 1 in 250 people in the United States. Immunologic response to these proteins triggers an inflammatory process in the enterocyte, which results in malabsorption of many nutrients, including protein, carbohydrate, fat, vitamin K, folate, vitamin B_{12}, iron, and calcium. These patients may present with diarrheal symptoms, but the diagnosis is usually made by endoscopic biopsy or the presence of positive serologic antiendomysial antibodies, antigliadin, or tissue transglutaminase antibodies.

Medical nutrition therapy for celiac sprue involves strict elimination of foods containing wheat, rye, and barley. This diet can be difficult to follow, as many prepared foods have these grains as hidden ingredients. Prepared food items, which are guaranteed to be gluten free, carry an international symbol on the package. Gluten-free bread, cereal, and pasta products are available.

Clinical Conditions That May Cause Malabsorption

Acute and Chronic Pancreatitis

Most patients admitted to the hospital for acute pancreatitis have mild disease, precipitated by gallstones or alcohol use. In this setting, patients are prescribed nothing by mouth (NPO) for a short period of time or clear liquids with intravenous fluid for hydration.

A second group have more severe disease, with complications of other organ dysfunction (renal, pulmonary, hemodynamic instability) and frank pancreatic necrosis on computed tomographic (CT) scan. The length of hospital stay and mortality are increased with severe pancreatic disease. The method of feeding varies on a case-by-case basis. As with other patients, if they can tolerate oral or enteral feedings, this route is preferred over parenteral to reduce the risk of catheter-related sepsis and any potential enhancement of bacterial translocation. The presence of proteins and fat in the duodenum stimulates the release of the hormones secretin and cholecystokinin, both of which stimulate the pancreas. Therefore, when an enteral feeding catheter can be placed below the duodenum, pancreatic secretion is stimulated to a lesser degree, thus allowing bowel rest. If severe hemodynamic instability develops, however, enteral feedings are not usually given and parenteral support is used.

For chronic pancreatitis, fat malabsorption and severe abdominal pain, which limits food intake, are common. If chronic pancreatitis is associated with alcohol abuse, abstention from alcohol is encouraged. A low-fat diet and oral pancreatic enzyme replacement may be helpful for symptom control.

Cystic Fibrosis

Cystic fibrosis (CF) is commonly associated with pancreatic dysfunction, resulting in inadequate digestive enzymes, pancreatic juice, and bile in the intestinal lumen. Up to 90% of patients with the disease have such severe malabsorption that oral replacement of pancreatic enzymes is needed. Energy requirements are commonly increased due to the disease-related increased work of breathing. Thus, medical nutrition therapy for patients with CF includes encouragement of a high calorie–high protein diet with pancreatic enzyme replacement and a multivitamin supplement. When nutrition occurs, nighttime enteral feedings using a low-fat formula may be needed to supplement daily nutrient intake (see Chapter 10, Case 2).

Inflammatory Bowel Disease

Inflammatory bowel disease (IBD) refers to idiopathic, chronic, inflammatory conditions affecting the GI tract, primarily Crohn's disease and ulcerative colitis. Because of the chronic involvement of the GI tract, most patients with IBD have some form of nutritional malabsorption. Therefore, careful attention to the diet can prevent nutritional deficiencies and help in the medical and surgical management of these diseases.

Protein-energy undernutrition is prevalent among patients with IBD. Nutritional assessment is essential because of the consequences of undernutrition, which include growth retardation in children, impaired healing of the inflamed and damaged bowel, and enhanced susceptibility to infection in children and adults. In addition, an undernourished patient with IBD may present with defects in GI function that further limit the absorption and utilization of nutrients.

Causes of Undernutrition

Undernutrition occurs in patients suffering from IBD as a consequence of

- Decreased dietary intake
- Increased nutrient losses
- Increased nutrient requirements

Decreased Dietary Intake

The most important factor contributing to the poor nutritional status seen in patients with IBD is inadequate dietary intake. GI symptoms, such as nausea, diarrhea, and recurrent abdominal pain at mealtimes, often decrease appetite and food intake. Also, eating certain foods, such as high-insoluble fiber foods, in Crohn's disease with strictures may precipitate an obstruction.

Increased Nutrient Losses

In Crohn's disease, small and large bowel inflammation, bacterial overgrowth, and multiple bowel resections can decrease the absorptive surface area of both the small and large intestine and cause malabsorption of essential nutrients. Resections of the ileum can cause bile salt deficiency, resulting in steatorrhea or fat malabsorption and subsequent deficiency of the fat-soluble vitamins (A, D, E, and K). Vitamin B_{12} binds with intrinsic factor, a protein that is secreted by the parietal cells of the stomach. Because the vitamin B_{12}-intrinsic factor complex is absorbed in the ileum, complete ileal resection produces a vitamin B_{12} deficiency that requires treatment with parenteral repletion (intramuscular injections of this vitamin or use of vitamin B_{12} nasal spray).

IBD also can result in protein-losing enteropathy or excessive intestinal secretion of protein-rich fluids through the inflamed bowel wall. Patients with IBD may also present with severe diarrhea or GI bleeding that can cause depletion of electrolytes, minerals such as iron, and trace elements such as zinc.

Increased Nutrient Requirements

The inflammatory process of IBD may increase resting energy expenditure, thereby contributing to weight loss and depleted fat stores if patients are not consuming adequate calories. Patients with fever or sepsis and those undergoing surgery also have greater requirements for protein, calories, and other nutrients than do patients who are less severely ill. Increased intestinal cell turnover can also raise nutrient requirements in patients with IBD.

Medical Nutrition Therapy for Inflammatory Bowel Disease

- Prevent symptoms associated with malabsorption
- Correct and prevent nutritional deficiencies
- Promote healing of the intestinal mucosa
- Minimize stress on inflamed and often narrowed segments of the bowel (Crohn's disease)
- In children, promote normal growth and development

Nutritional repletion by oral diet may be difficult to achieve during symptomatic, active IBD, since most patients' symptoms worsen during and after meals. To decrease the symptoms associated with eating and bowel activity during the healing process, patients hospitalized for IBD are sometimes placed on bowel rest. However, prolonged bowel rest without enteral or parenteral nutritional support can lead to nutritional depletion. An oral diet may be tolerated when active IBD is less severe. To control diarrhea and malabsorption, a low-fat, low-fiber, low-lactose diet is often prescribed. Small, frequent feedings may help to limit gastrointestinal secretions as well as reduce the volume of food that the damaged bowel must handle at any one time.

Calories

In adults, calories should be provided in amounts sufficient to maintain or restore body weight. In children, caloric supply should be adequate to support growth and development. Complications, such as sepsis and fistulas, may increase caloric requirements in adults to 35 to 45 kcal/kg per day, or approximately 1.5 to 1.7 times the basal energy expenditure according to the Harris-Benedict equation. Glucose polymers or medium-chain triglyceride (MCT) oil, which are undetectable when added to foods or beverages, can be used as caloric supplements.

Protein

Protein needs may be as high as 1.5 to 2.5 g/kg per day, compared with the recommended dietary allowance (RDA) of 0.8 g/kg per day in adults. The exact value depends on the degree of catabolism and protein losses in individual patients and can be evaluated in hospitalized patients by measurement of nitrogen balance.

Vitamins and Minerals

Because patients with IBD are at higher risk for vitamin, mineral, and trace element deficiencies, their diets should be supplemented with a multivitamin and mineral preparation that contains one to five times the normal recommended dietary allowance. Repletion doses of specific nutrients are indicated if clinical signs (such as anemia, peripheral neuropathy, or night blindness) or laboratory evidence show a deficiency. If the terminal ileum has been affected or resected, patients are likely to suffer from defective vitamin B_{12} absorption and require intramuscular administration or nasal spray supplements. IBD patients with persistent, watery diarrhea may require zinc and magnesium supplementation. Chronic blood loss and altered iron absorption, frequently observed in IBD, can cause iron-deficiency anemia. However, iron supplements in full therapeutic doses may exacerbate "GI distress." In particular, oral iron may cause symptoms of nausea, constipation, and abdominal cramping.

Long-term treatment with corticosteroids reduces the absorption and increases excretion of calcium. Oral calcium and vitamin D supplements are needed to avoid the development of osteoporosis. Patients treated with sulfasalazine (Azulfidine) should receive folate supplements because this medication inhibits uptake of folate by competitive inhibition of the enzyme, folate conjugase, in the jejunum.

Fiber

A low-fiber diet is often prescribed for patients with narrowed sections of bowel to decrease the possibility of intestinal obstruction, to minimize mechanical irritation to the inflamed bowel, to reduce stool weight and frequency, and to slow the rate of intestinal transit. The diet consists of white bread and refined cereals and avoidance of high-fiber fresh fruits and vegetables, nuts, skins, and seeds. Some controversy exists over the benefits of a low-fiber diet for these patients when their disease is quiescent. Research suggests that the short-chain fatty acids derived from bacterial digestion of fiber may be beneficial against IBD (see Appendix).

Lactose

Patients with IBD may malabsorb lactose because of decreased brush border epithelial cell lactase activity and rapid intestinal transit, although the incidence of lactose intolerance among those suffering from IBD is no greater than that of the general population. Patients may avoid lactose during or immediately after a disease flare but return to lactose-containing products a few weeks later.

Fat

Decreased fat intake may help control the symptoms of steatorrhea, especially in patients with Crohn's disease involving the small bowel. Omega-3 fatty acids to treat patients suffering from ulcerative colitis and Crohn's disease who are unresponsive to other treatment modalities are under investigation.

Nutrition Support for Inflammatory Bowel Disease

Enteral feedings by tube or oral formula may be indicated in severe flares of IBD to allow bowel rest during healing or to enhance absorption with minimal gastrointestinal symptoms. Liquid formulas used should be low in fat and fiber content and lactose-free. Tolerance and absorption may be enhanced with the use of a formula providing protein as peptides, rather than whole proteins. Formulas are also designed with the protein content as amino acids, called *elemental diets,* to eliminate the need for protein digestion (see Chapter 12). If the Crohn's disease flare is severe and includes the presence of a small bowel fistula (hole in the intestinal tract with leakage of intestinal fluids through the skin), a course of total parenteral nutrition can be considered to permit nutrient supply and to aid fistula healing (see Chapter 13).

Short Bowel Syndrome

The loss of intestinal length, due to surgical resection for thrombosis or disease, can severely limit the digestion and absorption of many nutrients. When less than 100 cm functional small intestine remains, the disorder is termed *short bowel syndrome,* and a course of total parenteral nutrition is usually necessary. Malabsorption of nutrients is most severe when no colon remains and when the disease process (often Crohn's disease or radiation enteritis) leaves the existing bowel with impaired functionality. With short bowel syndrome, a process of bowel adaptation may occur over 1 to 2 years in response to nutrient supply in the intestinal lumen, although the success of this process depends on the remaining length and type of bowel and its health. Some patients require parenteral nutrition support for the rest of their lives or until intestinal transplantation.

Medical Nutrition Therapy for Short Bowel Syndrome

Medical nutrition therapy for short bowel syndrome includes the provision of adequate amino acids, glucose, lipids, electrolytes, fluid, vitamins, and minerals to support nutrient needs by chronic total parenteral nutrition, usually delivered in the home setting. As the process of bowel adaptation proceeds, the supply of nutrients by the parenteral route is reduced. Continuation of oral food intake is a key factor in the promotion of bowel adaptation. Even though patients absorb less than 50% of all nutrients during the early days with short bowel syndrome, this percentage can increase over time. Ingestion of simple sugars is generally associated with increased diarrhea, but complex carbohydrates aid the process of adaptation. Fat malabsorption lags behind the absorption of carbohydrates and proteins because of the loss of bile acids in diarrhea or ileal resections limiting bile acid reabsorption. Oral fluids, such as soup broth, that contain sodium promote the absorption of fluid as well as sodium.

Gastric Disorders

Gastroesophageal Reflux Disease

Gastroesophageal reflux (GER) is the regurgitation of gastric contents into the esophagus through the lower esophageal sphincter (LES), typically due to transient, increased abdominal pressure or relaxation of the LES. When the gastric acid, bile, and pepsin in the stomach have frequent, prolonged contact with the esophagus, gastroesophageal reflux disease (GERD) may develop, and the patient becomes symptomatic. Heartburn, described as a burning epigastric or substernal pain, is a major symptom of GERD. Findings include a delayed esophageal clearing rate, weak or incompetent LES, delayed gastric emptying, and irritation of the esophageal mucosa. LES tone plays an important role in preventing GERD. If the pressure of the LES is not greater than the pressure in the stomach, the contents of the stomach will back up into the esophagus.

Medical Nutrition Therapy for Gastroesophageal Reflux Disease

Because the severity of symptoms varies greatly among individuals with GERD, medical nutrition therapy is based on the individual's tolerance to foods and beverages that may cause discomfort.

The goals of medical nutrition therapy for patients with GERD include:

* Avoiding decreases in LES pressure
* Decreasing the frequency and volume of the refluxate
* Reducing irritation of sensitive or inflamed esophageal tissue
* Improving esophageal clearing ability

Maintaining Lower Esophageal Sphincter Pressure A major goal in the treatment of GERD is to avoid decreasing LES pressure. From a nutritional standpoint, the following measures have proved to be helpful:

* *Limiting dietary fat intake:* High-fat meals tend to decrease LES pressure and delay gastric emptying time. As a consequence, the time that the esophagus is exposed to irritants increases, as does the gastric volume available for reflux.
* *Losing weight if obese:* Obesity affects GERD by increasing abdominal pressure and thus the likelihood of reflux.
* *Limiting alcohol, chocolate, and coffee:* These substances decrease LES pressure. Alcohol is also a powerful stimulus of gastric acid secretion.

Decreasing Reflux Frequency and Volume The following steps have proven useful to decrease the frequency and volume of GER:

- Eating small, frequent meals
- Drinking most fluids between meals rather than with meals
- Consuming adequate fiber to avoid constipation because straining increases intra-abdominal pressure

Decreasing Esophageal "Irritation" To decrease "irritation" in the esophagus, patients with GERD should monitor their dietary intake in the following ways:

- Limit intake of citrus fruits (oranges, grapefruits, lemons), tomato products, spicy foods, and carbonated beverages. Although most of these foods do not irritate the esophagus, they can cause heartburn and other GER symptoms in individuals with a sensitized esophagus.
- Avoid any other foods that regularly cause heartburn.

Improving Esophageal Clearing Time To improve clearing of food from the esophagus, patients should take the following precautions:

- Do not recline after eating. Sit upright or take a walk.
- Avoid eating for at least 2 to 3 hours before bedtime (or before assuming a supine position).
- Elevate the head of the bed.

Peptic Ulcer Disease

The goals of nutritional intervention in the treatment of peptic ulcer disease (PUD) are to reduce and neutralize the secretion of stomach acid and to maintain the resistance of the GI epithelial tissue to the acid. Traditionally, patients were prescribed special bland diets that restricted the intake of foods and beverages that were thought to irritate the gastric mucosa or produce excessive acid secretion.

Randomized, controlled clinical trials have shown no difference between unrestricted and therapeutic diets with regard to healing of the ulcer or remission of symptoms. In addition, foods with high protein content, such as milk and eggs, were found to be the most powerful stimuli of acid secretion, an outcome contrary to the goals of diet therapy in these patients. Therefore, current therapy is based on the individual's tolerance to foods and beverages that may cause discomfort. Nutritional advice is offered as an adjunct to conventional medical and pharmacologic therapy in order to reduce gastric acid secretion.

Medical Nutrition Therapy for Peptic Ulcer Disease

The acid-secreting parietal cells lie mostly in the fundus of the stomach. The sight or smell of food or distention of the stomach triggers neurally mediated reflexes, which stimulate acid secretion from the parietal cells. Caffeine and other alkaloids in coffee, polypeptides and amino acids (products of protein digestion), and alcohol stimulate the release of the hormone gastrin, thereby triggering gastric acid secretion. Although alcohol and caffeine consumption have not been directly implicated in the development of PUD, excessive intake of these substances may cause abdominal discomfort. In addition, individuals who abuse alcohol appear to have an increased risk of developing PUD. Therefore, patients with PUD should be advised to:

- Limit caffeine intake by reducing consumption of coffee, tea, cola, chocolate, and other foods and beverages that contain caffeine
- Limit alcohol intake and avoid drinking on an empty stomach
- Avoid cigarette smoking, which may increase gastric acid secretion and delay the healing process; cigarette smoking has also been associated with an increased frequency of duodenal ulcers
- Eat three meals daily, avoid skipping meals, and limit intake of spicy, fatty, or otherwise bothersome foods
- Avoid bedtime snacks to prevent acid secretion since symptoms often occur in the middle of the night

Dumping Syndrome

When surgical treatment for gastric disease results in removal or bypass of the pyloric sphincter, symptoms of dumping syndrome may occur as the food bolus enters the duodenum in a rapid, uncontrolled fashion. The symptoms include dizziness, diaphoresis, diarrhea, and sometimes hypoglycemia.

Medical Nutrition Therapy for Dumping Syndrome

- Limit simple sugar intake
- Emphasize high-protein, high-fat foods
- Eat small, frequent meals with snacks

Colonic Disorders

Constipation

Constipation describes the common symptom of infrequent bowel movements or the need to strain to have bowel movements. In addition to limited dietary fiber intake, this disorder can result from inadequate fluid intake for hydration of the fecal stream, side effect of medications, lack of physical activity, or severe electrolyte imbalances.

Medical Nutrition Therapy for Constipation

- Drink plenty of fluids daily (>64 oz per day)
- Gradually increase the fiber content of the diet to 25 g per day by increasing intake of whole grains, vegetables, fruits, and legumes; rapid increases in fiber intake are associated with abdominal discomfort (see Appendix)
- Take foods with a natural laxative effect, such as prunes, prune juice

Diarrhea

Diarrhea describes the common complaint of the passage of frequent, watery bowel movements. These symptoms can be related to medications, hospital procedures, nonabsorbable sugars such as sorbitol or lactulose, or overgrowth of *Clostridium difficile* in patients who are immunosuppressed or after antibiotic treatment. *C. difficile* bacteria grow out of proportion to usual bacteria and produce a toxin that causes diarrhea. It is usually not necessary to hold oral diets or enteral feedings, but antimotility medications should be avoided. *C. difficile* can progress to colonic perforation, although this is uncommon. If diarrhea is severe and prolonged, undernutrition and dehydration may result.

Medical Nutritional Therapy for Diarrhea

- Replace fluid and electrolytes losses with water, juices, Gatorade
- Discontinue (if possible) sorbitol- or lactulose-containing medications
- If solid foods are tolerated, encourage yogurt (to replace commensal gut flora) and avoid insoluble fiber (whole grains) to slow transit time
- If diarrhea is chronic, increasing soluble fiber intake may be helpful

Diverticulosis

Low-fiber diets and constipation have been associated with the development of colonic diverticulosis. The prevalence of this disorder increases with aging, with half of 60- to 80-year-olds and nearly 100% of people over 80 in the United States having this disorder. When the diverticuli burst and allow bowel contents to leak into the mesentery or peritoneal cavity, the disease is called *diverticulitis* and requires surgical intervention. When diverticulitis develops in an individual with diverticulosis, medical nutrition therapy changes. Instead of recommending a high-fiber diet, a low-fiber diet is advised. This allows the passage of stool through the inflamed, typically narrowed segment of the colon. Medical nutrition therapy for the prevention of future diverticuli encompasses increasing the insoluble fiber content of the diet. When diverticulitis occurs, the guidelines are to reduce fiber intake to avoid any mechanical obstruction of the bowel with undigested fiber. Drinking adequate fluids (64 oz per day) is important for both disorders, although the evidence to support how much is needed is limited.

Colorectal Cancer

Cancer of the colon or rectum is a disease process that is diagnosed more commonly after the age of 50 but is a chronic process that may take 10 years to develop (i.e., the progression from a polyp to a cancer). Inflammatory bowel diseases, both ulcerative colitis and Crohn's colitis (Crohn's disease involving the colon), are associated with an increased risk of colon cancer compared to the general population.

Epidemiologic data and experimental animal models suggest that a diet rich in fiber or wheat bran and low in fat is beneficial as a chemopreventive agent for the development of colon cancer. Short-term human trials, however, have not provided convincing evidence that these dietary changes are protective.

Liver Disease

The liver is involved in many of the body's metabolic processes, including regulation of protein, fat, and carbohydrate metabolism; vitamin storage and activation; and detoxification and excretion of waste products. Thus, impaired liver function can lead to nutrient deficiencies and, eventually, protein-energy undernutrition. Conversely, undernutrition can further impair liver function by affecting the liver's structural integrity. Of all active cases of cirrhosis in the United States, 90% are secondary to alcohol-related liver damage. Regardless of the cause, however, patients with cirrhosis usually present with some degree of muscle wasting and undernutrition.

Causes of Undernutrition in Patients with Liver Disease

- Poor dietary intake
- Maldigestion and malabsorption
- Abnormalities in the metabolism and storage of macro- and micronutrients

Poor Dietary Intake   Alcohol provides 7 kcal/g energy, but it contains no vitamins or minerals. Ingested alcohol is metabolized in preference to other nutrients and thus can use up vitamins needed for energy metabolism.

Patients with chronic liver disease frequently present with a poor dietary intake resulting from nausea, vomiting, diarrhea, abdominal pain, and early satiety. Ascites, resulting in distention of the abdominal cavity due to the accumulation of fluid, may also contribute to early satiety. Changes in mental status secondary to hepatic encephalopathy may also contribute to poor dietary intake in patients with advanced liver disease.

Maldigestion and Malabsorption   Individuals with chronic liver disease frequently present with both maldigestion and malabsorption of fat. High concentrations of alcohol can disrupt the gastric and duodenal mucosa, causing diarrhea and malabsorption of thiamine, folate, and vitamin B_{12}. Steatorrhea, the most common manifestation of malabsorption, occurs in approximately 50% of patients with cirrhosis. Cholestasis, which is associated with decreased bile salt secretion and pancreatic insufficiency, may contribute to fat malabsorption and subsequent fat-soluble vitamin (A, D, E, and K) deficiencies.

Abnormal Metabolism and Storage of Nutrients   Liver disease causes many metabolic problems and also affects the assessment parameters commonly used to evaluate a patient's nutritional status. Therefore, the severity of the patient's liver disease and the amount of fluid retention and ascites should always be taken into consideration when assessing nutritional status.

Medical Nutrition Therapy for Liver Disease

The goals of medical nutrition therapy for patients with liver disease are to provide adequate protein and calories to maintain nitrogen balance and support liver regeneration, while preventing such complications as encephalopathy. Abstinence from alcohol is an essential part of managing alcohol-related liver disease.

Calories An unrestricted diet is indicated for most patients with liver disease. Studies show no significant increase in energy requirements in liver disease. With ascites, calorie and protein requirements must be based on estimated "dry" weight, or total weight minus the estimated weight of the ascitic fluid. One liter of fluid is equivalent to approximately 1 kg body weight. When fluid is seen only in the abdominal cavity, the amount is at least 5 liters, or 5 kg body weight, and may be considerably more. If fluid is present in both the abdominal cavity and the lower extremities, the amount is estimated at 10 liters, or at least 10 kg body weight. Additional adjustments in energy needs must be made for superimposed infection, trauma, or surgery.

Fat Disturbances in fat metabolism can lead to decreased lipid clearance and increased serum triglyceride and cholesterol levels. Excessive alcohol consumption is associated with increased accumulation of triglycerides in hepatocytes, hepatic steatosis, or radiologic or biopsy studies.

Fat intake amounting to 20% to 40% of daily caloric requirements should be encouraged as tolerated in the absence of steatorrhea, because fat increases the palatability of the diet and adds calories. Providing fat calories in the form of oil composed solely of MCTs may be necessary in the presence of fat malabsorption. MCTs are more efficiently absorbed than long-chain triglycerides (LCTs) because they are absorbed directly into the portal vein by means of the lymphatics and subsequently are transported to the liver.

Protein Reduced hepatic synthesis of transport proteins may result in low serum albumin and transferrin values in these patients. Likewise, reduced synthesis of albumin can result in decreased serum oncotic pressure, the most probable cause of ascites and edema. Hepatic synthesis of clotting factors is also reduced, interfering with blood coagulation, as evidenced by a prolonged prothrombin time (PT) and partial thromboplastin time (PTT). Therefore, albumin and transferrin levels are not an accurate indicator of visceral protein status in advanced liver disease.

Positive nitrogen balance in patients with cirrhosis can be attained with an intake of 0.8 to 1.0 g/kg per day of estimated dry weight, or approximately 4 to 6 oz meat, fish, or chicken per day. At the onset of hepatic encephalopathy, precipitating factors, such as infection, electrolyte imbalance, and GI bleeding, should be identified and treated, but reduction in dietary protein intake should be initiated only if hepatic encephalopathy persists. Dietary protein intake may be restricted for a short period of time to 0.6 g/kg per day to reduce plasma ammonium production as a byproduct of protein metabolism. Drastic, long-term protein restriction is not indicated and may exacerbate protein malnutrition by promoting autocatabolism of muscle and reducing host defenses against infection. Protein restriction should be individualized and based on tolerance. Protein, 40 to 60 g per day (2 to 3 oz per day of meat, fish, or chicken) is the initial recommendation. With improvement in mental status, protein intake can be increased by increments of 10 to 15 g per day to attain the maintenance levels of 0.8 to 1.0 g/kg per day using estimated dry weight.

Carbohydrate Liver disease can also lead to disturbances in glucose metabolism, resulting in hypoglycemia or hyperglycemia. The hypoglycemia sometimes seen in acute liver disease may be due to impaired glycogenesis, glycogenolysis, and gluconeogenesis. Hyperglycemia, often observed in cirrhosis and chronic hepatitis, may be associated with increased glucagon levels and insulin resistance.

Sodium In the patient with ascites or edema, sodium and fluid should be restricted, but the extent to which sodium needs to be restricted is controversial. Some support the view that moderate sodium restriction (2 to 3 g per day), coupled with effective diuretics, can make the diet more palatable and nutritious. Cirrhotic patients have limited ability to excrete sodium, and some may require restriction initially to less than 1 g sodium per day. Once diuresis occurs, the diet can be liberalized.

Fluid By consensus, patients with hyponatremia (serum sodium under 130 mEq/L) require a fluid restriction of 1000 to 1500 mL per day. Fluid imbalances in liver disease generally make body weight and serum albumin levels unreliable indicators of nutritional status. Serum albumin levels may be falsely elevated if the patient is dehydrated or falsely decreased if the patient is in fluid overload. Massive fluid shifts result from edema, ascites, and diuretic therapy in these patients. Hypoalbuminemia is associated with a fluid shift from the intravascular space to the extravascular space.

Vitamins and Minerals Patients with chronic liver disease are at risk for vitamin and mineral deficiencies secondary to poor intake, malabsorption, impaired metabolism, and decreased storage. The physical examination therefore should include evaluation of the physical signs and symptoms of vitamin and mineral deficiencies. A combined multivitamin and mineral preparation should be routinely provided for patients with chronic liver disease. If the patient is still consuming alcohol, thiamine and folate supplements must be prescribed to prevent Wernicke's encephalopathy and macrocytic anemia, respectively. Patients with advanced chronic liver disease may have problems with vitamin storage, metabolism, and transport and thus may require subcutaneous injections of vitamins.

For a list of references for this chapter, please visit the University of Pennsylvania School of Medicine's Nutrition Education and Prevention Program web site: *http://www.med.upenn.edu/nutrimed/articles.html*

Case 1

Alcohol and Vitamin Deficiencies

Gail Morrison and Lisa D. Unger

Objectives

- Explain how excessive alcohol consumption contributes to nutritional deficiencies.
- Describe the biochemical and pathophysiologic abnormalities that occur with excessive alcohol intake.
- Recognize the importance of assessing a patient's alcohol intake during a routine social history.
- Describe the nutritional recommendations for patients who consume alcohol.

CT, a 52-year-old car salesman, presents to his family physician for his yearly physical examination reporting fatigue, burning in his feet, decreased memory, and heartburn. He has also noticed a recent weight gain and increased waist circumference and complains of increase in abdominal girth in association with weight gain and decreased endurance when exercising. He denies blurred vision, headaches, night sweats, or hearing loss.

Past Medical History

CT has no prior history of heart disease, stroke, or peripheral vascular disease. He has been told in the past that his liver is "damaged," but he has never received specific treatment for this. He is not taking any medications and has no known drug or food allergies.

Social History

CT states that he usually consumes three "healthy" meals every day, but his appetite has been poor for the past week. He has smoked one pack of cigarettes per day for 30 years (30 pack year history).

Family History

CT's family history is negative for the presence of heart disease, stroke, cholesterol and lipid disorders, or neurologic diseases.

Review of Systems

General: The patient reports lethargy, decreased appetite, and recent bloating; he relates that his pants are tighter in the waist than usual.

GI/abdomen: No vomiting or diarrhea.

Neurologic: No history of seizures, no tinnitus, no syncope. He has reported some memory loss.

Physical Examination

Vital Signs

Temperature: 98.2°F (36.8°C)

Heart rate: 104 beats per minute (BPM)

Respiratory rate: 16 BPM

Blood pressure: 120/90 mm Hg

Height: 5'8" (173 cm)

Current weight: 160 lb (73 kg)

Usual weight (1 month ago): 150 lb (68 kg)

BMI: 24 kg/m²

General: Well-dressed man who appears to be in mild distress

Skin: Jaundiced; spider angiomas on the upper chest (central blood vessels feeding small, dilated vessels, characteristic of chronic liver disease)

Eyes: Pale conjunctiva, sclera icteric; no ophthalmoplegia or nystagmus

Cardiac: Resting tachycardia; heart sounds are normal; no murmurs present

Chest/pulmonary: Lungs clear to auscultation and percussion bilaterally; mild gynecomastia (excessive development of male mammary glands)

Abdomen: Distended abdomen; presence of an abdominal fluid wave and shifting dullness, consistent with ascites (physical finding of fluid accumulation in the peritoneal cavity that can be associated with severe liver disease); enlarged liver size (14-cm span) with a firm, nontender edge; no splenomegaly

Extremities: Slight (1+) bilateral lower-extremity edema

Neurologic: Decreased vibratory sensation in the lower legs; bilaterally decreased knee reflexes; no asterixis; normal sensation and position sense in upper and lower extremities; cranial nerves II through XII grossly intact

Mental status: Alert; oriented to time, place, and person

Laboratory Data

Patient's Values	Normal Values
Red blood cells	
(RBC): 3.8 million/mm³	4.3–5.9 million/mm³
Hemoglobin: 10 g/dL	13.5–17.5 g/dL

Hematocrit: 35%	41%–53%
Mean corpuscular volume	
(MCV): 104 fL	80–100 fL
Albumin: 2.8 g/dL	3.5–5.8 g/dL
Prothrombin time: 15 s	11.0–13.2 seconds
International Normalized Ratio	
(INR): 1.3	1.0
Total bilirubin: 5 mg/dL	0.1–1.0 mg/dL
Aspartate aminotransferase	
(AST): 140 U/L	8–20 U/L
Alanine aminotransferase	
(ALT): 80 U/L	8–20 U/L
Sodium: 135 mmol/L	133–143 mmol/L

Case Questions

1. What additional information is important to obtain from a patient who presents with these symptoms?
2. What are the biochemical consequences of excessive alcohol consumption?
3. What is the prevalence of alcoholism in the United States, and what are the associated medical consequences?
4. What are the nutritional consequences of excessive alcohol consumption?
5. What evidence from CT's history, physical examination, and laboratory data suggests complications of alcoholism and nutritional deficiencies?
6. What does CT's serum albumin level indicate?
7. What additional laboratory tests would you request before giving CT a folate supplement?

Case Answers

1. **What additional information is important to obtain from a patient who presents with these symptoms?**

   Assessment of a patient's alcohol intake should always be included in the social history because many people who actively drink alcohol may not voluntarily admit to having a drinking problem. In addition, particular attention must be paid to those signs, symptoms, and laboratory tests that are likely to be abnormal in the alcoholic patient. Neurologic signs, combined with fatigue, gynecomastia, ascites, enlarged liver, possible gastroesophageal reflux, and abnormal liver function tests, all alert the clinician to probe for chronic alcohol ingestion. Once the patient admits to drinking, specific information regarding quantity, type, frequency, and duration of consumption should be obtained.

CT has been drinking heavily for 10 years. His daily routine consists of two cocktails before dinner, a few glasses of wine with dinner, and two cocktails after dinner, totaling six drinks per day. Considering that CT is a heavy drinker, as evidenced by his consumption of 42 drinks per week, he is a candidate for the CAGE test. The CAGE test was developed as a diagnostic tool for alcoholism. CT is asked the following questions, which are assigned a value of one point if answered "yes."

Have you ever felt you should Cut down on your drinking? _____(Yes)

Have people Annoyed you by criticizing your drinking? _____(No)

Have you ever felt bad or Guilty about your drinking? _____(Yes)

Have you ever had a drink the first thing in the morning

(Eye opener) to steady your nerves or to get rid of a hangover? _____(No)

When interpreting the CAGE test, one should take into account the patient's answers to the preliminary questions about alcohol use. A key question is, "When was the last time you had a drink?" Because CT reports drinking within the past 30 days and scored two on the CAGE test, he is very likely to have a current alcohol problem.

2. **What are the biochemical consequences of excessive alcohol consumption?**

    Excessive alcohol consumption can cause metabolic acidosis by interfering with the oxidation of acetyl coenzyme A (CoA) in the tricyclic antidepressant (TCA) cycle. Ethanol is oxidized to acetaldehyde by the enzyme alcohol dehydrogenase, which also simultaneously reduces nicotinamide adenine dinucleotide (NAD^+) to nicotinamide adenine dinucleotide (NADH) + H^+. Next, the enzyme acetylaldehyde dehydrogenase oxidizes acetaldehyde to acetyl CoA and reduces another NAD^+ to NADH + H^+. This enzyme requires NAD^+ to accept the hydrogen ions.

    The increased ratio of NADH to NAD^+ in the presence of excess alcohol, called an *altered redox state*, drives pyruvate to lactate instead of to acetyl CoA. High levels of lactate generated from pyruvate suggest an abnormality in the recycling of NADH to NAD^+ caused by excessive alcohol ingestion. In addition, instead of entering the TCA cycle, where more NADH is produced, acetyl CoA is converted to ketone bodies and fatty acids. As a result, a ketoacidotic state develops and fatty acids are converted to triglycerides. In turn, a significant rise in triglyceride levels can lead to fatty liver (Figure 8-1).

3. **What is the prevalence of alcoholism in the United States, and what are the associated medical consequences?**

    Alcoholism is a major problem in the United States. Each year, approximately 100,000 deaths in the United States are related to alcohol consumption. According to the 2000 National Household Survey on Drug

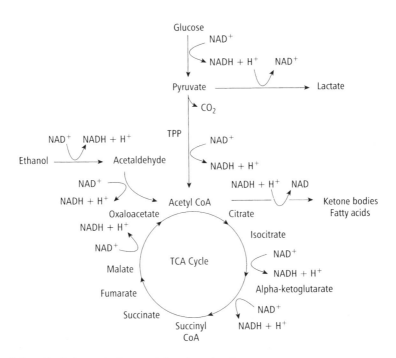

Figure 8-1 **Alcohol metabolism and the altered redox state.**

SOURCE: Adapted from Berg JM, Tymoczko JL, Stryer L. Biochemistry. 5th ed. New York: W.H. Freeman, 2002.

Abuse, almost half of Americans (46.6%) aged 12 and older reported being consumers of alcohol in some form or another. This translates into an estimated 103 million people. In addition, nearly 5.6% of people aged between 25 and 44 were heavy drinkers (5 or more drinks per day). The harm associated with the intake of large amounts of alcohol has been well documented.

Alcohol intake over 30 g per day (more than 2 drinks) has been associated with increased mortality due to hypertension, pancreatitis, gastrointestinal malignancies, stroke, cardiomyopathy, cirrhosis, motor vehicle accidents, and breast cancer. Alcoholics can also experience marital/family difficulties and also may lose their job as a result of work absenteeism. In addition, alcohol can interact with many different medications, affecting their potency.

4. **What are the nutritional consequences of excessive alcohol consumption?**

Alcohol provides 7 kcal/g, which can be used and metabolized when substituted for calories from food but provides no protein, vitamins, or minerals. Drinking causes a decrease in appetite that generally is proportional to the amount of ingested calories from alcohol and can significantly affect the nutritional adequacy of a patient's diet. High concentrations of alcohol can also disrupt the gastric and duodenal mucosa, affect the digestive and absorptive processes, and, as a consequence, reduce significantly the absorption of vitamins.

One of the most important vitamin supplements routinely given to alcoholics is thiamine (vitamin B_1), since alcohol interferes with thiamine absorption, even in healthy individuals. Thiamine is important in carbohydrate metabolism. Its predominant form, thiamine pyrophosphate (TPP), functions as a coenzyme for pyruvate dehydrogenase, which converts pyruvate to acetyl CoA. Inadequate thiamine intake forces pyruvate to be converted to lactate, further contributing to the development of lactic acidosis (see Figure 8-1). Thiamine deficiency manifests as anorexia, irritability, fatigue, and decreased memory. Later stages present with peripheral neuropathy, confusion, and tachycardia.

Chronic alcohol consumption has also been associated with folate deficiency; however, the etiology is unclear. Alcohol may affect folate levels by decreasing dietary intake, impairing absorption and metabolism and increasing urinary excretion of folate, and may also be directly toxic to bone marrow and other cells. Tetrahydrofolate (THF), the coenzyme derived from this vitamin, is involved in one-carbon-unit transfers, including amino acid interconversions and purine and pyrimidine biosynthesis. The interconversion of homocysteine to methionine requires methyl THF as the coenzyme for methionine synthase. Vitamin B_{12} also acts as a cofactor in the methylation of homocysteine to methionine, in which methyl THF is converted to THF. As a result, in vitamin B_{12} deficiency, the demethylation of methyl THF is prevented, blocking folate metabolism or trapping folate.

Folate is also required for normal purine and pyrimidine biosynthesis. The methylation of deoxyuridine monophosphate (dUMP) to thymidine monophosphate (dTMP,) catalyzed by thymidylate synthase, requires 5,10-methylene THF, which is synthesized from THF.

Folate deficiency alters RBC production, resulting in enlarged, oval erythrocytes, manifested as megaloblastic anemia. It often cannot be distinguished from the anemia associated with a vitamin B_{12} deficiency. However, the neurologic abnormalities that occur with a vitamin B_{12} deficiency are rarely seen in folate deficiency.

5. **What evidence from CT's history, physical examination, and laboratory data suggests complications of alcoholism and nutritional deficiencies?**

Decreased lower-extremity reflexes, decreased lower-extremity vibratory sensation, and paresthesias are all neurologic signs and symptoms associated with thiamine deficiency due to prolonged alcohol abuse. The diagnosis of thiamine deficiency is highly likely because this patient has been drinking heavily for 10 years. This condition is considered a medical emergency because, if left untreated, it can progress quickly and cause irreversible damage.

This patient's hematology laboratory data reveal that anemia is present, which may explain his fatigue. An elevated MCV indicates the presence of large RBCs, a characteristic finding in megaloblastic anemia. Megaloblastic anemia can be caused by either vitamin B_{12} or folate deficiency; however, alcoholics are not usually vitamin B_{12} deficient.

6. **What does CT's serum albumin level indicate?**

   CT's serum albumin value may reflect moderately depleted protein status. Decreased albumin, however, may not accurately reflect protein status in patients with severe liver disease because albumin is synthesized in the liver and is also influenced by hydration status. Usually, the liver retains its capacity to produce albumin until end-stage liver disease. The liver also synthesizes the vitamin K–dependent clotting factors, which explains CT's prolonged prothrombin time, since the liver's ability to produce factors II, VII, IX, and X can be affected early in liver disease.

7. **What additional laboratory tests would you request before giving CT a folate supplement?**

   Serum and RBC folate and serum vitamin B_{12} levels should be checked. Serum folate levels are greatly affected by current diet intake; however, RBC folate levels are a better measure of tissue folate status. Although alcoholics are not usually vitamin B_{12} deficient, it is important to check CT for vitamin B_{12} deficiency, because if his megaloblastic anemia is due to vitamin B_{12} deficiency, prescribing folate without vitamin B_{12} will improve the anemia but mask the vitamin B_{12} deficiency and its progression, with the associated neurologic damage. It is important to remember that neurologic impairments due to vitamin B_{12} deficiency do not respond to folate supplementation alone; however, hematologic abnormalities do respond both to folate and to vitamin B_{12}.

   CT's results from the recommended tests support the diagnosis of folate deficiency.

CT's Values	Normal Values
Vitamin B_{12}: 520 pg/mL	220–960 pg/mL
Serum folate: 2 ng/mL	3.0–17.0 ng/mL
RBC folate: 90 ng/mL	280–903 ng/mL

   Based on his clinical presentation and laboratory data, CT should receive thiamine, folate, and multivitamin supplements, especially if he continues to drink alcohol. He should be advised to eliminate drinking alcohol and enroll in an appropriate outpatient therapy program.

Case 2

Malabsorption

Gary R. Lichtenstein and Barbara Hopkins

> **Objectives**
>
> • Evaluate the clinical, anthropometric, and laboratory data of a patient with malabsorption.
> • Explain how dietary factors affect a patient with malabsorption.
> • Identify nutrient deficiencies associated with malabsorption and develop a nutritional care plan to treat these problems.

JR, a 27-year-old graduate student, sustained a gunshot wound to his abdomen 5 years ago and subsequently underwent resection of approximately 75% of his small intestine. Postoperatively, he noted about five liquid bowel movements daily, described as oily and foul smelling, which have persisted until the present time. After surgery he did not seek medical follow-up.

Past Medical History

JR's history is significant for a gunshot wound, requiring intestinal resection of the ileum and most of the jejunum with anastomosis (surgical connection) of the proximal jejunum to the cecum. JR takes no medications.

Social History

After surgery JR was instructed to eat five to six small meals per day; to follow a high-calorie, high-protein diet with 5 to 10 g soluble fiber and a limited intake of oxalates; and to take a daily multivitamin and mineral supplement. JR chose to discontinue the vitamin and mineral supplement 1 year ago. He does not smoke cigarettes, but he reports drinking two beers per week and three cups of coffee daily. He states that he does not have the energy to exercise.

Diet History

JR states that the following recall is his "typical" intake.

JR's 24-Hour Dietary Recall

Breakfast (diner)

Fried eggs with margarine	2 large
Bacon	3 slices
White toast	2 slices (enriched)
Butter	2 Tbsp.
Coffee with sugar	2 cups, 4 packets

Snack (food truck)

Coffee with sugar	2 cups, 4 packets
Jelly doughnut	1

Lunch (fast-food)

Cheeseburger	1
French fries	2 small orders
Soda (cola)	16 oz (480 mL)

Dinner (home)

Baked ham	8 oz (227 g)
Baked potato with butter	1 medium, 2 Tbsp.
White bread	2 slices (enriched)
Butter	2 Tbsp.
Apple pie	$1/6$ of 9-in. pie
Coffee with sugar	1 cup, 2 packets

Snack (home)

Corn chips	3-oz bag (85 g)
Beer	12 oz (360 mL)

Total calories: 4472 kcal

Protein: 134 g (12% of calories)

Fat: 229 g (46% of calories)

Carbohydrate: 470 g (42% of calories)

Review of Systems

General: Weight loss (10 lb, or 4.5 kg over the past year), fatigue, and weakness. Appetite good, but patient reports that he must eat "twice as much food" as he did before his operation and that he still continues to lose weight.

Skin: Dry and scaly

Eyes: Difficulty driving at night due to poor night vision

GI: Five liquid bowel movements daily, described as oily and foul smelling

Physical Examination

Vital Signs

Temperature: 98.0°F (37°C)

Heart rate: 80 beats per minute (BPM)

Respiration: 16 BPM

Blood pressure: 94/60 mm Hg

Height: 5'10" (178 cm)

Current weight: 125 lb (57 kg; lost 40 lb, or 18 kg, since surgery 5 years ago)

Usual body weight: 165 lb (75 kg)

BMI: 18 kg/m^2

General: 27-year-old man who appears very thin and wears loose-fitting clothes

Skin: Flaky dermatitis, ecchymosis

Head: Bilateral temporal muscle wasting

Mouth: Glossitis, cheilosis

GI/abdomen: Protuberant abdomen, bowel sounds with no activity, no hepatosplenomegaly

Extremities: Skeletal pain, interosseous muscle wasting, subcutaneous fat wasting, skeletal muscle wasting

Laboratory Data

Patient's Laboratory Values	Normal Values
Albumin: 2.5 g/dL	3.5–5.8 g/dL
Calcium: 5.5 mg/dL	9–11 mg/dL
Vitamin B$_{12}$: 100 pg/mL	>220–960 pg/mL
Vitamin A: 13 mg/dL	28–94 mg/dL
Vitamin E	
Alpha-tocopherol: 3 mg/L	4.6–14.5 mg/L
Beta-gamma–tocopherol: 0.6 mg/L	1.4–4.8 mg/L
PT: 16 seconds	<11–15 seconds
Serum folate: 2.5 ng/mL	>3–17 ng/mL
Zinc: 300 mg/dL	550–1400 mg/dL
Magnesium: 1.2 mg/dL	1.8–2.9 mg/dL
Fecal fat (72 hours): 28 g	<6 g per day

Case Questions

1. Explain why JR continues to lose weight even though he eats a large volume of food.

2. What is the cause of JR's steatorrhea?

3. What are the causes and associated clinical signs or symptoms of each laboratory abnormality with which JR presents?

4. Using JR's actual body weight, calculate the percentage change from his usual weight and interpret these results.

5. What conclusions can you draw regarding the fat, calorie, vitamin, and mineral content of JR's diet?

6. How does JR's current caloric intake compare with his requirements?

7. JR notes that his symptoms worsen when he eats fried or fatty foods. What should be done to correct these symptoms and his laboratory abnormalities?

Case Answers

Part 1: Diagnosis

1. **Explain why JR continues to lose weight even though he eats a large volume of food.**

   Profound weight loss may be a result of the fat malabsorption (steatorrhea). Moreover, although luminal digestion of starch into oligosaccharides and proteins into oligopeptides should be unaffected, decreased small bowel surface area interferes with brush border and cytoplasmic digestion, as well as transport across enterocytes. Transit time through the small intestine is decreased in patients who have undergone partial resection. Therefore, reduced exposure of nutrients to the intestinal mucosa also interferes with optimal absorption.

2. **What is the cause of JR's steatorrhea?**

   JR does not have an ileum and thus is unable to reabsorb bile salts. Bile salts are essential for the absorption of fats and fat-soluble vitamins. Normally, bile salts are reabsorbed through the ileum, transported to the liver via the enterohepatic circulation, and recycled back to the intestinal lumen to meet the need for bile salts. After ileal resection, bile salt loss through the stool increases because these salts are no longer being absorbed. The liver increases bile salt production in an attempt to compensate for the losses but often fails to accommodate them adequately. As a result, absorption of fat, fat-soluble vitamins (A, D, E, and K), and calcium and magnesium decreases as the bile salt pool becomes depleted. In spite of greatly increased hepatic synthesis of bile salts, a deficiency of conjugated bile salts may result.

   Bile salt deficiency leads to impairment in the body's ability to incorporate ingested dietary lipids (primarily LCTs) into the micellar phase. This inability leads to decreased mucosal absorption of ingested lipids and fat-soluble vitamins, resulting in subsequent steatorrhea, a condition called *cholerrheic enteropathy*.

   When dealing with patients who have undergone ileal resection, it is important to remember that, although bile salt absorption occurs passively through the upper small intestine, active sodium-coupled uptake of bile salts in the ileum normally is responsible for retrieval of more than 95% of the intraluminal bile salts.

Part 2: Laboratory Evaluation

Several laboratory abnormalities were observed in this patient. JR's nutritional problems reflect his decreased small bowel absorptive area, which renders him less able to absorb fat, protein, carbohydrate, vitamins, and minerals.

3. **What are the causes and associated clinical signs or symptoms of each laboratory abnormality with which JR presents?**

    Albumin JR's value: 2.5 g/dL Normal value: 3.5 to 5.8 g/dL
    A serum albumin level of 2.1 to 2.7 g/dL is associated with a moderate degree of visceral protein depletion caused by decreased protein absorption.

    Calcium JR's value: 5.5 mg/dL Normal value: 9 to 11 mg/dL
    Most calcium absorption occurs in the duodenum, but all small intestinal segments absorb calcium. When adjustments are made for transit time and the relative lengths of the different intestinal segments, both the jejunum and ileum therefore contribute substantially to overall calcium absorption. JR's resection has substantially reduced the available absorptive surface area of the small intestine and thus accounts in part for his low serum calcium value.

    A second cause for the low serum calcium seen in this patient is the reduction in the size of the bile salt pool with impairment of micellar solubilization. This condition leads to decreased calcium absorption due to intraluminal binding of dietary calcium to unabsorbed fatty acids (soap formation). Third, vitamin D malabsorption and deficiency also lead to calcium malabsorption.

    Because calcium is bound to albumin, it is always important to determine the corrected calcium based on the patient's albumin level to account for the ionization of calcium in serum, which is determined by an equilibrium between calcium and protein. We use the following equation to determine the corrected calcium:

    $$(\text{Normal albumin} - \text{serum albumin}) \times (\text{correction factor}) + \text{serum calcium}$$

    $$\text{Correction factor} = 0.8 \quad \text{Normal albumin} = 4.0 \text{ g/dL}$$

    Therefore, in JR's case

    $$\text{Corrected calcium} = (4.0 - 2.5)(0.8) + 5.5 = 6.7 \text{ mg/dL}$$

    This calcium value of 6.7 mg/dL, corrected for JR's albumin level, still is not in the normal range of 9 to 11 mg/dL. JR suffers from hypocalcemia, a low serum calcium level. Evaluation of ionized calcium would help in assessing the severity of calcium depletion. Clinical manifestations of calcium deficiency include skeletal pain, tetany, paresthesia, osteoporosis, and stunted growth in children. Dietary sources that are high in calcium are recommended.

Vitamin B$_{12}$ JR's value: 100 pg/mL Normal value: >220 to 960 pg/mL
After vitamin B$_{12}$ complexes with the binding protein, intrinsic factor (which is produced in the stomach), it is absorbed in the terminal ileum. Patients who have undergone removal of the terminal ileum thus cannot absorb vitamin B$_{12}$ and require intramuscular injections of this nutrient to prevent long-term deficiency and associated peripheral neuropathy, which generally first becomes apparent after 5 to 10 years. An intranasal form of vitamin B$_{12}$ has gained favor. Clinical manifestations of vitamin B$_{12}$ deficiency include megaloblastic anemia, peripheral neuropathy, glossitis, and cheilosis. The only dietary sources of vitamin B$_{12}$ are foods of animal origin, such as meat, chicken, fish, eggs, and dairy products. Because JR has no ileum, dietary sources are insignificant since absorption is not feasible.

Vitamin A JR's value: 13 mg/dL Normal value: 28 to 94 mg/dL
Vitamin A, in the form of dietary retinyl esters, is hydrolyzed to retinol by pancreatic and intestinal brush border esterases before uptake from the gut lumen. Absorption occurs in the proximal small intestine and is aided by the presence of bile salts. Another source of retinol is the vitamin precursor beta-carotene. After uptake and transport, vitamin A is stored in the liver cells called *stellate cells,* previously known as *Ito cells.* Clinical manifestations of vitamin A deficiency include xerophthalmia (with clinical findings ranging from night blindness to corneal ulceration and irreversible blindness), poor wound healing, and loss of epithelial integrity (in the skin, GI tract, and urinary and respiratory systems). Dietary sources of vitamin A and beta-carotene include dark-green, leafy vegetables and deep-yellow or orange fruits and vegetables. These nutrients also are found in meats, wheat and rice germ, nuts, and legumes.

Vitamin E   JR's alpha-tocopherol value: 3.0 mg/L
            Normal value: 4.6–14.5 mg/L
            JR's beta-gamma–tocopherol value: 0.6 mg/L
            Normal value: 1.4 to 4.8 mg/L
Vitamin E is absorbed passively in the proximal small intestine. Bile salts serve as an important factor in normal vitamin E absorption. Like other fat-soluble vitamins, vitamin E is packaged into chylomicrons and delivered into the mesenteric lymphatics. It is stored primarily in the liver and in the adipose tissue. Clinical manifestations of vitamin E deficiency include neurologic dysfunction in the form of cerebellar ataxia, loss of deep tendon reflexes, and diminished vibratory and position sense. Hemolytic anemia is another significant consequence of vitamin E deficiency. Dietary sources of vitamin E are whole grains, vegetables, vegetable oils, and meats.

Vitamin K JR's PT: 16 seconds Normal PT: <11 to 15 seconds
Vitamin K is obtained from dietary sources and also produced by colonic flora. Absorption of vitamin K occurs primarily in the proximal small bowel and requires bile salts. Following intestinal absorption, vitamin K is taken up largely by the liver and accumulated in the microsomal fraction. In the liver, vitamin K is a required cofactor for the enzymatic gamma-carboxylation of glutamic acid on vitamin K–dependent coagulation proenzymes [factors II (prothrombin), VII, IX, and X] and other proteins involved in coagulation and fibrinolysis (proteins C, S, M, and Z). Clinical manifestations of vitamin K deficiency include prolonged clotting time, resulting in bleeding problems (oral, genitourinary, gastrointestinal, and skin). Long-term antibiotics may eliminate bacterial production of vitamin K for patients, rendering them prone to clinical deficiency if they do not receive exogenous sources of vitamin K. Dietary sources of vitamin K are the green leafy vegetables (spinach and kale), whole grains, liver, and nuts.

Folate JR's value: 2.5 ng/mL Normal value: >3 to 17 ng/mL
The jejunum absorbs folate for subsequent delivery into the portal circulation. After intestinal resection, the remaining portions of the small intestine may increase their uptake of folate to compensate for poor absorption. Serum folate levels reflect very recent dietary ingestion rather than total body folate stores. Therefore, a normal serum folate test does not exclude folate deficiency. A better reflection of total body folate stores would be an erythrocyte folate level. Clinical manifestations of folate deficiency include megaloblastic anemia and glossitis. Dietary sources of folate are dark-green leafy vegetables, oranges, orange juice, potatoes, yeast, red meat, eggs, and whole grains. Folate is easily destroyed in cooking or processing.

Zinc JR's value: 300 mg/dL Normal value: 550 to 1400 mg/dL
Zinc absorption occurs throughout the small intestine, but its rate of absorption is greater in the jejunum than in the ileum or duodenum. In patients who have undergone intestinal resection, transit time and surface area for absorption decrease, especially for zinc absorption. Intestinal reabsorption of zinc is impaired further in these patients because the jejunum and ileum have been removed. Clinical manifestations of zinc deficiency include anorexia, hypogeusia, alopecia, delayed onset of puberty, dermatitis, and poor wound healing. Oysters, meats, nuts, and legumes all constitute excellent dietary sources of zinc.

Magnesium JR's value: 1.2 mg/dL Normal value: 1.8 to 2.9 mg/dL
Magnesium is absorbed primarily in the jejunum and ileum by a passive mechanism. In patients with steatorrhea, unabsorbed fatty acids inhibit magnesium absorption by forming insoluble complexes in a reaction called *chelation*. Magnesium absorption is reduced in patients who have undergone small intestinal resections because of the decreased surface area available for this process. Clinical manifestations of magnesium deficiency

may include neuromuscular weakness, confusion, fatigue, tetany, and paresthesias. Dietary sources of magnesium include milk, cheese, yogurt, fruits, legumes, cereals, vegetables, fish, poultry, and meats.

Fecal Fat 28 g over 72 hours Normal <6 g per day
Normal fat excretion on a diet of 80 to 100 g fat is usually up to 6 g fat per day. A larger amount of fat excretion is associated with a disorder of fat digestion or fat malabsorption, or both.

Part 3: Clinical Assessment

4. **Using JR's current body weight, calculate the percentage change from his usual weight and interpret these results.**

$$\% \text{ Weight changes} = \frac{\text{usual weight} - \text{current weight}}{\text{usual weight}} \times 100$$

$$\% \text{ Weight changes} = \frac{165 \text{ lb} - 125 \text{ lb}}{165 \text{ lb}} \times 100 = 24\%$$

   A value of this magnitude indicates a clinically significant and severe weight loss.

5. **What conclusions can you draw regarding the fat, calorie, vitamin, and mineral content of JR's diet?**

   According to JR's 24-hour dietary recall, his diet is high in fatty and salty foods and sweets. JR's diet lacks foods from three major food groups: fruits, vegetables, and dairy products. The fact that he rarely selects foods from these food groups places him at high risk for vitamin and mineral deficiencies compounded by malabsorption of several vitamins and minerals.

6. **How does JR's current caloric intake compare with his requirements?**

   According to the Harris-Benedict and 35 kcal/kg equations, JR should consume 2700 to 2800 kcal per day to achieve a weight of 166 lb (75 kg). However, according to JR's actual intake, he is consuming 4472 kcal per day. Normally, fat weight gain can be expected even when excess intake amounts to only a few hundred calories, but JR's significant malabsorption problem has resulted in weight loss instead.

Part 4: Treatment

7. **JR notes that his symptoms worsen when he eats fried or fatty foods. What should be done to correct these symptoms and his laboratory abnormalities?**

   JR is experiencing fat malabsorption secondary to his surgery. Because his ileum was resected, JR cannot reabsorb the bile acids required for fat digestion. Thus, his dietary fat intake, at 46% of total calories, far exceeds his ability to digest and absorb fat properly. Referral to a registered dietitian for individualized counseling and reinforcement of the following suggestions are highly recommended in JR's case.

JR should be encouraged to eat small frequent meals and to decrease intake of fat at meals by limiting intake of fried and fast foods. However, because JR may find gaining weight difficult if his diet is too low in fat, monitoring his weight carefully is important. It should be noted, too, that not all patients with malabsorption require a low-fat diet. JR should consume a wide variety of foods and increase his intake of soluble fiber (e.g., legumes, fruits, oats). Because many patients with malabsorption due to intestinal resection tend to be lactose intolerant as a consequence of their reduced levels of lactase enzyme, a lactose-free diet may be beneficial.

Vitamin and mineral supplementation is indicated, since his surgery has significantly increased his intestinal motility and decreased transit time and the available absorptive area for the vitamins and minerals described previously. In addition, as a result of bile salt depletion, his absorption of fat and fat-soluble vitamins A, D, E, and K also has decreased. Other food factors that are troublesome in patients with resected small intestines include insoluble fiber (whole-wheat products), oxalates (chocolate, cocoa, coffee, and most berries, especially strawberries and cranberries), most nuts (especially peanuts), beans, beets, bell peppers, black pepper, parsley, rhubarb, spinach, Swiss chard, summer squash, sweet potatoes, tea, and concentrated sweets.

Case 3

Acquired Immunodeficiency Syndrome with Opportunistic Infection

Cade Fields-Gardner and Janet Hines

Objectives

- Assess the nutritional status of a patient with advanced human immunodeficiency virus (HIV) disease.
- Explain the nutritional consequences of weight loss, diarrhea, and malabsorption in patients with HIV disease.
- Develop appropriate medical nutrition therapy goals for patients with HIV disease.
- Describe the role of medications in supporting nutritional status in HIV disease.

MD is a 38-year-old man who presented to the outpatient clinic with weight loss. He was in his usual state of health until 3 years ago, when he presented to an AIDS Service organization (ASO) for an HIV test, shortly after his brother died of acquired immunodeficiency syndrome (AIDS). When the results came back positive, he was provided with a list of physicians and clinics for follow-up care. However, he stated that he felt well at that time and remained without complaints until 6 months before this presentation.

MD works in the construction industry as a finish carpenter. His daily activities were becoming increasingly limited by the several bouts of watery diarrhea, which was associated with nausea. MD compensated by reducing his food intake. After several days of decreased intake, his diarrhea would decrease, but he became weak and ultimately lost his appetite. His job was threatened by frequent absenteeism because of weakness and diarrhea.

MD noted additional weight loss and loose-fitting clothes. He denied fever, chills, night sweats, or muscle or joint pain.

Usual Dietary Intake

Food intake: Primarily crackers, rehydrating sports drinks, and juices, approximately 500 calories per day over the past 2 weeks

Alcohol intake: None recently

Tobacco: None

Intravenous (IV) drug use: None

Table 8-1   Body composition data.

PARAMETER	PATIENT'S VALUE	NORMAL VALUE
Fat-free mass (kg)	105.7	>102.3
Body cell mass (kg)	48.1	>55.4
Extracellular tissue (kg)	54.1	47–53
Fat (kg)	15	12–24
Mid-upper arm circumference (percentile)	27.5 cm (<5th percentile)	30.5–34.2 cm (25th–75th percentile)
Triceps fatfold (percentile)	4 mm (<5th percentile)	8–16 mm (25th–75th percentile)

Physical Examination

Vital Signs

Temperature: 97.0°F (36.1°C)

Heart rate: 100 beats per minute (BPM)

Respiration: 15 BPM

Blood pressure: 100/60 mm Hg

Height: 5'6" (173 cm)

Current weight: 117 lb (53 kg)

Usual weight (6 weeks ago): 145 lb (66 kg)

Percent weight change: 19% [145 to 117/145]

BMI: 18.9 kg/m²

General: Thin, cachectic man in no apparent distress

Skin: Cold, dry

Head/neck: Bilateral temporal wasting and nasolabial fat loss, thin hair

Mouth: Gums red around tooth edges

Cardiac: Normal

Abdomen: Bowel sounds present, scaphoid, soft, nontender, no organomegaly

Extremities: Interosseous muscle wasting bilaterally

Neurologic: Nonfocal grossly

Body Composition Data

See Table 8-1.

Laboratory Data

Patient's Laboratory Values	Normal Values
HIV viral load: >500,000 copies/mL	0 copies/mL
CD4 count: 50 cells/mm³	600–1800 cells/mm³
Albumin: 3.4 g/dL	3.5–5.8 g/dL
Hemoglobin: 10.0 g/dL	13.5–17.5 g/dL

Hematocrit: 31%	41%–53%
ALT: 22 U/L	0–35 U/L
AST: 22 U/L	0–35 U/L
Alkaline phosphatase (ALP): 160 IU/L	53–128 IU/L
Total cholesterol: 85 mg/dL	<200 mg/dL
Low-density lipoprotein (LDL) cholesterol: 60 mg/dL	<160 mg/dL
High-density lipoprotein (HDL) cholesterol: 20 mg/dL	>40 mg/dL
Triglycerides: 300 mg/dL	<150 mg/dL
Glucose: 120 mg/dL	70–110 mg/dL
Testosterone (total): 300 ng/dL	500–1000 ng/dL

Case Questions

1. Compare MD's weight and body composition to appropriate goal levels. What do the results suggest for his level of wasting and medical problems?
2. What factors have contributed to MD's wasting?
3. What is your overall impression of MD's nutritional status, and what intervention strategies should be initiated?
4. Based on MD's nutritional evaluation, what medical nutrition therapy is appropriate at this time?
5. What medical therapies may be necessary to improve MD's nutritional status?
6. Once MD is being treated with antiviral medications, what follow-up recommendations would be appropriate?

Case Answers

Part I: Nutrition Assessment

1. **Compare MD's weight and body composition to goal levels. What do the results suggest for his level of wasting and medical problems?**

   The Centers for Disease Control and Prevention (CDC) case reporting definition of AIDS includes a weight loss of greater than 10% with diarrhea or fever for more than 30 days. MD qualifies for that definition, but, of even more concern, his body composition suggests that he also qualifies for a more evidence-based definition of wasting that is associated with a significant decline in health and functional capacity (Table 8-2). MD has lost 28 lb (12.7 kg) or nearly 20% of his usual body weight. Although the fat-free mass level is adequate, the body cell mass compartment (muscle

Table 8-2   Definition of wasting.

- \>10% loss of weight over a 12-mo period
- \>7.5% loss of weight over a 6-mo period
- Body mass index (BMI) <20 kg/m^2
- 5% loss of body cell mass over a 6-mo period
- Body cell mass $<35\%$ of weight in men (if BMI <27 kg/m^2)
- Body cell mass $<23\%$ of weight in women (if BMI <27 kg/m^2)

SOURCE: Reprinted with permission from Polsky B, Kotler D, Steinhart C. HIV-associated wasting in the HAART era: guidelines for assessment, diagnosis, and treatment. AIDS Patient Care 2001;15:411–423.

and organ tissues) has been depleted by more than 16 lb (7.3 kg), or nearly 15% from ideal. The other portion of the fat-free mass, extracellular tissues (representing bone, collagen, and fluids outside of body cell mass), is slightly elevated. These values are calculated using Kotter's equations for body mass composition.

We would expect that with poor appetite and decreased food intake, along with diarrhea, MD would present with a picture of starvation in which all body compartments decline. In MD's case, even though there has been significant diarrhea, extracellular fluids are elevated, which is a common finding in the state of infection or injury. It may be suspected that in the absence of injury, the lack of fever with fluid shifts may indicate the presence of an underlying infection with severe body cell mass depletion and the inability to mount an adequate inflammatory response.

2. **What factors have contributed to MD's wasting?**

A combination of several factors contributed to wasting in MD's case. High HIV viral load and low CD4 counts increase his risk for an opportunistic infection, which can initiate weight loss and body cell mass wasting. Opportunistic infections are commonly complicated by the development of anorexia. Diarrhea can increase fluid and nutrient losses leading to wasting. Although serum testosterone levels are commonly low in HIV infection, a large weight loss can also lead to reduced testosterone synthesis, compromising the maintenance of body cell mass. In addition to total testosterone, free testosterone levels should be documented because globulin levels in HIV are frequently elevated, leading to an artificially normal testosterone.

3. **What is your overall impression of MD's nutritional status and what strategies should be initiated?**

MD's nutritional status is quite poor based on his weight, BMI, and body composition. Although his triglycerides are high, as would be expected during nonspecific inflammation or stress, the low-normal albumin and low cholesterol levels combined with anemia are findings consistent with the presence of advanced HIV disease. Intervention to improve nutritional status and reduce mortality includes both medical and nutritional management. MD's high viral load and very low CD4 count require treatment to limit the effects of HIV infection, immune suppression, and opportunistic infection on his poor nutritional status.

Simultaneously, expediting nutritional status restoration will be important to support both survival and adequate tissue stores to process and support the efficacy of anti-HIV and other medications. Additional support for the restoration of weight and body composition will be essential to improving MD's health status. These interventions may include adequate oral intake or enteral or parenteral nutrition support, additional medications, and social support strategies.

Part 2: Treatment and Management

4. **Based on MD's nutritional evaluation, what medical nutrition therapy is appropriate at this time?**

    Establishing a goal weight of 140 to 145 lb (64 to 66 kg) and restoration of body composition levels will help MD and his health care team formulate appropriate goals. These include adherence to anti-HIV therapies, diet adequacy, and increased physical activity. Dietary intervention should include both a personalized plan of action and education. Personalized exercise recommendations can be based on an evaluation by a physical therapist to evaluate capabilities and limitations or risks.

    In this case, nutritional repletion strategies should be approached with caution since the risks associated with refeeding include restoration of a capacity for mounting a difficult-to-control inflammatory response. Combined with the reconstitution of immunity after initiation of anti-HIV therapy, the ensuing inflammatory response can be substantial.

    Malabsorption may be an issue, and in severe cases, parenteral nutrition and fluid resuscitation can be considered. Some form of oral intake should be maintained, as it will be important to maintain gut integrity, particularly with HIV infection. Oral feeding strategies may include a low-residue diet in small, frequent meals to improve digestibility and possibly a lactose-free diet if he is lactose intolerant.

    Because MD is significantly underweight, it may be counterproductive to rely on an extremely restrictive diet (such as the "BRAT" diet: bananas, rice, apples, and toast) to help in controlling diarrhea. If such a diet is used, it should be followed for just a few days and replaced as quickly as possible with more calorically dense foods.

5. **What medical therapies may be necessary to improve MD's nutritional status?**

    Highly active antiretroviral therapy (HAART) should be introduced and may reduce the influence of HIV infection and immune suppression on nutritional status. A significant incidence of transient and intermittent side effects occurs with the introduction of antiretrovirals that can compromise nutritional status and therefore should be carefully monitored and treated as needed. Diarrhea should be worked up, and any appropriate treatments should be initiated for infection or other medical problems that contribute to diarrhea. In the case of general or fat malabsorption, diet strategies may include the use of lactase and pancreatic enzyme supplements to limit malabsorption. In select cases, antidiarrheal medications can be used to overcome short-term diarrhea problems, particularly if no pathogen is found and the abdominal examination is benign.

Because nearly 20% of baseline weight was lost and body cell mass is at a critically low level, one would expect a lower level of testosterone. Physiologic testosterone replacement strategies may include the use of topical gel, patches, or injections of testosterone. Levels of total and free testosterone should be monitored occasionally to assure maintenance of appropriate levels to improve well-being and restore normal muscle mass. Additional therapies that can be used as required include antinausea and appetite stimulation medications, growth hormone, anabolic steroids, and other symptom management and anabolic agents (Table 8-3).

Table 8-3   Examples of commonly used therapies to restore nutritional status.

CATEGORIES OF INTERVENTIONS

Nutrition	Diet therapy, supplements, enteral nutrition, parenteral nutrition
Exercise	Aerobic exercise, progressive resistance exercise
Appetite stimulants	Dronabinol (Marinol)
	Megestrol acetate (Megace)
Hormonal therapy	Replacement testosterone:
	Injection: testosterone cypionate
	Patch: Testoderm, Androderm
	Gel: Androgel
	Anabolic steroid: oxandrolone (Oxandrin), oxymetholone (Anadrol)
	Growth hormone: Serostim
Others	Insulin sensitizers: metformin (Glucophage), rosiglitazone (Avandia)
	Anticytokines: thalidomide (Thalidomid; not commonly used)

SOURCE: Cade Fields-Gardner, MS, RD, LD, CD, The Cutting Edge, 2002. Used with permission.

6. **Once MD is being treated with antiviral medications, what follow-up recommendations would be appropriate?**

MD initiated combination antiretroviral (anti-HIV) therapy and is monitored closely for symptom management. He continues to gain weight and body cell mass and has returned to a normal diet. MD is back on his construction job and doing well at this time.

MD's immune and nutritional recovery will require close monitoring to make sure he responds appropriately. For instance, while it is normal to replenish some fat tissues during the initial phases of nutrition intervention, body cell mass should return toward normal as body weight is increased. In addition, restored function of tissues should be monitored. MD should be encouraged to self-monitor weight and other body measures as well as to maintain an adequate nutrient intake in spite of bouts of diarrhea, should they continue. The normalization of testosterone levels and any need for additional anabolic therapies should be carefully monitored every few months. To enhance the efficacy of both nutrient and testosterone or other therapies, exercise should be encouraged.

Antiretroviral medications in all classes have been required by the Food and Drug Administration (FDA) to carry in their labeling the fact that use of the drugs may lead to altered fat metabolism and deposition, known as *lipodystrophy*. These complications are still a poorly understood disorder that entails the deposition or loss of fat in a number of body sites. Such alterations can have profound implications for the patient's health maintenance and well-being.

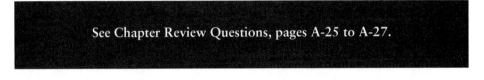

See Chapter Review Questions, pages A-25 to A-27.

9

Endocrine Disease: Diabetes Mellitus

Marion J. Franz and Stephen Havas

Objectives*

- Describe the most common macrovascular and microvascular complications associated with diabetes mellitus and describe the role of glycemic control, nutrition therapy, and exercise in reducing these complications.

- Summarize the current nutrition principles and recommendations for diabetes developed by the American Diabetes Association, and compare and contrast the nutrition strategies for persons with type 1 versus type 2 diabetes.

- Identify the minimum components of a healthy eating pattern and lifestyle for the prevention of type 2 diabetes.

- Take a thorough history of a person with diabetes, including an assessment of the 1) family history of diabetes; 2) onset and duration of diabetes symptoms; 3) evidence of complications; 4) weight history; 5) usual food intake; 6) frequency, intensity, and duration of physical activity; 7) use of medications; and 8) alcohol consumption. Identify any problem areas.

- Recognize the central importance of nutrition and physical activity in the maintenance of health, and demonstrate a commitment to support patient adherence to the American Diabetes Association nutrition recommendations.

- Recognize the value of using a team approach in the treatment of diabetes mellitus.

* SOURCE: Objectives for chapter and cases adapted from the *NIH Nutrition Curriculum Guide for Training Physicians* (*http://www.nhlbi.nih.gov/funding/training/naa*).

Diabetes mellitus is manifested in three primary forms: type 1 diabetes, type 2 diabetes, and gestational diabetes. The disease is characterized by high blood glucose concentrations resulting from defects in insulin secretion or insulin action, or both. Insulin, a hormone produced by the beta cells of the pancreas, is necessary for the use or storage of body fuels.

Without sufficient effective insulin action, hyperglycemia occurs, resulting in short-term and long-term macrovascular and microvascular complications. Macrovascular complications include an increased risk of coronary heart diseases, congestive heart failure, stroke, and amputations, leading to increased all-cause mortality. Microvascular complications include retinopathy, nephropathy, and neuropathy.

Approximately 15 million US adults have diagnosed diabetes, an increase from 4.9% of the adult population in 1990 to 7.3% in 2000. If undiagnosed diabetes is included, almost 10% of US adults have diabetes. Diabetes prevalence increases with increasing age, affecting 18.4% of those 65 years of age or older, and is particularly prevalent in high-risk ethnic populations, such as African-Americans, Hispanic populations (Latinos and Mexican-Americans), Native Americans and Alaska Natives, Asian-Americans, and Pacific Islanders. Among children with newly diagnosed diabetes, the prevalence of type 2 diabetes increased from less than 4% before 1990 to as high as 45% in certain racial/ethnic groups in recent years.

In addition, greater than 20 million adults have impaired glucose tolerance (IGT), 13 to 14 million impaired fasting glucose (IFG), and 40 to 50 million metabolic syndrome (see Chapter 1, Case 1; Chapter 7). These individuals are at high risk for type 2 diabetes and cardiovascular disease compared to persons with normal blood glucose concentrations if lifestyle prevention strategies are not implemented.

Diagnosis of Diabetes Mellitus

Three ways to diagnose diabetes are available. Any of the following glucose values are diagnostic of diabetes:

- Fasting plasma glucose (FPG) $\geq$126 mg/dL (7.0 mmol/L)
- Casual plasma glucose $\geq$200 mg/dL (11.1 mmol/L) plus the classic symptoms of polyuria, polydipsia, and unexplained weight loss *or*
- 2-hour plasma glucose (PG) $\geq$200 mg/dL (11.1 mmol/L) during an oral glucose tolerance test (OGTT) using a glucose load containing the equivalent of 75 g anhydrous glucose dissolved in water

Fasting plasma glucose is the preferred test because of ease of use, acceptability to patients, and lower cost.

Screening Recommendations

Testing or screening for diabetes should be considered in all individuals aged 45 years and older, and, if normal, it should be repeated at 3-year intervals.

Testing should be considered at a younger age or be carried out more frequently if individuals have any of the following risk factors:

- Family history of diabetes (i.e., parents or siblings with diabetes)
- Body mass index (BMI) ≥ 25 kg/m^2
- Member of a high-risk ethnic population, including African-Americans, Latinos, Asian-Americans, and American Indians
- Women diagnosed with gestational diabetes mellitus (GDM) during pregnancy or a history of having a baby weighing greater than 9 lb (4 kg) at birth
- Hypertension (blood pressure $\geq 140/90$ mm Hg)
- High-density lipoprotein (HDL) cholesterol level ≤ 35 mg/dL or triglyceride level ≥ 250 mg/dL, or both
- IGT or IFG on previous testing
- Polycystic ovary syndrome

Consistent with screening recommendations for adults, children and youth at increased risk for type 2 diabetes should be screened if

- Overweight (BMI greater than eighty-fifth percentile for age and sex)
- Two of the following risk factors are present: family history of type 2 diabetes, member of high-risk ethnic populations, signs of insulin resistance (such as acanthosis nigricans, gray-brown skin pigmentations)

Pathophysiology of Diabetes

Type 1 Diabetes

Type 1 diabetes accounts for 5% to 10% of all diagnosed cases of diabetes. The primary defect is pancreatic beta-cell destruction, usually leading to absolute insulin deficiency (insulinopenia) and resulting in hyperglycemia, polyuria, polydipsia, weight loss, dehydration, electrolyte disturbance, and ketoacidosis. The capacity of a healthy pancreas to secrete insulin is far in excess of what is needed normally; therefore, the clinical onset of diabetes may be preceded by an extensive asymptomatic period (months to years), during which beta cells are undergoing gradual destruction. Persons with type 1 diabetes are dependent on exogenous insulin to prevent ketoacidosis and death. Although it can occur at any age, even in the eighth and ninth decades of life, most cases are diagnosed in people younger than 30 years of age, with peak incidence between 10 and 12 years in girls and 12 and 14 years in boys.

Type 1 diabetes is a result of a genetic predisposition combined with autoimmune destruction of the islet beta cells. At diagnosis, 85% to 90% of persons with type 1 diabetes have one or more circulating autoantibodies. Antibodies identified as contributing to the destruction of beta cells are 1) islet cell autoantibodies (ICAs); 2) insulin autoantibodies (IAAs), which may occur in persons who have never received insulin therapy; and 3) autoantibodies to glutamic acid decarboxylase (GAD), a protein on the surface of beta cells. GAD autoantibodies appear to provoke an attack by the T cells (killer T lymphocytes), which may be what destroys the beta cells in diabetes.

Frequently, after diagnosis and the correction of hyperglycemia, metabolic acidosis, and ketoacidosis, endogenous insulin secretion recovers. During this "honeymoon phase," exogenous insulin requirements decrease dramatically. However, the need for exogenous insulin is inevitable, and within 8 to 10 years after clinical onset, beta-cell loss is complete and insulin deficiency is absolute.

Type 2 Diabetes

Type 2 diabetes accounts for 90% to 95% of all diagnosed cases of diabetes and is a progressive disease that is often present long before it is diagnosed. Affected individuals may or may not experience the classic symptoms of uncontrolled diabetes, and they are not prone to development of ketoacidosis. Although persons with type 2 diabetes do not require exogenous insulin for survival, approximately 40% or more eventually require exogenous insulin for adequate glycemic control. Insulin may also be needed during periods of stress-induced hyperglycemia such as during illness or surgery.

Risk factors include genetic and environmental factors. Although approximately 50% of men and 70% of women are obese at the time of diagnosis, type 2 diabetes also occurs in nonobese individuals, especially the elderly.

Type 2 diabetes results from a combination of insulin resistance and relative insulin deficiency. Endogenous insulin levels may be normal, depressed, or elevated, but they are inadequate to overcome concomitant insulin resistance (decreased tissue sensitivity or responsiveness to insulin); as a result, hyperglycemia ensues. Hyperglycemia is first exhibited as an elevation of postprandial glucose due to insulin resistance at the cellular (muscle and liver) level and is followed by an elevation in fasting glucose concentrations. As insulin secretion decreases, hepatic glucose production increases, causing elevations in fasting glucose levels. Compounding the problem is the deleterious effect of hyperglycemia itself—glucotoxicity—on both insulin sensitivity and insulin secretion: hence, the importance of achieving near-euglycemia in persons with type 2 diabetes.

Insulin resistance is also demonstrated in adipocytes, leading to lipolysis and an elevation in circulating free fatty acids. Increased free fatty acids cause a further decrease in insulin sensitivity at the cellular level, impair insulin secretion, and augment hepatic glucose production (lipotoxicity). All the defects (cellular, hepatic, and beta cell) contribute to the development and progression of type 2 diabetes.

Treatment of Diabetes

Optimal control of diabetes requires the restoration of normal carbohydrate, protein, and fat metabolism. Insulin is both anticatabolic and anabolic and facilitates cellular transport. In general, the counterregulatory hormones—glucagon, growth hormone, cortisol, epinephrine, and norepinephrine—have the opposite effect of insulin.

Diabetes is a chronic disease that requires lifetime changes in lifestyle. The management of diabetes includes appropriate medical nutrition therapy, increasing physical activity, regular self-management education, and, for many, medications. An important goal is to provide the individual with the necessary tools to achieve the best possible control of glycemia, lipids, and blood pressure to prevent, delay, or arrest the microvascular and macrovascular complications of diabetes while minimizing hypoglycemic and excess weight gain.

Two large, long-term studies demonstrated the clear link between glycemic control and the development of microvascular complications in persons with type 1 and type 2 diabetes. They also provided strong evidence for the role of medical nutrition therapy in the management of diabetes. The Diabetes Control and Complications Trial (DCCT) was a long-term, randomized, controlled, multicenter trial that studied approximately 800 young adults (aged 13 to 39 years) with type 1 diabetes who were treated with either intensive therapy (multiple injections of insulin or use of insulin pumps guided by blood glucose monitoring data) or conventional therapy (1 or 2 insulin injections per day). Both groups received diet and exercise counseling. The DCCT clearly showed that even small improvements reduced the rate of microvascular complications. Patients in the intensive treatment group showed a 50% to 75% reduction in the risk of progression to retinopathy, nephropathy, and neuropathy. Subjects in the intensive therapy arm who reported following their meal plan greater than 90% of the time had hemoglobin A1C (A1C) levels 1% lower than those who reported following their meal plan only 40% of the time.

The United Kingdom Prospective Diabetes Study (UKPDS) demonstrated that reduction of elevated blood glucose levels reduced microvascular complications in type 2 diabetes just as in type 1 diabetes. The UKPDS followed 5102 newly diagnosed individuals with type 2 diabetes for an average of 10 to 11 years who were randomized into a group treated conventionally or an intensively treated group. The intensively treated group experienced a 25% reduction in the rate of retinopathy and nephropathy; however, only patients taking metformin alone experienced reductions in heart attack, diabetes-related death, or all-cause mortality. In contrast, improved blood pressure control resulted in a 34% reduction in all macrovascular endpoints, which included a 56% reduction in the risk of heart failure and 44% reduction in the risk of stroke; improved blood pressure control also resulted in a 37% reduction in all microvascular endpoints.

The UKPDS also illustrated the progressive nature of type 2 diabetes. At diagnosis and before randomization into intensive or conventional treatment, subjects received individualized intensive nutrition therapy for 3 months. During this period A1C levels decreased by approximately 2% (9% to 7%) and patients lost an average of 3.5 kg (8 lb). Researchers concluded that a reduction of energy intake was at least as important, if not more important, than the actual weight lost in determining glucose improvements. However, as the study progressed nutrition therapy alone was not enough to keep the majority of the patients' A1C levels at 7%. Medication(s) and, for many, insulin, needed to be combined with nutrition therapy. It was not the "diet" failing but instead was the pancreas failing to secrete enough insulin to maintain adequate glucose control.

Monitoring of Metabolic Outcomes

Individuals can assess day-to-day glycemic control by self-monitoring of blood glucose (SMBG). SMBG is essential for patients to determine the impact that food choices and physical activity have on their blood glucose levels, to guide them in modifying these choices, and to make the adjustments required to achieve glycemic goals. SMBG should be done three to four times a day by patients who are taking insulin and less frequently by those taking oral medications.

Complementing day-to-day testing are measurements of glycosylated hemoglobin (simplified as A1C), reflecting a weighted average of plasma glucose over the preceding 6 to 8 weeks, and long-term glycemic control. When hemoglobin and other proteins are exposed to glucose, the glucose becomes attached to the protein in a slow, nonenzymatic, and concentration-dependent manner. In nondiabetic persons, A1C values are 4.0% to 6.0%; these values correspond to mean plasma glucose levels of approximately 90 mg/dL (5.0 mmol/L).

Lipid levels and blood pressure should also be monitored. Lipids should be measured annually and blood pressure at every visit. The American Diabetes Association (ADA) glycemic, lipid, and blood pressure goals are listed in Tables 9-1 and 9-2.

Medical Nutrition Therapy

The primary goal of medical nutrition therapy for diabetes mellitus is to assist in attaining and maintaining optimal metabolic outcomes, including

- Blood glucose levels in the normal range to the greatest extent possible to prevent the microvascular complications of diabetes
- A lipid and lipoprotein profile that reduces the risk for cardiovascular diseases
- A blood pressure level that reduces the risk for vascular diseases

Outcome studies support medical nutrition therapy as an effective therapy in reaching treatment goals. Research studies show that medical nutrition therapy delivered by registered dietitians lowers A1C by approximately 1% in newly diagnosed type 1 diabetes, by about 2% in newly diagnosed type 2 diabetes, and by about 1% in type 2 diabetes of 4 years' duration. These outcomes are similar to those from oral glucose-lowering medications.

Reducing saturated fat to less than 7% of daily energy intake and dietary cholesterol to 200 mg per day lowers low-density lipoprotein (LDL) cholesterol on average by 16% (~25 mg/dL). In hypertensive patients who consume excessive sodium, reducing intake to approximately 2400 mg per day can lower systolic blood pressure by 6 mm Hg and diastolic blood pressure by 2 mm Hg.

The outcomes of nutrition interventions on glycemia, lipids, and blood pressure are usually evident by 6 weeks to 3 months. At this point, whether or not to continue nutrition therapy alone or add medications needs to be determined.

Before 1994, the ADA nutrition recommendations attempted to define "ideal" macronutrient percentages for a diabetes nutrition prescription. Then, by determining an individual's energy needs based on theoretic calorie requirements and

Table 9-1   Clinical goals for medical nutrition therapy in diabetes: glycemic control for people with diabetes.

	NORMAL	GOAL	ADDITIONAL ACTION SUGGESTED
Plasma values			
Average preprandial glucose (mg/dL)[a]	<110	90–130	<90/>150
Average bedtime glucose (mg/dL)[a]	<120	110–150	<110/>180
Average postprandial glucose (mg/dL)[a,b]	<140	<160	>180
Whole blood values			
Average preprandial glucose (mg/dL)[c]	<100	80–120	<80/>140
Average bedtime glucose (mg/dL)[c]	<110	100–140	<100/>160
Average postprandial glucose (mg/dL)[b,c]	<130	<150	<170
A1C (%)[d]	<6	<7	>8

[a] Values calibrated to plasma glucose.

[b] Measurement of capillary blood glucose.

[c] Two hours after the start of the meal. These recommendations come from consensus among diabetes care providers. No American Diabetes Association recommendations exist for postprandial glucose levels.

[d] A1C is referenced to a nondiabetic range of 4.0% to 6.0%.

SOURCE: Adapted from American Diabetes Association. Standards of medical care for patients with diabetes mellitus (position statement). Diabetes Care 2002;25(Suppl 1):S33–S49.

Table 9-2   Clinical goals for medical nutrition therapy in diabetes: target lipid and blood pressure goals for adults with diabetes.

Total cholesterol, mg/dL	<200
LDL cholesterol, mg/dL	<100
HDL cholesterol, mg/dL	>45 for men >55 for women
Triglycerides, mg/dL	<150
Blood pressure, mm Hg	<130/<80

LDL, low-density lipoprotein; HDL, high-density lipoprotein.

SOURCE: Adapted from American Diabetes Association. Standards of medical care for patients with diabetes mellitus (position statement). Diabetes Care 2002;25(Suppl 1):S33–S49.

using the ideal percentages of carbohydrate, protein, and fat, a nutrition prescription was ordered. This approach limited individualization. In 1994, the ADA recommended a different approach. Instead of rigid percentages, the nutrition prescription was to be based on an assessment of lifestyle changes required to assist the individual with diabetes in achieving and maintaining therapeutic goals employing changes that the patient was able and willing to make.

This transition to a more flexible and realistic approach to medical nutrition therapy continues in the 2002 ADA diabetes nutrition principles and recommendations. To achieve nutrition-related objectives requires a coordinated team effort that includes physicians, registered dietitians, diabetes educators, and the person with diabetes, who must be involved in problem solving. A system of care that provides ongoing support and education is essential.

Prioritizing Nutrition Strategies for Diabetes

Historically, nutrition advice, such as "don't eat foods with sugar," has been given to patients with diabetes. This advice has often been accompanied by a calorie-level "diet sheet" or a pamphlet or brochure with general guidelines. Patients often find such information difficult to understand and implement. To achieve positive outcomes, appropriate priorities should be set with the patient.

Type 1 Diabetes

The first priority for persons requiring insulin therapy is to integrate an insulin regimen into their lifestyle. After an initial food/meal plan is determined (with the patient's input), it should be discussed with the professional who is planning the insulin regimen. With the many insulin options now available, an insulin regimen can usually be developed that conforms to the patient's preferred meal times and food choices. Flexible insulin regimens using background (basal) insulin and premeal (bolus) insulin give the patient freedom in timing and composition of meals and are the preferred mode of therapy to maximize blood glucose control and minimize complications.

The total amount of carbohydrate in the meal (and snacks) is the major determinant of the premeal rapid-acting insulin dose and postprandial glucose response. After the amount of insulin required to cover their usual meal carbohydrate is determined, patients can be taught how to adjust premeal insulin doses based on the amount of carbohydrate they are planning to eat (insulin-carbohydrate ratio). For persons who are receiving fixed insulin regimens and not adjusting premeal insulin doses, consistency of day-to-day carbohydrate amounts at meals is recommended.

Type 2 Diabetes

Previously, nutrition advice focused on losing weight and avoiding sugars. Today the focus of medical nutrition therapy for type 2 diabetes is to implement lifestyle strategies that will reduce hyperglycemia, lipid levels, and blood pressure. Because many persons with type 2 diabetes are insulin resistant and overweight, medical nutrition therapy often begins with lifestyle strategies that reduce energy intake and increase energy expenditure through physical activity. Many individuals have already tried unsuccessfully to lose weight, and it is important to note that other lifestyle strategies, even without weight loss, can improve glycemia. Teaching individuals how to make appropriate food choices, often through the use of carbohydrate counting in routine and special occasions, encouraging physical activity, and using data from blood glucose monitoring to evaluate effectiveness, will improve success for type 2 diabetes. These strategies should be implemented as soon as the diagnosis of diabetes (or prediabetes) is made.

Short-term studies lasting 6 months or less demonstrate that modest amounts of weight loss improve metabolic abnormalities in many individuals, but not in all. Weight loss, especially of intra-abdominal fat, reduces insulin resistance and helps correct dyslipidemias in the short term. However, long-term data assessing the extent to which these improvements can be maintained are not available, as long-term weight loss is difficult to achieve. When used alone, standard weight reduction diets providing 500 to 1000 fewer calories than estimated energy requirements rarely lead to long-term weight loss. Data from the Finnish Diabetes Programs and the Diabetes Prevention Program demonstrate that to sustain a 5% to 7% weight loss over a period of 2 to 3 years requires structured, intensive lifestyle programs that include low-fat diets, increased physical activity, ongoing educational sessions, and monthly patient contact.

Physical activity improves insulin sensitivity, can acutely lower blood glucose concentrations, and improves cardiovascular status but by itself has only a modest effect on short-term weight loss. Physical activity is useful as an adjunct to other weight-loss strategies and is important for long-term weight maintenance.

Nutrition Recommendations

Carbohydrate

Because carbohydrate and adequacy of insulin determine postprandial glucose response, it is addressed first. With the continued popularity of low-carbohydrate diets, it should be remembered that foods containing carbohydrate—grains, fruits, vegetables, and low-fat milk—are important components of a healthy diet and should be included in a food/meal plan for persons with diabetes. All patients can benefit from basic information about carbohydrates—what foods contain carbohydrate (starches, fruit, starchy vegetables, milk, sweets and desserts), the fact that one average serving is equivalent to 15 g, and how many servings to select for meals (and snacks if desired). The following are other recommendations for food carbohydrates:

- With regard to the effects of carbohydrate on glucose concentrations, the total amount of carbohydrate in meals is as important as the source (starch or sugar) or the type (high- or low-glycemic index—the incremental area under the blood glucose response curve).
- Although differing carbohydrates have different glycemic responses (glycemic index), there is limited evidence to show long-term benefit when low-glycemic index diets are compared to high-glycemic index diets. The concept of the glycemic index is best used for fine-tuning postprandial responses after first focusing on total carbohydrate.
- Although very large amounts of fiber (50 g) can have beneficial effects on postprandial glycemia, insulin, and lipid levels, it is unknown if the majority of patients can regularly consume enough dietary fiber to see this benefit.
- Sucrose does not increase glycemia to a greater extent than isocaloric amounts of starch. Therefore, sucrose and sucrose-containing foods do not need to be limited by people with diabetes based on concern about aggravating hyperglycemia. However,

these foods should be substituted for other carbohydrate sources or, if added, covered with additional insulin or other glucose-lowering medications.

- Nonnutritive sweeteners are safe when consumed within the accepted daily intake levels established by the Food and Drug Administration.
- Eating five servings of fruits and vegetables a day is recommended for both prevention and treatment of high blood pressure.

Protein

No evidence has been found to suggest that usual intake of protein (15% to 20% of energy intake) be changed in persons who do not have renal disease. Some evidence has been shown that lowering protein intake to 0.8 to 1.0 g/kg per day in patients with microalbuminuria and to 0.8 g/kg per day with overt nephropathy will slow the progression of renal disease.

Aside from sugars, protein is probably the most misunderstood nutrient, with inaccurate advice frequently given to persons with diabetes. Although nonessential amino acids serve as substrates for gluconeogenesis, in subjects with controlled diabetes, this glucose does not enter the general circulation. Protein does not slow the absorption of carbohydrate, and therefore, adding protein to the treatment of hypoglycemia does not prevent subsequent hypoglycemia. The ADA recommendations make the following statements:

- Ingested protein does not increase plasma glucose concentrations, although it is just as potent a stimulant of insulin as carbohydrate.
- The long-term effects of diets that are high in protein and low in carbohydrate are unknown. Although initially blood glucose levels may improve and weight may be lost, it is unknown whether long-term weight loss is maintained any better with these diets than with other low-calorie diets. Because these diets are usually high in saturated fat, the long-term effect of these diets on LDL cholesterol is also a concern.

Dietary Fat

Limiting intake of saturated fatty acids, trans-fatty acids, and dietary cholesterol is recommended, especially in individuals with LDL cholesterol greater than 100 mg/dL (see Chapter 6). The ADA recommendations are somewhat cautious in recommending increased intake of monounsaturated or polyunsaturated fats. The concern is that a high monounsaturated fat (MUFA) diet selected *ad libitum* may lead to higher energy intakes and weight gain. The ADA recommendations are the following:

- Reduced-fat diets when maintained long term contribute to modest weight loss and improvement in dyslipidemia.
- To lower LDL cholesterol, the calories from saturated fat can be reduced if weight loss is desirable or the calories from saturated fat are replaced with carbohydrates or MUFA if weight loss is not the goal.
- Trans-unsaturated fatty acids from stick margarines, fried foods, and processed baked goods should also be limited to reduce LDL cholesterol.

- For individuals with metabolic syndrome, improved glycemic control, modest weight loss, dietary saturated fat restriction, increased physical activity, and the incorporation of MUFAs may be beneficial.

Alcohol

Recommendations for alcohol intake are similar to those for the general public. If individuals choose to drink, alcoholic beverage consumption should be limited to no more than two per day for men and no more than one drink for women. One drink is defined as a 12-oz beer, 5-oz wine, or 1.5-oz distilled spirits, each of which contains approximately 15 g alcohol. For individuals who use insulin or insulin secretagogues, alcohol should be consumed with food to reduce the risk of hypoglycemia.

Sodium

For both normotensive and hypertensive individuals, a reduction in sodium intake lowers blood pressure. The goal should be to reduce sodium intake to 2400 mg per day.

Micronutrients

No evidence has been found of benefit from vitamin or mineral supplementation in persons with diabetes who do not have underlying deficiencies. Exceptions are folate for the prevention of birth defects and calcium for the prevention of bone disease. Routine supplementation of the diet with antioxidants has not proven beneficial, and therefore these supplements are not recommended.

Physical Activity

Physical activity should be an integral part of the treatment plan for persons with diabetes. Exercise helps improve insulin sensitivity, reduce cardiovascular risk factors, control weight, and bring about a healthier outlook. People with diabetes can exercise safely. The exercise plan will vary depending on age, general health, and level of physical fitness. A minimum of 30 minutes all or most days of the week is recommended. Persons taking insulin or insulin secretagogues should monitor their blood glucose and take appropriate precautions to avoid hypoglycemia.

Treatment of Hypoglycemia

Any available carbohydrate-containing food, including glucose tablets, sucrose, juice, regular soda, and syrup, will raise glucose levels. Glucose is the preferred treatment, and commercially available glucose tablets have the advantage of being premeasured to help prevent overtreatment. Treatment begins with 15 to 20 g glucose, and an initial response should be seen in approximately 10 to 20 minutes. Blood glucose should be evaluated again in approximately 60 minutes, as additional treatment may be necessary. The form of carbohydrate does not assist in treatment or in prevention of subsequent hypoglycemia.

Medications

Oral Glucose-Lowering Medications

If metabolic parameters do not improve with nutrition therapy and physical activity, medication(s) must be combined with nutrition therapy. The use of newer oral glucose-lowering medications, alone or in combinations, provides numerous options for achieving euglycemia in persons with type 2 diabetes. However, eventually many patients with type 2 diabetes will require two or more daily insulin injections to achieve glycemic control.

Currently, there are four classes of oral medications: 1) biguanides (metformin), which suppress hepatic glucose production and lower insulin resistance but do not stimulate insulin secretion; 2) insulin secretagogues, which include the sulfonylureas (first and second generation) and the meglitinides (repaglinide and nateglinide), whose actions are to promote insulin secretion by the beta cells of the pancreas; 3) thiazolidinediones (pioglitazone, rosiglitazone), which decrease insulin resistance in peripheral tissues and thus enhance the ability of muscle and adipose cells to take up glucose; and 4) alpha-glucosidase inhibitors (acarbose, miglitol), which work in the small intestine to inhibit enzymes that digest carbohydrates, thereby delaying carbohydrate absorption and lowering postprandial glycemia. With the exception of metformin and the sulfonylureas, no long-term data are available on safety or reduction of complications. Table 9-3 lists the recommended dose, principal site of action, and average decrease in A1C for oral glucose-lowering medications.

Insulin

All persons with type 1 diabetes and patients with type 2 diabetes who no longer produce adequate endogenous insulin need replacement of insulin that mimics normal insulin action. After eating, plasma glucose and insulin concentrations increase rapidly, peak in 30 to 60 minutes, and return to basal concentrations within 2 to 3 hours in nondiabetics. To mimic this, rapid-acting insulin, such as lispro, or aspart, is given before meals. Premeal insulin doses are adjusted based on the amount of carbohydrate in the meal.

Background or basal insulin, such as glargine, neutral protamine Hagedorn (NPH), or ultralente, is required in the postabsorptive state to restrain endogenous glucose output primarily from the liver and to limit lipolysis and excess flux of free fatty acids to the liver. Glargine, an insulin analog of 24-hour duration and with no peak action time, can be used as a background insulin and is given at bedtime. It cannot be mixed with other insulins. NPH or ultralente insulin can also be used as background insulin but may have to be given twice a day, usually at bedtime to control fasting glucose levels and before breakfast. These types of flexible insulin regimens give the patient freedom in timing and composition of meals.

Table 9-3 Oral glucose-lowering medications.

CLASS AND GENERIC NAMES	PRINCIPAL SITE OF ACTION	MEAN DECREASE IN A1C
Biguanide	Decrease hepatic glucose	1.5%–2.0%
Metformin (Glucophage)	production	
Metformin extended release	Also increase insulin secretion	
(Glucophage XR)		
Glyburide/metformin		
(Glucovance; 1.25/250 mg)		
Sulfonylureas (second generation)	Stimulate insulin secretion from	1%–2%
Glipizide (Glucotrol)	the beta cells	
Glipizide (Glucotrol XL)		
Glyburide (Glynase Prestabs)		
Glimepiride (Amaryl)		
Meglitinide	Stimulate insulin secretion from	1%–2%
Repaglinide (Prandin)	beta cells	
Nateglinide (Starlix)		
Thiazolidinediones	Improve peripheral insulin	1%–2%
Pioglitazone (Actos)	sensitivity	
Rosiglitazone (Avandia)		
Alpha-glucosidase inhibitor	Delay carbohydrate absorption	0.5%–1.0%
Acarbose (Precose)		
Miglitol (Glyset)		

SOURCE: Adapted with permission from Franz MJ, Reader D, Monk A. Implementing Group and Individual Medical Nutrition Therapy for Diabetes. Alexandria, VA: American Diabetes Association, 2002:66.

Table 9-4 is a listing of human insulins, their onset of action, peak action time, usual effective duration, and when to test for their effect on blood glucose levels.

Because of the potential for hypoglycemia with insulin therapy, physicians and patients should be aware of the onset, peak, and durations of insulin being used. Food intake and physical activity should be adjusted appropriately to minimize the occurrence of hypoglycemia. The type and timing of insulin regimens should be individualized, based on eating and exercise habits and blood glucose concentrations.

Insulin pump therapy provides basal rapid-acting or short-acting insulin pumped continuously by a mechanical device in micro amounts through a subcutaneous catheter that is monitored 24 hours a day. Boluses of insulin are then given before meals. Pump therapy requires a committed and motivated person who is willing to do a minimum of four blood glucose tests per day, keep blood glucose and food records, and learn the technical features of pump usage.

Self-Management Education

For metabolic goals to be achieved, open communication and self-management education are required. With chronic illnesses such as diabetes, the role of

Table 9-4   Action times of human insulin preparations.

TYPE OF INSULIN	ONSET OF ACTION	PEAK ACTION	USUAL EFFECTIVE DURATION	MONITOR EFFECT IN:
Rapid-acting	<15 min	0.5–1.5 hr	2–4 h	2 h
Lispro				
Aspart				
Short-acting	0.5 to 1.0 h	2–4 h	3–6 h	4 h
Regular				
Intermediate-acting	2–4 h	6–8 h	10–16 h	8–12 h
NPH				
Long-acting	6–10 h	10–16 h	18–20 h	10–12 h
Ultralente				
Glargine	1.1 h		24 h	10–12 h
Mixtures	0.5–1.0 h	Dual	10–16 h	
70/30 (70% NPH, 30% regular)				
50/50 (50% NPH, 50% regular)				
75/25 (75% NPL, 25% lispro)				

NPH, neutral protamine Hagedorn; NPL, neutral protamine lispro.

SOURCE: Adapted from Franz MJ, Reader D, Monk A. Implementing Group and Individual Medical Nutrition Therapy for Diabetes. Alexandria, VA: American Diabetes Association, 2002:70; and Havas S. Educational guidelines for achieving tight control and minimizing complications of type 1 diabetes. Am Fam Phys 1999;60:1985–1992.

health care providers shifts from providing direct medical care to facilitating self-management by individuals with diabetes and their families. Although some physicians provide their own nutrition and physical activity education, it is a time-consuming process. Many choose to use a team approach with registered dietitians (as well as other team members) in their medical center or clinic or delegate the educational and skill-building components by referring to a registered dietitian or a diabetes education center, or both.

It is reported that individuals who hold two important beliefs are more likely to engage in effective self-management behaviors than are those who do not hold these beliefs: 1) consider diabetes to be serious and 2) believe that their own actions make a difference. An individual's self-efficacy and self-confidence in making and maintaining a change are significant predictors of later adherence. A simple but effective role that physicians can provide is to endorse and support lifestyle changes and to express confidence in the patient's ability to make change.

Nutrition Recommendations for the Prevention of Diabetes

The development of type 2 diabetes is strongly related to lifestyle factors, thus suggesting that onset might be prevented. Observational studies provided evidence that increased physical activity, modest weight loss, and increased dietary intake of whole grains/fiber and decreased dietary fat might delay or prevent type 2 diabetes. The Finnish Diabetes Prevention Study and the Diabetes

Prevention Program investigated the effects of lifestyle interventions on the prevention of diabetes in those at high risk (impaired glucose tolerance): In both studies the incidence of diabetes was reduced by 58% in the intensive lifestyle intervention group. Based on the evidence the following are recommendations for prevention of diabetes:

- Structured programs that emphasize lifestyle changes, including education, reduced fat and energy intake, regular physical activity, and regular participant contact, can produce a long-term weight loss of 5% to 7% of starting weight and reduce the risk of developing diabetes.

- All individuals, especially family members of individuals with type 2 diabetes, should be encouraged to engage in regular physical activity to decrease the risk of developing type 2 diabetes.

For a list of references for this chapter, please visit the University of Pennsylvania School of Medicine's Nutrition Education and Prevention Program web site: *http://www.med.upenn.edu/nutrimed/articles.html*

Case 1

Diabetic Ketoacidosis in Type 1 Diabetes Mellitus

Brian W. Tobin, Judith Wylie-Rosett, and Balint Kacsoh

Objectives

- Describe the role of exogenous insulin and medical nutrition therapy in the management of type 1 diabetes and in the prevention or treatment, or both, of secondary complications.
- Explain the current ADA nutrition priorities, principles, and recommended practices for type 1 diabetes.
- Take an appropriate medical history of a person with type 1 diabetes.
- Recognize the importance of behavioral and lifestyle modifications in medical nutrition therapy.
- Evaluate and identify potential metabolic complications of diabetes mellitus based on nutritional and physical activity history, use of medications, and alcohol consumption.

MN, a 33-year-old Hispanic woman with type 1 diabetes, is brought to the clinic by her mother in a semicomatose state. MN is 5'4" (163 cm) and currently weighs 112 lb (51 kg). Her mother reports that she was unable to wake MN after Thanksgiving dinner and was concerned that she might not be receiving enough insulin. She reports that MN has lost 9 lb (4.1 kg) in the last 2 days after coming down with a cold. According to her mother, she complained of dizziness, fatigue, frequent urination, and being excessively thirsty and hungry. She often fell asleep after meals.

Past Medical History

MN has been a type 1 diabetic for the past 3 years. Except for the current illness, she has been well but has been more sedentary and recently reported a decreased exercise capacity. Recent assessment of her kidney function and an eye examination were normal.

MN's usual schedule and food intake consist of the following:

1. Biosynthetic human insulin (Humulin) given subcutaneously as 16 units NPH and 6 units regular before breakfast and 5 units NPH and 5 units regular before dinner. She takes no other medications.

2. A 2000-calorie food plan distributed among three meals and three snacks that she received from the nutritionist at the hospital when she was first diagnosed 3 years ago. It consists of 50% carbohydrate, 20% protein, and 30% fat. MN has noted that "sticking to her diet" is one of the most difficult aspects of her diabetes self-care.

3. Monitoring and recording capillary glucose by means of a home glucose monitor before breakfast and dinner. Her goal is to maintain her fasting capillary glucose levels between 80 and 150 mg/dL, but they are above 150 mg/dL approximately 50% of the time. Her morning readings are usually elevated. Her glucose self-monitoring results are rarely below 60 mg/dL.

Family History

MN's mother developed type 1 diabetes in her late 30s and is currently treated with daily insulin injections. Her paternal grandfather developed diabetes in his sixties and was treated initially with oral medication.

Social History

MN has a hectic schedule during the week. She works long hours at a law firm and attends classes two nights a week. MN tries to go to the gym before work but is often too tired. She does not smoke and drinks alcohol only socially on weekends when she occasionally goes dancing with friends. On these nights, she may have two or three frozen margaritas but feels weak shortly after drinking and reports that she "is just too tired to dance the way she used to."

MN's Usual Intake

Breakfast (office, 7:30 a.m.)

Instant oatmeal (flavored, apple-cinnamon)	1 package
Coffee	12 oz (360 mL)
Whole milk	2 Tbsp.
Sugar	2 packets
Orange juice	12 oz (360 mL)

Lunch (fast-food restaurant, 1:00 p.m.)

Hamburger	4 oz (113 g)
Roll	1
Lettuce	1 leaf
Tomato	2 slices
Apple juice	12 oz (360 mL)

Snack (vending machine, 5:00 p.m.)

Pretzels	1 oz (28 g)
Cola	20 oz (600 mL)

Dinner (home, 8:00 p.m.)

Chicken breast (baked)	6 oz (170 g)
Rice	1 cup
Black beans	1 cup
Olive oil	1 Tbsp.
Mixed salad	1 cup
French dressing	2 Tbsp.
Iced tea (sweetened)	16 oz (480 mL)

Snack (home, 11:00 p.m.)

Chocolate chip cookies	3 small
Whole milk	8 oz (240 mL)

Total calories: 2863 kcal
Protein: 124 g (17% of total calories)
Carbohydrate: 403 g (56% of total calories)
Total fat: 87 g (27% of total calories)
Saturated fat: 27 g (8% of total calories)
Monounsaturated fat: 35 g (11% of total calories)
Cholesterol: 287 mg
Dietary fiber: 25 g
Sodium: 2386 mg

Physical Examination

Vital signs

Temperature: 101.3°F (38.5°C)
Heart rate: 120 beats per minute (BPM)
Respiratory rate: 28 BPM
Blood pressure: 120/60 mm Hg
Height: 5'4" (163 cm)
Weight: 112 lb (51 kg)
Body mass index (BMI): 19.2 kg/m^2

General appearance: Sick-looking woman with deep and rapid respirations. Acetone was noted on her breath. By examination she was assessed to have lost at least 10% of her body weight as fluids.
Eyes: Dry conjunctivae. Normal fundoscopy.
Throat: Erythematous, but tonsils were neither large nor pustular. Her buccal mucous membranes were dry.
Neck: No thyromegaly.
Heart and lung examination: Normal.

Abdomen: Soft but generally mildly tender. No hepatosplenomegaly.

Extremities: Cool and mottled in the periphery, with weak but equal pulses.

Neurologic: Lethargic but easily aroused. Once aroused, she was able to provide a coherent history. She responded to verbal orders and was oriented to time, place, and person.

The rest of her examination was normal.

Laboratory Tests

Patient's Laboratory Values	Normal Values
White blood cell: 20,800/mm³	4500–11,000/mm³
Segmented neutrophils: 7.2 (10³/L)	2.5–7.5 (10³/L)
Hematocrit: 47%	36%–46%
Glucose: 720 mg/dL	70–110 mg/dL
Sodium (Na): 128 mEq/L	133–143 mEq/L
Potassium (K): 4.5 mEq/L	3.5–5.3 mEq/L
Chloride (Cl): 95 mEq/L	98–108 mEq/L
Bicarbonate: 7 mEq/L	22–28 mEq/L
Blood urea nitrogen (BUN): 35 mg/dL	7–18 mg/dL
Creatinine: 2.0 mg/dL	0.6–1.2 mg/dL
Calcium (Ca): 9.2 mg/dL	9.0–11.0 mg/dL
Phosphate (PO_4): 2.4 mg/dL	2.5–4.6 mg/dL
Acetone: 4+	Negative
Venous pH: 7.10	7.35–7.45
Triglyceride: 300 mg/dL	<150 mg/dL
Cholesterol: 220 mg/dL	<200 mg/dL
A1C: 8.5%	4%–6%

Patient's Urinary Laboratory Values	Normal Values
Specific gravity: 1.031	1.002–1.030
pH: 4.5	5–6
Glucose (Chem strip): 4+	Negative
Ketone bodies (Chem strip): 4+	Negative
Protein (Chem strip): negative	Negative

Treatment and Course

MN was diagnosed with diabetic ketoacidosis (DKA) and transported to the hospital for treatment. Immediate management for DKA was aimed at replacing her past and ongoing fluid and electrolyte losses and decreasing her plasma glucose level at a rate of 50 to 100 mg/dL per hour. Sodium chloride–containing intravenous fluids and a continuous infusion of insulin were started. Potassium chloride and potassium phosphorus were added to intravenous fluids as MN's serum potassium decreased further. Glucose was also added to intravenous fluids when plasma glucose decreased to below 250 mg/dL.

Clinically, she improved gradually: She became more alert, polyuria and polydipsia decreased, appetite improved, and her fever abated. Twenty-four hours after admission her laboratory tests were as follows: plasma glucose: 160 mg/dL, Na: 138 mEq/L, K: 4.2 mEq/L, Cl: 108 mEq/L, bicarbonate: 20 mEq/L, creatinine: 1.0 mg/dL, PO_4: 3.2 mg/dL, venous pH: 7.35, and triglycerides: 200 mg/dL. Her urine had only 1+ glucose and trace ketones.

New Insulin Regimen

Subsequently, MN's usual subcutaneous insulin dose and diabetic diet were restarted. Because of the high A1C, her total insulin dose was changed to 24 units of long-acting glargine at bedtime for background and, depending on her carbohydrate intake, 5 to 10 units of rapid-acting lispro before meals to give her more flexibility in her lifestyle. Glargine provides basal insulin without peaks and is proven to decrease the incidence of both hypoglycemia and prebreakfast hyperglygemia caused by the Somogyi effect.

Case Questions

1. Explain how MN's symptoms and laboratory tests are related to the absence of insulin.
2. How are macrovascular and microvascular complications associated with diabetes control?
3. Why is medical nutrition therapy a vital component of managing patients with type 1 diabetes?
4. What are the goals of medical nutrition therapy in patients with type 1 diabetes?
5. How should carbohydrate intake be adjusted before and after exercise?
6. How can diabetic ketoacidosis be prevented in this patient?

Case Answers

Part 1: Diagnosis and Pathophysiology

1. **Explain how MN's symptoms and laboratory tests are related to the absence of insulin.**

    Insulin-dependent tissues require insulin for glucose uptake and normal energy metabolism. Type 1 diabetes develops after approximately 80% to 90% of the beta cells of the pancreas have been destroyed (usually as the result of an autoimmune inflammatory reaction involving primary insulitis, cytotoxic T-lymphocytes, and secretion of interleukins and tumor necrosis factor-alpha). The insulin secretory capacity of the pancreas normally exceeds the body's need. The decline of the islet cell mass, therefore, remains nonsymptomatic for a long time, unless the body's insulin requirements increase, such as during infection or stress. When insulin secretory capacity becomes insufficient to regulate hepatic glucose output and glucose uptake by peripheral tissues, hyperglycemia occurs.

MN begins to excrete glucose in her urine when her plasma glucose has exceeded the reabsorption capacity of her kidneys. The kidney threshold for glucose is approximately 180 to 220 mg/dL. Above this plasma glucose level, osmotic diuresis begins. As her kidneys begin to filter more glucose, urinary volume and water loss increase. Hyperglycemia results in polyuria (increased urinary volume and frequency) that in turn leads to hypovolemia (decreased volume of circulating plasma) and secondary polydipsia (increased thirst prompting fluid intake). Polyphagia (increased appetite) presents concurrently because insulin-dependent cells are in a "starved state," despite hyperglycemia.

In the absence of insulin, the body releases fatty acids from adipose tissue because of increased adenylate cyclase activation and decreased inhibition of hormone-sensitive lipase. The liver produces ketone bodies (beta-hydroxybutyrate, acetoacetate, acetone) from the increased levels of acetyl coenzyme A (CoA) formed from the oxidation of free fatty acids. Ketone bodies accumulate in the blood (ketonemia) and are excreted in the urine (ketonuria). Ketonemia is a normal response to starvation; in starvation-induced ketonemia blood glucose is low-normal.

In DKA, blood glucose levels are elevated. The primary source of blood glucose in DKA is hepatic gluconeogenesis. Gluconeogenesis is a process whereby certain amino acids, pyruvate, lactate, and intermediates of the TCA (tricarboxylic acid) cycle are converted to glucose. Gluconeogenesis is directly stimulated by stress-induced hormones (cortisol, adrenaline, glucagon). These hormones, in antagonism with insulin, increase lipolysis in adipose tissue and raise free fatty acid levels in plasma. The increased levels of free fatty acids provide energy [adenosine triphosphate (ATP), nicotinamide adenine dinucleotide (NADH)] and reducing equivalents for gluconeogenesis. Insulin primarily inhibits hepatic gluconeogenesis by its antilipolytic action in adipose tissue.

Ketone bodies are relatively weak acids that generate large numbers of hydrogen ions by dissociation, causing metabolic acidosis. The serum bicarbonate level, an indicator of the partial pressure of carbon dioxide (CO_2), decreases as hyperventilation decreases CO_2 in alveolar air and in arterial blood and as the excess hydrogen ions are buffered by bicarbonate and eliminated with urine. Acidosis means the accumulation of protons. These protons in the extracellular fluid are exchanged with intracellular potassium. The potassium and other electrolytes are lost in the urine. A patient in DKA may display hypokalemia, hyperkalemia, or normokalemia depending on the stage of the condition and fluxes of potassium.

Regardless of plasma potassium concentration, total body potassium stores are significantly decreased.

With insulin deficiency, weight loss can occur as body fat and protein stores are reduced because of increased rates of lipolysis and proteolysis. MN's rapid weight loss (9 lb in 2 days) is likely to occur in severe insulinopenia and hyperglycemia despite an increase in appetite and caloric intake. This weight loss is due to fluid loss and not from loss of muscle mass and adipose tissue.

2. **How are macrovascular and microvascular complications associated with diabetes control?**

Diabetic complications that affect smaller blood vessels in the eyes and kidneys and neurologic functioning are closely related to elevation of blood glucose. The Diabetes Control and Complications Trial (DCCT) demonstrated that intensive treatment of patients with type 1 diabetes dramatically reduces the risk of progression to retinopathy, nephropathy, and neuropathy by 50% to 75%. The DCCT-intensified diabetes management included self-monitoring blood glucose at least four times a day and the use of multiple insulin injections or the use of a continuous insulin infusion pump to reduce A1C from approximately 9% to 7%. Use of nutritional strategies, such as more regular meal times, use of snacks, and adjustments to match carbohydrate to insulin dosage were stressed as an essential component of behavior modification. The DCCT intensive treatment was, however, associated with an increased risk of hypoglycemia and weight gain. Because weight gain will adversely affect glycemia, lipid levels, blood pressure, and general health, prevention of weight gain should be advised.

The duration of diabetes is an important component in the development of diabetic complications. The longer the patient has had diabetes, the less adequate the glucose control and the higher the risk for development of complications. Some of these are related to the direct impact of high glucose levels; others are associated with the abnormal plasma lipoprotein profile. Diabetes is associated with increased triglycerides and cholesterol [very-low-density lipoprotein (VLDL) and LDL], a constellation that predisposes to macrovascular complications, including atherosclerosis, ischemic heart disease, and stroke. The DCCT showed 25% less hypercholesterolemia with tight control.

Control of blood pressure and lipid levels is essential to prevent or ameliorate the macrovascular complications of diabetes. The improvement of glycemic control resulted in a borderline significant reduction in macrovascular complications during the 7 to 10 years of follow-up in the DCCT, most likely because the cohort was below the age of 40 years on study entry and too young.

Microalbuminuria is an indication of increased risk for both atherosclerosis and diabetic nephropathy, and the ADA recommends the use of angiotensin-converting enzyme (ACE) inhibitors as a means to slow down the progression of nephropathy.

Part 2: Medical Nutrition Therapy

3. **Why is medical nutrition therapy a vital component of managing patients with type 1 diabetes?**

   Medical nutrition therapy (MNT) is vital to achieving more stable glycemic control. The goals of MNT are to match insulin regimens to the patient's usual schedule of meals, carbohydrate intake, physical activity, and energy needs. The timing and dosage of insulin therapy need to "mimic" how the beta cells of the pancreas normally secrete insulin in response to food intake. Insulin needs to be provided for basal needs [long-acting such as glargine (Lantus) or intermediate such as NPH or lente] and mealtime bolus insulin from rapid-acting insulins such as lispro (Humalog) or aspart (Novolog) or regular insulin (Humulin). Insulin pumps can also be programmed to provide basal and bolus insulin.

   The amount of rapid-acting insulin is based on the carbohydrate content of meals. If the patient prefers snacks with more than 15 g carbohydrate, rapid-acting insulin may also be needed before the snack. If the patient prefers snacks on a daily basis, regular insulin before meals may work better than a rapid-acting insulin, since this would cover those carbohydrates. Patients who have a fixed insulin dose and schedule must be consistent with both the amount of carbohydrate eaten and the timing of meals and snacks. However, patients on flexible insulin regimens can adjust their bolus insulin and accommodate changes in the times and amounts of carbohydrate eaten. Adjustments in insulin or carbohydrate intake, or both, are also important for planning physical activity and in managing sick days. For planned physical activity, it may be necessary to decrease bolus insulin doses or to consume additional carbohydrates.

   To reduce her long-term risk for cardiovascular disease, MN's diabetes goals include an LDL cholesterol of less than 100 mg/dL and a blood pressure goal of less than 130/85 mm Hg. To achieve this goal, cholesterol synthesis inhibitor drugs ("statins") and hypertensive medications are often needed in addition to increased physical activity and a diet low in saturated fat, cholesterol, and sodium.

4. **What are the goals of medical nutrition therapy in patients with type 1 diabetes?**

   The process of intensifying type 1 diabetes management to improve glycemic control involves several stages and individualization. At the time of diagnosis, the insulin dose can be calculated based on current body weight with approximately 0.5 to 0.6 units of insulin per kilogram per day, with approximately half for basal needs and half as boluses for meals and snacks. During this initial stage, which is usually three to four visits, diabetes management and MNT will focus on basic skills. Nutrition counseling should emphasize tailoring insulin therapy to carbohydrate intake and eating times. Blood glucose monitoring data can be used to refine the dosage of basal insulin and meal-related insulin boluses. Patients need to master a basic understanding of the relationship between insulin action and lifestyle before moving on to more complex planning to achieve better glycemic control and a more flexible lifestyle.

Guidelines for Coordinating Insulin Therapy and Dietary Carbohydrate

1. Make adjustments to reduce elevated glucose based on self-monitoring blood glucose. Obtain self-monitoring blood glucose at 2 a.m. if the patient encounters difficulty sleeping or evidence of hypoglycemia overnight (especially for intermediate-acting insulin at dinnertime).

2. Individualize adjustment of insulin for changes in carbohydrate (when information is limited, try 1 unit of regular insulin for 15 g carbohydrate).

3. Increase self-monitoring blood glucose to four or more times per day to intensify therapy and improve glycemic control.

4. Try to evaluate the effects of one change for 3 days before making another change in carbohydrates or insulin therapy.

MN's current weight is 112 lb, but her normal weight is 121 lb. She is very likely to be dehydrated at presentation to the clinic. Improving her glycemic control and electrolyte infusion will restore fluid balance, which will help her restore her normal body weight. However, MN could be at risk for excessive weight gain if she overeats to prevent or treat hypoglycemia.

Patients learn to adjust insulin or carbohydrate intake, or both, based on blood glucose levels. This estimate can be based on the number of carbohydrate exchanges or servings from the food groups that contain approximately 15 g carbohydrate per carbohydrate serving [milk and yogurt (1 cup); starches–rice ($^1/_3$ cup cooked); potatoes, pasta, starchy vegetables ($^1/_2$ cup); breads (1 slice or 1 oz); cereals ($^3/_4$ cup dry); and fruit and fruit juices ($^1/_2$ cup or 1 small).] A more precise estimate can be made from a detailed listing of the carbohydrate content of foods (Table 9-5).

MN eats approximately 90 g carbohydrate at breakfast, 75 g at lunch, and 120 g at dinner. Her afternoon snack contains 97 g carbohydrate, and her nighttime snack contains 30 g carbohydrate. It may be difficult to match insulin dosage for the carbohydrate at meals and snacks without some alternations in her carbohydrate intake. MN increased her juice intake, assuming it was "healthy" to treat her cold.

Reducing her carbohydrate intake from beverages (fruit juices and sugar-containing beverages) may help in synchronizing carbohydrate and insulin intake. If nutritional needs are met, sugar can be incorporated into a diabetic meal plan, substituting for other carbohydrates on a gram-for-gram basis.

Table 9-5   Carbohydrate content of food.

TIME	FOOD INTAKE	CARBOHYDRATE SERVING	CARBOHYDRATE (g)
Breakfast	Orange juice, 12 oz	3	45
	Instant oatmeal	2	30
	Coffee, milk, and 2 packets sugars	1	15
Meal total			(90)
Lunch	Hamburger with roll	2	30
	Lettuce and tomato		
	Apple juice, 12 oz	3	45
Meal total			(75)
Snack, 5 p.m.	Pretzels, 1 oz	1.5	22
	Cola, 20 oz (regular)	5	75
Snack total			(97)
Dinner	Chicken		
	Rice, 1 cup	3	45
	Spicy black beans, 1 cup	2	30
	Green salad		
	Bottle of ice tea (sweetened), 16 oz	3	45
Meal total			(120)
Snack	Cookies, 2 small	1	15
	Milk, 8 oz	1	15
Snack total			(30)

5.   How should carbohydrate intake be adjusted before and after exercise?

Patients with type 1 diabetes should be advised to monitor their blood glucose before and after exercise in order to detect and prevent hypoglycemia. Insulin dosage may need to be reduced when exercise is planned to prevent hypoglycemia. Additional carbohydrates may be needed for unplanned exercise, depending on the glucose levels.

If blood glucose is less than 100 mg/dL, approximately 15 g carbohydrate is needed for 30 minutes of walking or other low- to moderate-intensity activities. About 30 to 60 g carbohydrate is needed for 1 hour of moderate to strenuous activity (glucose should be monitored accordingly).

If blood glucose is 100 to 200 mg/dL, no additional carbohydrate is usually needed for 30 minutes of walking or low-intensity activity; approximately 15 g carbohydrate is needed for 1 hour of moderate activity. If glucose is 200 to 300 mg/dL, about 15 g additional carbohydrate is needed for strenuous activity. If glucose is greater than 300 mg/dL, physical activity should wait until blood glucose is lower.

6. **How can diabetic ketoacidosis be prevented in this patient?**

    An effective diabetes education program includes counseling on sick day management, which includes the use of short-acting insulin, monitoring of blood glucose and urinary ketones, and consumption of fluids containing sugar and salt (i.e., sports drinks that contain glucose and electrolytes). Patients should be taught to continue taking their insulin and to contact their physician early in their illness. Guidelines should be provided as to when to seek medical treatment, including a weight loss of 5% or more of body weight, a persistent elevation in blood glucose concentration, respiration rate of greater than 35 BPM, uncontrolled fever, nausea, or vomiting.

Case 2

Type 2 Diabetes

Samuel N. Grief, Linda Snetselaar, and Fran Burke

Objectives

- Describe the role of glycemic control and medical nutrition therapy in reducing the complications of type 2 diabetes.
- Identify the minimum components of a healthy lifestyle for the prevention of type 2 diabetes.
- Take an appropriate medical history, including family, social, nutritional/dietary, physical activity, and weight histories of a person with type 2 diabetes.
- Provide effective medical nutrition therapy for patients with type 2 diabetes.

DM, a 45-year-old man, presents to his family physician with a 6-month history of fatigue and lethargy. He also periodically experiences transient blurry vision that lasts a few minutes. He denies any recent change in weight or appetite, shortness of breath, increased frequency of urination, or numbness of his extremities.

Past Medical History

DM denies any personal history of diabetes, high blood pressure, high cholesterol, or heart disease. He has no history of previous hospitalizations or other illnesses.

Family History

DM has one sibling, a 49-year-old brother, who has no known medical problems. Both his parents have high blood pressure and are overweight.

Social History

DM is married with two children. He is an engineer who spends the majority of his workday sitting at the computer. He occasionally plays doubles tennis on the weekend. DM is not taking any medication or other vitamin, nutritional, or herbal supplements. He drinks alcohol on social occasions, which average twice per month. He has smoked up to one pack of cigarettes a day for 25 years

(25 pack year history). At his physician's request, DM provided the following 24-hour dietary recall.

Breakfast (office)

Large plain bagel	4 oz (113 g)
Cream cheese	2 Tbsp.
Orange juice	8 oz (240 mL)

Snack (office)

Doughnut	1 medium
Coffee	20 oz (360 mL)
Creamer (half-and-half)	2 oz (60 mL)

Lunch (deli restaurant)

Salami	4 oz (113 g)
Swiss cheese	1 oz (28 g)
Mayonnaise, regular	2 Tbsp.
White bread	2 slices
Cranberry juice cocktail	16-oz bottle (480 mL)
Potato chips	1.5 oz (42 g)

Dinner (Chinese restaurant)

Shrimp egg roll	2
Sweet and sour chicken thigh	2 (5.5 oz/156 g)
Vegetable fried rice	2 cups
Beer, ale	24 fluid oz (720 mL)
Fortune cookie	2
Sherbet	1 cup

Total calories: 3757 kcal
Protein: 93 g (10% of total calories)
Carbohydrate: 448 g (47% of total calories)
Total fat: 160 g (38% of total calories)
Saturated fat: 49 g (12% of total calories)
Monounsaturated fats: 54 g (13% of total calories)
Cholesterol: 446 mg
Dietary fiber: 14 g
Alcohol: 26 g
Sodium: 5737 mg

Review of Systems

General: Fatigue, lethargy, and blurred vision.

Endocrine: Negative polyuria, polydipsia, or changes in appetite.

Genitourinary: DM admits to decreased strength and duration of erections on several occasions over the past 6 months. He has no pain with intercourse.

Neurologic: Negative for headache, tinnitus, eye pain, numbness, or tingling in extremities.

Physical Examination

General: Obese man in no acute distress

Head, ears, eyes, nose, throat (HEENT): Normal, visual acuity 20/25 bilaterally, normal fundoscopic examination

Neck: No carotid bruits, thyromegaly, or lymphadenopathy

Lungs: Clear

Heart: Regular rate and rhythm, no murmurs

Abdomen: Obese, nontender without organomegaly; no femoral bruits

Genitourinary: Uncircumcised penis without fibrosis, normal testicles, no hernias

Vital Signs

Temperature: 98.8°F (37.1°C)

Heart rate: 92 beats per minute (BPM)

Respiration: 16 BPM

Blood pressure: 145/90 mm Hg

Height: 5'8" (172 cm)

Current weight: 216 lb (98 kg)

BMI: 33 kg/m^2

Waist circumference: 42 in. (108 cm)

Weight history: DM describes a gradual weight gain since he stopped playing sports in college, at which time he weighed 160 lb (72.6 kg).

Laboratory Data

Random capillary glucose: 200 mg/dL (normal: 70 to 110 mg/dL)

DM returned the following day for fasting blood work and came back the following week to review and discuss his test results with his family physician.

Patient's Values (Fasting)	Normal Values
Plasma glucose: 145 mg/dL	70–110 mg/dL
A1C: 8.0%	4%–6%
Total cholesterol: 230 mg/dL	<200 mg/dL
HDL: 38 mg/dL	>40 mg/dL
LDL: 140 mg/dL	<100 mg/dL
Triglycerides: 220 mg/dL	<150 mg/dL

Based on his history and laboratory data, DM was diagnosed with type 2 diabetes. He was counseled to lose weight, begin a regular exercise program, and return for a follow-up appointment in 3 months. Smoking cessation was strongly encouraged as one of the most important lifestyle changes that DM could make. DM was referred to an ophthalmologist for further evaluation and treatment of his blurred vision and a complete eye examination.

Three months later, DM returned to the office. He did not make any lifestyle changes as prescribed. He reported a slight improvement in his fatigue but worsening of his erectile dysfunction. His physical examination was unchanged. Laboratory data obtained 1 week before this visit were essentially unchanged as well.

DM was referred to a registered dietitian for nutrition counseling and to a nurse practitioner to begin a smoking-cessation program. He was started on the following medications:

Metformin: 500 mg twice a day with meals
Atorvastatin: 10 mg once a day
Enalapril: 2.5 mg once a day
Enteric coated aspirin: 325 mg once a day
Sildenafil: 50 mg prn

Case Questions

1. What do DM's symptoms and laboratory values indicate about his glycemic and lipid control?
2. Define and describe insulin resistance in type 2 diabetes mellitus.
3. What specific evidenced-based food/nutrition recommendations would you offer DM given his current diagnosis?
4. What is the role of exercise in patients with type 2 diabetes?
5. What evidence exists regarding the prevention of type 2 diabetes for patients with impaired glucose tolerance?

Case Answers

Part 1: Assessment

1. **What do DM's symptoms and laboratory values indicate about his glycemic and lipid control?**

    DM came to his family physician complaining of fatigue, blurry vision, and admitted erectile dysfunction (ED). DM's fatigue and transient blurry vision are most likely caused by his fluctuating plasma glucose levels, consistent with his diabetes. Blurry vision may also represent transient ischemic attacks and other vascular diseases, warranting an ophthalmology referral.

DM's laboratory values indicate that his glycemic control is poor. The A1C goal for patients with diabetes is less than 7%. DM's A1C is 8.2%, which indicates that his average blood glucose during the previous 3-month period was in the range of 180 to 200 mg/dL. The United Kingdom Prospective Diabetes Study (UKPDS) demonstrated that a 0.9% reduction in A1C (A1C reduced from 7.9% to 7.0%) resulted in a 25% reduction in microvascular complications.

Because lipid abnormalities are often associated with poor glycemic control, the treatment plan would be to optimize DM's diabetes control with medical nutrition therapy aimed at reducing energy intake and increasing physical activity. Pharmacologic therapy can be added as needed. The dyslipidemia often seen in patients with type 2 diabetes is characterized by high triglycerides, low HDL, and small, dense LDL particles. DM presents with abdominal obesity as indicated by a waist circumference greater than 42 in. (107 cm). He is relatively physically inactive. DM's 25 pack year smoking history puts him at increased risk of cardiovascular disease (CVD) by reducing his HDL levels, inhibiting platelet aggregation, increasing LDL oxidation, and contributing to endothelial dysfunction.

Diabetes confers a similar risk of disease and death from cardiovascular disease compared to that of someone with known cardiovascular disease. A major focus of the National Cholesterol Education Program Adult Treatment Panel (ATP) III Guidelines is the identification and treatment of patients with metabolic syndrome. DM meets all five of the criteria for diagnosis of metabolic syndrome: hypertension (>130/85 mm Hg), high triglycerides, low HDL, diabetes (or insulin resistance and glucose intolerance), and abdominal obesity [indicated by a waist circumference >40 in. (102 cm)]. DM's stage 1 hypertension places him in the Risk Group C classification according to the Joint National Committee (JNC) VI, which recommends immediate antihypertensive drug therapy as the standard of care (see Chapter 7).

DM's ED is a common problem in men with diabetes, who have a threefold increase in the prevalence of ED compared with nondiabetic men. Sildenafil and other newer medicines are less effective in men with diabetes than in nondiabetic men.

2. **Define and describe insulin resistance in type 2 diabetes mellitus.**

Insulin resistance is associated with type 2 diabetes, hypertension, dyslipidemia, central abdominal obesity, hyperinsulinemia, and other abnormalities. Insulin resistance can be defined as the diminished sensitivity of cells to the action of insulin. Since insulin resistance usually develops before the onset of the disease, treating insulin-resistant individuals may help to possibly delay or prevent type 2 diabetes.

The reasons for the development of insulin resistance are becoming more defined, as genetics, diet, and level of physical activity all play a vital role. Individuals in whom insulin resistance is more likely to develop have a personal history of impaired glucose tolerance, a first-degree relative with type 2 diabetes, and, in women, a history of gestational diabetes or polycystic ovary disease. The condition is also associated with obesity, especially abdominal or central obesity.

Type 2 diabetes is characterized by both a progressive decrease in insulin production by the pancreas and the development of insulin resistance in both skeletal muscle and the liver. The effect of insulin resistance in muscle tissue is postprandial hyperglycemia and impaired glucose tolerance. Over time, insulin resistance may worsen. Insulin resistance has five stages. Stage I is characterized by increased insulin production by the pancreas; stages II and III present with increased hepatic glucose production and A1C levels and elevated fasting plasma glucose concentrations (110 to 125 mg/dL for stage II and 126 to 160 mg/dL for stage III). Eventually, insulin resistance becomes moderate to severe, insulin secretion declines, and fasting plasma glucose concentrations range from 161 to 240 mg/dL (stage IV) and more than 240 mg/dL (stage V).

Medical nutrition therapy and regular physical activity can be very effective and may be sufficient treatment when insulin resistance is moderate or in the prediabetic stage, when the pancreatic beta cells are still producing insulin. However, as the disease progresses nutrition and pharmacologic therapy may need to be combined to achieve the desired glucose and lipid outcomes.

Since DM did not make any food or physical activity changes during the previous 3 months when his diagnosis was confirmed, it would be worthwhile to spend time assessing his readiness for change. Clinicians often find that when patients focus on "what they can eat" rather than "what they cannot eat" they are more likely to lose weight. Motivational interviewing should be used to identify what the patient wants to learn and what he feels are areas of difficulty and to help him identify problem-solving strategies to successfully implement lifestyle changes. Involving DM's wife in these discussions would also be helpful (see Chapter 1).

Part 2: Medical Nutrition Therapy

3. **What specific evidence-based food/nutrition recommendations would you offer DM given his current diagnosis?**

DM presents with type 2 diabetes, dyslipidemia, hypertension, and obesity. His A1C goal is less than 7%, and his LDL and triglyceride goals are less than 100 mg/dL and less than 150 mg/dL, respectively. The goals of medical nutrition therapy for patients with diabetes are to achieve and maintain normal or near normal glucose, blood pressure, and lipid levels to prevent or reduce the complications of diabetes and risk for CVD. The analysis of DM's diet indicates excessive calories, saturated fat, cholesterol, and sodium. Since DM is considered obese with a BMI of 33 kg/m^2, reducing his total calories, carbohydrate, and fat intake is important. Because he is a smoker and his LDL and total cholesterol are elevated, DM should be advised to reduce his saturated fat intake to less than 7% of his total caloric intake.

Carbohydrate counting is probably the best meal-planning approach for DM. One carbohydrate serving is equal to the amount of food providing 15 g carbohydrate. Foods that contain carbohydrate include, for example, fruit and fruit juice, milk and yogurt, starches, and baked desserts. To reduce his carbohydrate calories at breakfast, DM could cut his orange juice serving in half, skip the doughnuts, and opt for smaller bagels. Store-bought bagels are 4 oz (113 g) each and may contain up to 400 calories, the equivalent of four servings of carbohydrate. By purchasing smaller, frozen bagels (2 oz, or 57 g) or eating one-half of a regular bagel, he can save up to 200 calories every day. Replacing regular cream cheese with a low-fat variety will also cut the calories by one-half; alternatively, a low-sugar jelly can be used. Substituting a small piece of fresh fruit for fruit juice will also decrease carbohydrates and increase soluble fiber.

For his snack, DM can use low-fat or skim milk in his coffee. Instead of eating the blueberry muffin, which can contain up to 400 calories from saturated fat and sugar, DM can choose a low-fat sugar-free yogurt. For lunch DM can eat a lean meat sandwich, such as turkey or grilled salmon on wheat bread instead of white bread, if he is eating out. Using mustard that is fat free and substituting low-salt pretzels, fresh fruit, or carrots for the potato chips will help to reduce the calorie, fat, and sodium content of DM's meal.

For dinner, DM should be made aware that the choices he has selected in the Chinese restaurant are all fried and therefore high in both total and saturated fat. In addition, Chinese food is usually high in sodium. Better choices would be steamed white rice; steamed vegetables with shrimp, scallops, or white-meat chicken; and an additional vegetable dish, such as string beans with garlic sauce. DM should be instructed that every one-third of a cup of rice is equivalent to one carbohydrate serving. Other ethnic foods can be prepared in a low-fat manner as well. Since DM is married, it would be helpful to include his wife in the discussions related to dinner.

Adding more fiber from whole grains, fresh fruit, and vegetables is also advisable; however, fiber's effect on plasma blood glucose stability has not been confirmed. It appears that very high intakes of dietary fiber, particularly soluble fiber, above levels recommended by the ADA (20 to 35 g per day) improve glycemic control in some patients. However, the palatability and gastrointestinal side effects may make this an impractical recommendation. DM's current dietary fiber intake is 14 g.

The following recommended sample diet increases his dietary fiber intake to 38 g by adding a banana and oatmeal for breakfast, more vegetables for lunch and dinner, and fresh fruit and nuts instead of juices and baked products for snacks. These dietary changes will decrease DM's caloric intake from 3757 to 2484 kcal per day. By reducing his calories by approximately 1000 kcal per day, DM may lose 1 to 2 lb per week. These changes also reduced his saturated fat intake to 22 g per day, or 7.8% of his total calories, which is consistent with the ADA and ATP III Guidelines. Below is a revised menu for DM.

DM's Recommended Sample Diet

Breakfast (home)

Banana	$^1/_2$ medium
Oatmeal	1 cup cooked
2% low-fat milk	4 oz (120 mL)
Light cream cheese	1 Tbsp.
Plain bagel	2 oz (57 g)

Snack (office)

Non-fat yogurt with NutraSweet	8 oz (226 g)
Aspartame sweetener	1 packet
2% low-fat milk	2 oz (60 mL)
Coffee, brewed	12 oz (360 mL)

Lunch (deli)

Turkey breast	4 oz (113 g)
Low-fat Swiss cheese	1 oz (28 g)
Whole-grain wheat bread	2 slices
Mustard	1 tsp.
Raw carrots	3 oz (85 g)
Low-fat ranch dressing	2 Tbsp.
Water or diet beverage	12 oz (240 mL)

Dinner (Mexican restaurant)

Chicken fajita (chicken, pepper, onions) (No cheese or sour cream)	2 large
Nacho tortilla chips	1 oz (28 g)
Salsa	$^1/_2$ cup
Beer, ale	12 oz (360 mL)

Snack (home)

Dry-roasted mixed nuts, unsalted	$^1/_2$ cup
Fresh apple	1 medium

Total calories: 2484 kcal
Protein: 120 g (19% of total calories)
Carbohydrate: 288 g (46% of total calories)

Total fat: 90 g (32% of total calories)

Saturated fat: 22 g (7.8% of total calories)

Monounsaturated fats: 40 g (15% of total calories)
Cholesterol: 174 mg

Dietary fiber: 38 g

Alcohol: 13 g

Sodium: 4239 mg

4. **What is the role of exercise in patients with type 2 diabetes?**

All patients with diabetes or prediabetes should be physically active and encouraged to begin a regular exercise program if they are sedentary. The American College of Sports Medicine (ASCM)/Centers for Disease Control and Prevention (CDC) and the Surgeon General recommend 30 minutes per day of moderate-intensity exercise. The definition of moderate-intensity physical activity is 50% to 70% of one's maximal heart rate for age. However, before starting an exercise program the patient should consult with his/her physician.

Exercise improves overall well-being and has been proven to lower postprandial glucose levels by increasing peripheral insulin uptake and increasing insulin sensitivity. Exercise may not contribute to a greater short-term weight reduction than diet alone, but it has been shown to be the single best predictor of long-term weight loss in overweight or obese people.

For all individuals with diabetes, the benefits of exercise include decreasing the risk of cardiovascular disease, improving one's lipoprotein profile, and increased cardiovascular fitness. It is likely that the beneficial effects of exercise on the prevention of cardiovascular disease are associated with improvements in the metabolic syndrome. In hypertensive patients with hyperinsulinemia, regular exercise has consistently demonstrated a reduction in blood pressure levels. Regular exercise has also been shown to reduce levels of triglyceride-rich VLDL particles. However, its effects on HDL levels have not been as favorable, probably due to the lack of intensive activity used in most studies.

Since DM does not engage in a regular exercise program, walking at least 3 nonconsecutive days a week to start (increasing up to 5 to 7 days) for 30 minutes a day is a reasonable initial exercise program. Ideally, DM would eventually incorporate some physical activity into each day. DM might start out with just 10 minutes every day during lunch, after work or in the evening, and work up to this optimum level gradually. Tailoring exercise to each patient's needs is very important to maximize adherence. Motivating patients to maintain a physically active lifestyle is not a simple task, but it is a worthwhile endeavor.

5. **What evidence exists regarding the prevention of type 2 diabetes for patients with impaired glucose tolerance?**

Strong evidence has shown that type 2 diabetes can be prevented or delayed. Therefore, individuals at high risk of developing diabetes (those individuals who are overweight or obese or who have a family history of diabetes) need to be aware of the benefits of modest weight loss and participation in regular physical activity. In the Diabetes Prevention Program (DPP), 3234 subjects with impaired glucose tolerance and a mean BMI of 34 kg/m^2 were randomly assigned to one of three intervention groups that included intensive lifestyle modification or one of the medicine treatment groups (metformin vs. placebo). After an average follow-up of 2.8 years, the lifestyle group reduced the onset of diabetes by 58% and the metformin group reduced the onset of diabetes by 31% compared to placebo. The goals of the lifestyle intervention were at least a 7% weight reduction and a total of 150 minutes per week of physical activity. On average, 50% of the lifestyle group achieved this weight reduction goal and 74% maintained the required amount of physical activity.

In the DPP, the lifestyle group lost about 12 lb after 2 years and 9 lb after 3 years. Clearly, follow-up was very important to the success of these patients, who met with a counselor very often during the first 6 months of the study and by telephone thereafter, which is not an available option in most physician practices. Additional research confirms the potential for moderate weight loss (5% to 7%) in reducing the risk of developing diabetes. An active lifestyle has also been shown to prevent or delay the development of type 2 diabetes, since both moderate and vigorous exercise decrease the risk of impaired glucose tolerance and type 2 diabetes.

See Chapter Review Questions, pages A-27 to A-30.

10

Pulmonary Disease

Gregg Lipschik, Jennifer Williams, and Maria R. Mascarenhas

Objectives*

- Define the nutritional deficits, requirements, and medical nutrition therapy in patients with chronic obstructive pulmonary disease (COPD) and cystic fibrosis.
- Examine available feeding options and their indications for mechanically ventilated patients and the risk associated with nutritional support.
- Identify the association between obstructive sleep apnea syndrome and obesity, and outline the nutritional regimen recommendations for these patients.
- Recognize the importance of incorporating nutrition into the history, review of systems, and physical examinations of patients with pulmonary diseases.

Chronic Obstructive Pulmonary Disease

Between 25% and 50% of patients with COPD have some degree of nutritional depletion. Weight loss is exceedingly common among patients with COPD, as are reductions in fat reserves and muscle mass. Patients who experience progressive weight loss with 15% or more weight change in 1 year are at risk for undernutrition. Patients at normal body weight may also be undernourished. More severe COPD is associated with an increased risk of undernutrition and weight loss. The greater the weight loss, the smaller the mass of the respiratory muscles and diaphragm. Malnourished patients with COPD have a poor prognosis.

* SOURCE: Objectives for chapter and cases adapted from the *NIH Nutrition Curriculum Guide for Training Physicians* (*http://www.nhlbi.nih.gov/funding/training/naa*).

Patients with COPD benefit from nutritional assessment because the consequences of undernutrition include adverse effects on respiratory muscle mass and function that result in decreased respiratory muscle strength. Furthermore, because undernutrition is also associated with decreased cell-mediated immunity, altered immunoglobulin production, and impaired cellular resistance of the tracheobronchial mucosa to bacterial infection, undernourished patients are at increased risk for respiratory infections, especially pneumonia and bronchitis. Patients with advanced COPD are also at risk for osteoporosis, another nutrition-related complication. Low body mass index (BMI) is an independent predictor of osteoporosis. Interestingly, recent studies suggest that foods high in antioxidants, including fruits and vegetables, as well as whole grains and alcohol, may have protective or ameliorative effects on the development of COPD.

Causes of Weight Loss

Hypermetabolism

Two major causes of hypermetabolism result in increased energy requirements in patients with COPD.

Increased Work of Breathing In patients with normal lung function, breathing expends 36 to 72 calories per day. Patients with COPD may have up to a 10-fold increase in their daily energy expenditure from breathing. Both the increased resistive load and the reduced respiratory muscle efficiency experienced by these patients contribute to this increased daily energy expenditure from breathing. This increased work of breathing results in an increased daily energy requirement. If patients do not ingest additional calories to meet these increased needs, they lose weight.

Frequent, Recurrent Respiratory Infections Respiratory infections may increase metabolic rate, depending on the severity of the illness, further contributing to weight loss.

Poor Nutritional Intake

Factors that may result in inadequate intake in patients with COPD include:

- Chronic sputum production and frequent coughing, which may alter the desire for and taste of food, as well as interfere with swallowing.
- Severe dyspnea and fatigue, which can interfere with the ability to prepare and ingest adequate meals.
- Depression from the illness, a possible cause of anorexia.
- Overinflation of the lungs, causing flattening of the diaphragm and pressure on the abdominal cavity during eating, resulting in early satiety and swallowing problems (dysglutition).
- Oxyhemoglobin desaturation during eating, resulting in increased dyspnea, which further limits dietary intake.

- Side effects of medications, such as nausea, vomiting, diarrhea, dysgeusia, dry mouth, and gastric irritation, which may limit dietary intake. Medications may also increase the need for protein, calcium, vitamin A, and folic acid or result in altered serum levels of potassium, magnesium, vitamins, or cholesterol.

Other Factors

Recent studies suggest that elevated levels of the cytokine, tumor necrosis factor (TNF)-alpha, and low levels of the fat cell–derived protein, leptin, contribute to weight loss, skeletal muscle loss, and increased resting energy requirement in patients with COPD.

Several studies suggest that metabolism of the amino acid leucine is abnormal in patients with severe COPD. The clinical significance of this is not known.

Medical Nutrition Therapy for Chronic Obstructive Pulmonary Disease

Because patients with COPD have increased energy requirements combined with poor nutritional intake, they have difficulty meeting their caloric requirements and frequently lose weight. It is safe to assume that patients who are not ingesting their caloric requirements and present with weight loss may also suffer from vitamin and mineral deficiencies. Certain electrolytes (calcium, magnesium, potassium, and phosphorus) are especially important in undernourished COPD patients because depletion of these electrolytes may contribute to the impairment of respiratory muscle function. When severely undernourished COPD patients are rapidly refed with glucose infusions, careful attention must be paid to these electrolytes because the need for them increases during anabolism (see Chapter 5, Case 2).

Inadequate electrolyte repletion in this setting can result in severe metabolic consequences and, thus, refeeding syndrome. Therefore, the goals of medical nutrition therapy for COPD patients are to:

- Supply adequate calories, protein, vitamins, and minerals to maintain desirable body weight (BMI 20 to 24 kg/m^2), energy level, and nutritional status.
- Provide small, frequent meals with nutrient-dense foods, such as peanut butter and jelly sandwiches, and soft-textured, easily consumed foods, such as omelets, yogurt, cottage cheese, and casseroles.
- Add high-calorie, high-protein, liquid or pudding nutritional supplements or milk shakes to the diet.
- Recommend foods that require little preparation, such as frozen dinners heated in a microwave oven.
- Follow the Food Guide Pyramid recommendations, with specific emphasis on high milk, fruit, and whole-grain consumption (Appendix).
- Limit alcohol consumption to fewer than two drinks (30 g alcohol) per day.
- Time the main daily meal when the patient's energy level is the highest.
- Encourage patients to rest before mealtime.
- Prescribe a daily multivitamin and mineral supplement.

Mechanical Ventilation

Rationale for Nutrition Support

Patients with respiratory failure requiring mechanical ventilation cannot ingest food through the mouth because of the endotracheal tube, unless a tracheostomy (transcutaneous airway direct into the trachea) has been placed. Because many patients require mechanical ventilation for prolonged periods, nutrition support is necessary to prevent undernutrition.

Undernutrition associated with critical illness impairs cell-mediated immunity, alters immunoglobulin production, and impairs cellular resistance to infection. Therefore, patients who are not fed for more than 7 to 10 days are at increased risk of infection. In addition, undernutrition causes difficulty in weaning from the ventilator, presumably due to respiratory muscle weakness. Conversely, ventilated patients with preexisting undernutrition who are fed have improved respiratory muscle strength and function, which may hasten weaning from the ventilator.

Feeding Options

Most patients who require mechanical ventilation for more than several days should receive enteral nutrition via a nasoenteral feeding tube as long as the GI tract is functioning (see Chapter 12). Parenteral nutrition should be reserved for patients who do not have a functioning gut (e.g., those with bowel obstruction or ileus; see Chapter 13). A recent prospective controlled trial in mechanically ventilated patients suggests that early (day 1) enteral provision of total nutritional requirements is associated with an increase in ventilator-associated pneumonia, diarrhea, and length of stay. Thus, initiation of enteral feeding probably should be delayed several days. The decision to begin parenteral nutritional support is made if the patient is severely undernourished, is not a candidate for enteral feedings, and will be unable to eat for more than 7 to 10 days.

Minimizing Effects of Nutrition Support on Carbon Dioxide Production

The caloric and nutrient composition of the diet has a profound effect on gas exchange, especially carbon dioxide (CO_2) production. The respiratory quotient (RQ) is expressed as the ratio of CO_2 produced to oxygen consumed.

$$RQ = \frac{CO_2 \text{ produced}}{O_2 \text{ consumed}}$$

The RQ of carbohydrates is 1.0, while the RQ of fat is 0.7 and of a mixed meal is 0.83. Thus, CO_2 production is greater during carbohydrate metabolism than during fat metabolism. A diet high in carbohydrate thus requires increased ventilation to eliminate the excess CO_2 and might conceivably complicate weaning from the ventilator. Consequently, high-fat, low-carbohydrate enteral feeding products have been formulated and recommended for feeding mechanically ventilated patients with severe COPD. These have not been proven effective, however, probably because excess CO_2 production associated with mixed or high-carbohydrate diets is not clinically relevant unless caloric requirements are exceeded. Thus, it is essential to avoid overfeeding these patients because this can result in excessive CO_2 production, increased RQ, and difficulty in weaning from mechanical ventilation. If indirect calorimetry is available to determine caloric expenditure, this should be recommended; otherwise, 100% to 120% of predicted caloric expenditure should be used.

Cystic Fibrosis

Cystic fibrosis (CF), a life-threatening genetic disorder usually seen in children and young adults, presents with profuse, abnormally thick exocrine gland secretions. These excessive secretions may obstruct the pancreatic and bile ducts, intestines, and bronchi, resulting in a variety of clinical problems. Chronic lung disease and pancreatic insufficiency are the two most common problems in patients with CF. A definite association has been found between worsening lung disease and undernutrition. The degree of undernutrition seen in these patients may vary considerably. Nutritional deficiencies of specific micronutrients may be subclinical initially and may progress to clinically evident symptoms and signs if not recognized and treated. Deficiencies of calories, protein, essential fatty acids, fat-soluble vitamins (A, K, E, and D), beta-carotene, zinc, iron, and sodium have been described. Bone disease, such as osteoporosis, is also being increasingly recognized (see Case 2).

Causes of Weight Loss and Undernutrition

The causes of weight loss and undernutrition in patients with CF are multifactorial. These include maldigestion or malabsorption (due to pancreatic insufficiency), or both; inadequate oral caloric intake; increased caloric and nutrient needs and the development of CF-related organ system disease, particularly pulmonary disease; liver disease; intestinal resection; and CF-related diabetes mellitus (CFRD).

Maldigestion and Malabsorption

Most patients with CF (80% to 85%) have pancreatic insufficiency and consequent malabsorption of fat, protein, carbohydrate, vitamins, and minerals, which, if untreated, leads to undernutrition. Pancreatic enzyme supplements are administered with meals and snacks to assist with the absorption of nutrients. The amount and type of enzyme supplements depend on the degree of malabsorption and the fat content of the diet. Steatorrhea is considered a clinical indicator of fat malabsorption (see Chapter 8, Case 2).

Increased Nutritional Needs

Despite pancreatic enzyme supplementation, the energy and protein needs of CF patients are significantly increased by their loss of nutrients due to malabsorption and by higher than normal protein catabolism and energy expenditure due to frequent infections.

Increased Work of Breathing

Patients with CF commonly suffer from chronic bronchitis, airway obstruction, and recurrent infections. These increase the work of breathing, resulting in a higher energy expenditure. The effects of muscle wasting and undernutrition on respiratory muscles contribute as well.

Other Factors

Gastroesophageal reflux, abdominal pain, and psychosocial stresses may also contribute to poor caloric intake. Liver disease with decreased bile salt excretion worsens the malabsorption. CFRD with glucosuria results in increased energy loss. Patients who undergo significant intestinal resection may have decreased intestinal surface area for absorption of nutrients.

Medical Nutrition Therapy for Cystic Fibrosis

Because of their increased nutrient needs and losses and often inadequate intake, patients with CF usually are unable to meet their caloric and protein require-ments and maintain their weight. CF is usually diagnosed in infancy or early childhood, and monitoring growth and development in these patients is particu-larly important. Not uncommonly, CF patients remain at or fall below the fifth percentile in both weight and height for their age on the pediatric growth charts. The goals of nutrition therapy for CF patients are:

- Routine nutritional assessment to include height, weight, BMI, weight change, pediatric growth parameters, dietary history, physical examination, and evaluation of laboratory values.
- Dietary counseling to provide adequate intake of calories, protein, vitamins, and minerals. This will include education about high-calorie balanced meals with added salt, nutrient-dense snacks two to three times a day, and nutritional supplements.
- Adequate pancreatic enzyme replacement therapy adjusted to avoid malabsorption for all patients with pancreatic insufficiency.
- Adequate vitamin and mineral supplements as per the CF Foundation Guidelines.

If patients continue to experience weight loss to such an extent that they fall below 85% of their ideal body weight, or if they have difficulty maintaining their weight, additional nutrition support may be necessary. Both enteral (using nasogastric or gastrostomy tubes) and parenteral feedings can be employed, as clinically indicated.

Obstructive Sleep Apnea Syndrome

Obstructive sleep apnea syndrome (OSAS) is defined as recurrent episodes of apnea during sleep caused by occlusion of the upper airway. A primary risk factor for OSAS is obesity. Up to two-thirds of all patients who present with OSAS are obese. OSAS may be caused by an increased amount of fat surrounding the structures of the upper airway. Although not all obese patients have OSAS, and occasionally nonobese patients may have it, it is clear that weight loss in obese patients with OSAS improves signs and symptoms. Symptoms of sleep apnea, such as snoring and excessive daytime sleepiness, should always be ascertained as part of the medical history in obese patients. In addition to weight loss, patients with OSAS are most commonly treated with continuous positive airway pressure therapy (CPAP). Recent studies have suggested a role for the fat cell protein, leptin, in the pathogenesis of respiratory dysfunction in OSAS.

Causes of Weight Gain and Obesity

Fatigue due to chronic sleep disruption, a common symptom of patients with OSAS, may influence patients' eating behaviors. Often too tired and lacking in motivation to exercise, they tend to lead sedentary lifestyles. In addition, many patients with OSAS report falling asleep often after eating, which further decreases their energy expenditure. Certain overweight patients with OSAS also may be prone to binge eating as a result of depression about their illness and their body image. Whatever the exact causes, a combination of decreased physical activity and increased caloric consumption contributes to weight gain in these patients.

Nutrition Components of the Medical History

The following topics should be covered during the medical history of any obese patient with diagnosed or suspected OSAS: weight history and previous dieting experience; sleep patterns; frequency of meals and snacks, especially after dinner; binge eating during the day or night; assessment of nutritional content (e.g., high fat, high sugar) of the diet; exercise habits; alcohol intake, including frequency and amount; and other medical problems the patient reports that may respond to dietary modification (e.g., hypertension, diabetes mellitus, cardiovascular disease).

Medical Nutrition Therapy for Sleep Apnea

Weight Loss

Because obesity contributes to the pathogenesis of OSAS, weight loss is of primary importance in obese patients with OSAS. Weight loss as small as 10 lb (4.5 kg) can dramatically improve breathing and sleep patterns. Once CPAP treatment has been initiated, patients would benefit from a referral to a registered dietitian for either individual or group nutritional counseling.

Increasing Activity

Once patients begin to feel better and have more energy, they should be encouraged to begin a low-intensity exercise program, such as walking 15 minutes once or twice a day.

Lung Transplantation

Lung transplantation has become a viable alternative for some patients with severe pulmonary disease, including COPD, cystic fibrosis, and pulmonary hypertension. The nutritional implications for lung transplantation patients vary depending on whether they are awaiting or have received a transplant, and whether they are breathing spontaneously or mechanically ventilated following surgery. The following recommendations are listed accordingly.

Nutrition Assessment before Lung Transplantation

Routine nutrition assessment before lung transplantation entails the following steps:

- Assess nutritional status using the patient's weight history.
- Assess nutritional status using visceral protein status, such as albumin, transferrin, and prealbumin (half-life: 2 days). If protein status is depleted, supplement the diet with high-protein milk shakes and snacks.
- Assess serum lipid levels. If cholesterol (normal: <200 mg/dL) and triglyceride (normal: <150 mg/dL) levels are elevated, appropriate modifications include substituting foods low in saturated fat and cholesterol into the diet and limiting concentrated sweets and alcohol.
- Monitor the patient's satiety level and gastrointestinal symptoms, such as bloating and gas, that could interfere with adequate dietary intake.
- Assess bone density. Supplement calcium if signs of osteoporosis exist.

Medical Nutrition Therapy after Lung Transplantation

Appropriate medical nutrition therapy immediately following lung transplantation involves the following measures:

- Increase protein and calories to promote repletion as clinically indicated and assist with wound healing during the catabolic state following surgery.
- Decrease sodium intake if fluid retention develops.
- Monitor glucose control and lipids in patients on corticosteroids.

Medical Nutrition Therapy on Discharge

Several of the drugs used for immunosuppression after lung transplantation have an impact on nutrition. Cyclosporine can cause hyperkalemia and may also elevate serum cholesterol and triglyceride levels. These changes may require limitation of dietary potassium or a decrease in dietary saturated fat and cholesterol.

Tacrolimus, often substituted for cyclosporine, causes hyperglycemia. The antimetabolite, azathioprine, causes nausea, vomiting, and diarrhea. The similarly acting mycophenolate, mofetil, may produce diarrhea and dyspepsia. These problems may interfere with the provision of adequate calories and must be addressed.

Corticosteroids (e.g., prednisone) cause hyperglycemia and increased appetite and may result in weight gain and obesity. Thus, weight and calorie and fat intake should be monitored following lung transplantation. Patients taking corticosteroids also may experience fluid retention, requiring limitation of dietary sodium intake.

For a list of references for this chapter, please visit the University of Pennsylvania School of Medicine's Nutrition Education and Prevention Program web site: *http://www.med.upenn.edu/nutrimed/articles.html*

Case 1

Chronic Obstructive Pulmonary Disease

Darwin Deen and Jennifer M. Williams

Objectives

- Review those factors in the history and physical examination that are important to the nutritional assessment of a patient with COPD.
- Assess the relevance of routine nutritional assessment parameters in a patient with pulmonary disease.
- Explain the causes of weight loss in patients with COPD.
- Outline the appropriate dietary interventions for a COPD patient with weight loss.

PD, a 53-year-old woman diagnosed with COPD 8 years ago, visits her physician reporting dyspnea. This has worsened progressively over the last 3 days since she caught a cold from her grandchildren. She explains that her customary shortness of breath worsens when she is sick or under increased stress, when the humidity is high, when the temperature is extremely cold, or when she eats a large meal. Currently, PD has two-pillow orthopnea and bilateral lower-extremity edema. She reports a loss of 18 lb (8.2 kg) within the last year and denies trying to lose weight. Pulmonary function tests from last year confirmed severe COPD with a forced expiratory volume (FEV_1) of 36% of predicted, a forced vital capacity (FVC) of 1.65 liters, and a ratio of FEV to FVC of 39%. A recent chest x-ray revealed hyperinflation of lung fields, with diminished lung markings in the upper lung fields.

Past Medical History

PD has been treated for hypertension for 12 years and for hypercholesterolemia for the past 2 years. She has no previous history of diabetes mellitus, thyroid disease, or liver disease.

Medications

PD is currently taking verapamil (Calan SR), furosemide (Lasix), potassium chloride (K-Lyte/Cl), atorvastatin (Lipitor), prednisone, ipratropium bromide (Atrovent), alendronate (Fosamax), and albuterol (Ventolin). She does not take any vitamin/mineral or herbal supplements. PD has no known food allergies.

Family History

PD's mother died at age 70 of a heart attack. Her father also died of a heart attack, at age 73.

Social History

PD lives with her husband in a two-story home. They have four children and 14 grandchildren. PD worked in a local department store as a salesperson until last year, when she retired because of her illness. She formerly attended church regularly with her husband but lately has been too tired to go. Her husband has also recently taken over the food shopping. PD usually follows a low-salt, low-fat diet at home. She reports the following substance use:

> *Alcohol intake*: None
>
> *Tobacco*: 45 pack year smoking history (1½ packs per day for 30 years); quit 5 years ago
>
> *Caffeine*: One cup of coffee per day

Diet History

PD is on a low-fat, low-cholesterol, low-salt diet for elevated cholesterol and hypertension. She provided the following 24-hour dietary recall that reportedly reflects her typical daily intake. She does not add salt to her food or use salt in cooking.

PD's 24-Hour Dietary Recall

Breakfast (home)	Farina	1.5 cup
	White toast	1 slice
	Jelly	2 Tbsp.
	Coffee	1 cup
	1% milk	4 oz (120 mL)
Lunch (home)	Low-fat yogurt	1 cup
	Apple juice	6 oz (180 mL)
Dinner (home)	Chicken breast	4 oz (114 g)
	Baked potato	1 medium
	Cooked carrots	½ cup
	Diet margarine	1 Tbsp.
	Water	1 glass
Snack (home)	Banana	1 medium

Total calories: 1262 kcal

Protein: 63 g (20% of calories)

Fat: 21 g (15% of calories)
Saturated fat: 7.0 g (5% of calories)
Monounsaturated fat: 5.0 g (4% of calories)
Carbohydrate: 209 g (66% of calories)
Sodium: 1036 mg
Cholesterol: 112 mg
Fiber: 11 g

Review of Systems

General: Weakness, fatigue, and weight loss [18 lb (8.2 kg) in the last year]
Mouth: Wears dentures (top and bottom; loose fitting)
Gastrointestinal (GI): Poor appetite; no diarrhea, nausea, or vomiting
Extremities: No joint pain; has difficulty walking without a walker

Physical Examination

Vital Signs

Temperature: 97°F (36°C)
Heart rate: 94 beats per minute (BPM)
Respiration: 20 BPM
Blood pressure: 150/80 mm Hg
Height: 5'6" (168 cm)
Current weight: 169 lb (77 kg)
Estimated dry weight: 147 lb (67 kg) [Dry weight is estimated by subtracting the weight of the fluid from the current weight. Fluid weight is estimated at 22 lb (10 kg) since she has 2+ pitting edema on both ankles. Eleven pounds (5 kg) can be used to estimate fluid in patients with ascites and no peripheral edema.]
Usual weight: 187 lb (85 kg)
BMI using estimated dry weight: 24 kg/m^2
Percent weight change using estimated dry weight (>1 year): 21% decrease [(85–67)/85]
General: Frail woman in no acute distress
Skin: Ecchymoses
Head/neck: Normal palpable thyroid
Mouth: Loose-fitting dentures; no sores; symmetric soft palate and uvula
Cardiac: Regular rate and rhythm; normal first and second heart sounds; a third heart sound is present as well; jugular venous distention and hepatojugular reflux noted
Lung: Increased anteroposterior (A-P) diameter, decreased breath sounds; diffuse mild expiratory wheezing throughout the chest with a prolonged expiratory phase

Abdomen: Nondistended, nontender; enlarged liver 12 cm in span; no splenomegaly; normal bowel sounds

Extremities: 2+ pitting edema on both ankles

Rectal: Soft, brown stool in vault; heme negative

Neurologic: Alert; appropriate reactions; good memory; no evidence of sensory loss

Laboratory Data

Patient's Values	Normal Values
Albumin: 4.3 g/dL	3.5–5.8 g/dL
Hemoglobin: 10.8 g/dL	12.0–16.0 g/dL
Hematocrit: 35%	36%–46%
Mean corpuscular volume (MCV): 78 fL	80–100 fL
Cholesterol: 265 mg/dL	<200 mg/dL
Low-density lipoprotein (LDL) cholesterol: 173 mg/dL	<130 mg/dL
High-density lipoprotein (HDL) cholesterol: 42 mg/dL	>40 mg/dL
Triglycerides: 150 mg/dL	<150 mg/dL
Arterial blood gases (ABG)	
pH 7.43	7.35–7.45
pO_2 84 mm Hg	75–105 mm Hg
pCO_2 46 mm Hg	33–45 mm Hg

Case Questions

1. Does PD's percent weight change indicate a significant weight loss?
2. What factors have contributed to PD's weight loss?
3. Estimate PD's caloric needs using the Harris-Benedict equation, including a stress factor for COPD.
4. Based on PD's history, what may account for her severe fatigue?
5. How does poor nutritional status compromise pulmonary function?
6. Discuss the impact of current medications on nutritional status.
7. What is the appropriate medical nutrition therapy for PD, including specific recommendations to improve her nutritional and fluid status?

Case Answers

Part 1: Nutrition Assessment

1. **Does PD's percent weight change indicate a significant weight loss?**

   Determining whether her weight loss is intentional or unintentional is critical. Since PD states that she has lost weight without trying, it can be assumed that this was an unintentional weight loss. Progressive, unintentional weight change of greater than 5% in 1 month or greater than 15% of body weight within a 1-year period is considered a severe weight loss and represents a significant risk for undernutrition. PD had an unintentional weight change of 21% over the past year.

2. **What factors have contributed to PD's weight loss?**

    PD's diet history reveals that her calorie intake meets only two-thirds of her nutritional requirements (see answer to question 3). Her low-calorie intake is due in part to the low-fat, low-cholesterol diet originally prescribed to manage her hypertension and hypercholesterolemia. Because of reduced lung function, PD requires more energy to breathe; the normal daily intake of calories required to maintain body weight is insufficient to meet the excessive demands of breathing for COPD patients. Also, patients with pulmonary disease may ingest even fewer calories because they are too tired to prepare food or to eat a meal. Such patients report dyspnea while chewing and swallowing food, preventing them from breathing adequately and thereby increasing the amount of hemoglobin desaturation.

    Because PD is currently retaining fluid, her actual "dry" weight is 22 lb (10 kg) lower than her reported weight. PD should be asked about recent lifestyle changes and possible depression, which could be contributing to her reduced appetite and unintentional weight loss. Also, her weight loss likely contributed to the ill-fitting dentures, thus increasing the risk of inadequate ingestion of meat or other foods that require chewing.

3. **Estimate PD's calorie needs using the Harris-Benedict equation, including a stress factor for COPD.**

    The Harris-Benedict equation for women:

    Resting energy expenditure (REE) = [655 + (9.7 × wt* in kg)
    $$+ (1.8 \times \text{ht in cm}) - (4.7 \times \text{age})]$$

    *Use estimated dry weight in this patient with bilateral pitting edema.

    Total energy expenditure** (TEE) = [655 + (9.7 × 67 kg)
    $$+ (1.8 \times 168 \text{ cm}) - (4.7 \times 53)]$$
    × 1.3 (sedentary) or (pulmonary disease)

    TEE = (1358 × 1.3) = 1765 kcal per day

    **When defining TEE by Harris-Benedict for activity and stress factors, use one correction only (the highest appropriate). In this case both are 1.3. Compared to PD's current intake, which totals 1262 calories on the day analyzed, it is understandable why she is losing weight.

4. **Based on PD's history, what may account for her severe fatigue?**

    COPD can cause arterial hypercapnia that limits exercise tolerance. Similarly, arterial hypoxemia reduces the amount of oxygen available to the tissues and other organs. PD has fluid overload, probably due to cor pulmonale (right ventricular failure). Patients with COPD typically have elevated hemoglobin and hematocrit levels because of chronic hypoxia. PD's hemoglobin and hematocrit are low, further reducing her body's ability to transport oxygen. Her low MCV may reflect an iron deficiency or inadequate heme synthesis due to protein-calorie undernutrition. Again, recent lifestyle changes and possible depression may also contribute to her fatigue. PD's current calorie intake is inadequate, adding to her fatigue. Liberalizing the monounsaturated and polyunsaturated fat content in PD's diet will provide additional calories without the potential to increase her lipids.

5. **How does poor nutritional status compromise pulmonary function?**

Unintentional weight loss is very common in patients with COPD, and progressive weight loss resulting in a BMI of less than 18.5 kg/m^2 is considered a risk for undernutrition. Poor nutritional status can further compromise a patient with COPD by impeding pulmonary defense mechanisms and altering respiratory muscle structure and function. Limitations of pulmonary defense mechanisms include decreased surfactant production, decreased immunoglobulin levels, and impaired cellular resistance of the tracheobronchial mucosa to bacterial infection. Poor protein status, mineral deficiencies (calcium, magnesium, and phosphorus), and electrolyte (potassium) wasting can decrease the diaphragmatic muscle mass or function, reduce diaphragmatic strength and contractility, diminish the vital capacity, and depress ventilatory responses even to minimal exertion such as walking.

6. **Discuss the impact of current medications on nutritional status and the need for medical nutrition therapy.**

The impact of nutritional status and dietary intake on the use of medication can be complex. Drug-nutrient interactions may be trivial or significant. Patients with protein-calorie undernutrition have impaired drug metabolism. In this case, a patient with COPD who has lost a significant amount of weight and who is consuming an inadequate diet can be expected to have significant alterations in her drug metabolism, increasing the possibility of drug toxicity. For example, energy deficiency reduces theophylline clearance and adding protein to the diet can increase theophylline elimination. Added dietary fat may reduce the tremulousness caused by high-dose theophylline. Reducing dietary protein intake and increasing carbohydrates can reduce theophylline clearance and prolong its serum half-life. The blood pressure–lowering effects of verapamil have been shown not to be dependent on dietary sodium intake, but verapamil absorption is lower with increased sodium intake. Corticosteroids increase hepatic glycogen storage to protect glucose-sensitive tissues (heart and brain), resulting in gluconeogenesis and increased protein turnover. This could have the result of increasing the patient's protein requirements. Drug-drug interactions also must be considered: Prednisone can increase the hypokalemia produced by furosemide, and thus the dose of potassium replacement should be monitored closely. With this in mind, the following considerations apply to the specific medications being used by this patient. They may have an important impact or none at all but should be kept in mind if problems arise.

Slow-release forms of **verapamil SR** need to be swallowed whole with food or milk. Other formulations can be ingested without regard to food. This drug may cause constipation. Alcohol should be avoided. A diet low in sodium with limited caffeine may also be recommended. Verapamil SR may cause elevations of liver enzymes.

Furosemide is best if taken on an empty stomach but can be taken with food or milk to reduce abdominal distress. Furosemide can produce anorexia, increased thirst, or nausea and should be administered with caution to diabetic patients. It lowers serum potassium, magnesium, sodium, chloride, and calcium; it raises glucose and blood urea nitrogen and may transiently elevate cholesterol levels. High intake of dietary sodium makes furosemide less effective. Supplements of potassium, magnesium, and calcium may be recommended.

K-Lyte/Cl should be taken with meals and 8 oz (240 mL) liquid. Possible side effects include gastric irritation, nausea, and iatrogenic elevations in serum potassium and chloride levels.

Prednisone should be taken with meals to avoid GI intolerance. Side effects include esophagitis, nausea, dyspepsia, increased appetite, weight gain, negative nitrogen balance, osteoporosis, fluid retention, hypertension, bruising, and slow wound healing. Hypercholesterolemia and reductions in serum zinc, vitamin A, and vitamin C levels can result from prednisone therapy. It reduces the absorption of calcium and phosphate (PO_4) and antagonizes the action of insulin resulting in hyperglycemia. Alcohol should be avoided. Appropriate nutritional supplements while being treated with prednisone include potassium, calcium, and phosphorus; folate; and vitamins A, C, and D.

The inhalation of **ipratropium bromide** may cause dry mouth, bitter taste, nausea, dyspepsia, constipation, cough, headache, or dyspnea.

Patients who take **albuterol** (nebulized or inhaled) should be cautioned to limit caffeine intake. Albuterol should be taken with food if GI upset occurs. Side effects include anorexia, peculiar taste, sore/dry throat, nausea, tremor, headache, dizziness, and increased glucose levels.

Patients who take **atorvastatin (Lipitor)** should avoid grapefruit juice and limit alcohol consumption. Side effects include nausea, dyspepsia, abdominal pain, constipation, flatulence, and increased liver function tests. 5-Hydroxy-3-methyl-glutaryl coenzyme A (HMG CoA) reductase inhibitors decrease coenzyme Q_{10} synthesis, which may cause fatigue in some patients; this may respond to CoQ_{10} supplements.

Alendronate (Fosamax) should be taken before meals with lots of water. The patient should not lie down for 30 minutes after the dose.

Part 2: Recommendations

7. **What is the appropriate medical nutrition therapy for PD, including specific recommendations to improve her nutrition and fluid status?**

Providing adequate calories and protein for weight and skeletal muscle maintenance is a major goal of medical nutrition therapy. By liberalizing her monounsaturated fat intake, she will increase her calories (see PD's recommended sample diet). The acute risks of weight loss and undernutrition at this time exceed the long-term risks associated with hypercholesterolemia, which can be pharmacologically managed if needed by increasing her dose of atorvastatin or waiting until prednisone can be discontinued and rechecking her cholesterol level. Fluid balance is also an important consideration to prevent dehydration or hyponatremia (too much fluid). One should consider referring PD and her husband to a dietitian, because he will be shopping and cooking and would benefit from nutritional guidance. Medical nutrition therapy should be aimed at maintaining a BMI between 20 and 25 kg/m^2 and an albumin level of 3.5 to 5.8 g/dL. Since PD has microcytic anemia, she should be evaluated for iron deficiency. Medical nutrition therapy should also include the following:

- Rest before mealtime.
- Eat foods that are easy to chew, such as soft meats and casseroles.
- Avoid eating in bed; sit upright when eating.
- Drink Carnation Instant Breakfast, Boost, or Ensure, at least one can per day, for additional calories, protein, vitamins, and minerals.
- Include milk, which does not usually contribute to mucus/sputum production.
- Use a microwave oven to prepare convenience foods and decrease cooking time.
- Consume small, frequent meals consisting of nutrient-dense foods, such as peanut butter and jelly sandwiches.
- Use additional margarine (tub or liquid) on bread, potatoes, and vegetables as a calorie supplement.
- Consume the main meal at a time of the day when her energy level is highest.
- Avoid foods that cause gas or bloating, which makes breathing more difficult. Examples include cauliflower, broccoli, cabbage, brussels sprouts, onions, beans, and melons.
- Gradually increase intake of fiber-rich foods to enhance GI motility.
- Limit fluid intake during meals. Instead, drink fluids between meals.
- Avoid salty foods, such as canned, smoked, or cured products, to minimize fluid retention and bloating.
- Take a multivitamin/mineral supplement and 500 mg per day calcium.
- Patients on home oxygen should be advised to use oxygen when preparing and eating meals and to avoid cooking on a gas stove. The microwave oven is a safer option.

Recommended Revised Diet for PD

Breakfast (home)	Coffee	1 cup
	Instant oatmeal	1 packet
	2% milk	6 oz (180 mL)
	Raisins	$1/4$ cup
	Regular margarine	1 Tbsp.
Snack (home)	Apple	1 medium
Lunch (home)	Tuna salad	3 oz (85 g)
	Whole-wheat bread	1 slice
Snack (home)	2% milk	$1/2$ cup
	Saltines (low sodium)	6
	Peanut butter	1 Tbsp.
	Jelly	2 Tbsp.
Dinner (home)	Lean ground beef patty	4 oz (113 g)
	Brown rice	$1/2$ cup
	Tossed salad	1 cup
	Olive oil	2 Tbsp.
	Balsamic vinegar	1 Tbsp.
Snack (home)	Low-fat yogurt	4 oz (113 g)
	Orange	1 medium

Total calories: 1919 kcal

Protein: 76 g (16% of calories)

Fat: 89 g (42% of calories)

Saturated fat: 22 g (10% of calories)

Monounsaturated fat: 45 g (21% of calories)

Carbohydrate: 213 g (44% of calories)

Sodium: 1346 mg

Cholesterol: 143 mg

Fiber: 21 g

Case 2

Cystic Fibrosis

Maria R. Mascarenhas and Marianne S. Aloupis

Objectives

- Explain the nutritional abnormalities commonly observed in patients with cystic fibrosis.
- Conduct a nutritional assessment of patients with cystic fibrosis.
- Develop an appropriate nutritional care plan for patients with cystic fibrosis.
- Recognize the importance of medical nutrition therapy in the long-term survival and well-being of patients with cystic fibrosis.

FC, a 21-year-old woman with CF, presents to the pulmonary clinic with a 1-week history of increased cough, shortness of breath, and a 3-lb weight loss. She reports increased mucus production with a change in color from yellow to green. She has also been passing three or four foul-smelling, floating stools daily.

Past Medical History

FC's CF was diagnosed at 5 years of age based on recurrent upper respiratory tract infections, bulky foul-smelling stools, and hepatomegaly. In addition, FC has scoliosis, diagnosed 2 years ago, and hearing loss due to frequent intravenous antibiotic therapy. She has been hospitalized two times over the past year for acute exacerbations of CF. FC has no known food or drug allergies.

Medications

FC's current medication regimen includes pancrealipase (Pancrease MT 10; 4 capsules per meal, 2 capsules with snacks), cotrimoxazole (Bactrim), cefaclor (Ceclor), albuterol (Ventolin), and acetylcysteine (Mucomyst) solutions via nebulizer, cromolyn sodium (Intal metered-dose inhalers), triamcinolone acetonide (Azmacort metered-dose inhaler), rhDNase (Pulmozyme via inhalation), and ranitidine (Zantac). She also receives frequent chest percussion therapy.

Diet History/Vitamin and Mineral Supplements

FC follows a high-calorie, high-protein, high-fat, extra-salt diet that includes three meals and three snacks daily. She also drinks two servings per day of a high-calorie, high-protein powder supplement that is mixed with whole milk. FC's current vitamin/mineral therapy includes a multivitamin with iron twice a day, vitamin E (400 IU) once a day, and vitamin K (5 mg 3 times per week). FC prepares her breakfast and lunch, and her mother prepares dinner.

Social History

FC is a junior in college and lives at home with her parents. She denies smoking, alcohol, drug use, and sexual activity.

Review of Systems

The remainder of the review of systems was unremarkable except for poor appetite, shortness of breath, and increased frequency of bulky, foul-smelling stools.

Physical Examination

Vital Signs

Temperature: 101.4°F (40°C)
Heart rate: 110 beats per minute (BPM) (tachycardia)
Respiration: 24 BPM (tachypnea)
Blood pressure: 134/74 mm Hg
Height: 5'2" (158 cm)
Current weight: 88 lb (40 kg)
Usual weight: 91 lb (41 kg)
BMI: 16 kg/m^2
Triceps skinfold (TSF): 13 mm (<25th percentile)
Midarm muscle circumference (MAMC): 200 mm (20 cm; <25th percentile)

The patient's physical examination is normal except for the following observations:

General: Thin, ill-appearing woman
Skin: Warm to the touch
Head, ears, eyes, nose, throat (HEENT): Right nasal polyp
Chest: New rales and rhonchi in right upper lung zone, no wheezing or dullness to percussion
Cardiac: Elevated rate, normal rhythm, no murmurs

Laboratory Data

Patient's Values	Normal Values
Albumin: 4.2 g/L	3.5–5.8 g/L
Hemoglobin: 13.4 g/dL	12.0–16.0 g/dL
Prothrombin time: 14 seconds	<15 seconds
Random glucose: 220 mg/dL	70–110 mg/dL

Go to questions 1 to 5.

Treatment

Because of her worsening symptoms, abnormal physical examination, and decreasing pulmonary function, FC is diagnosed with an acute exacerbation of CF and admitted to the hospital. During her 1-week hospital admission, she has received intravenous antibiotics, respiratory treatments, vigorous chest percussion to help mobilize her secretions, and a dual-energy x-ray absorptiometry (DEXA) scan. The DEXA scan was ordered to get additional body composition data to diagnose bone disease. It is recommended that all children 8 years of age and older at nutritional risk have a DEXA scan.

Despite these therapies, FC's appetite has remained poor, and she has lost an additional 4 lb (1.8 kg). In addition, random blood glucose levels have been consistently elevated, suggesting CF-related diabetes. After consultation with Endocrinology, an insulin regimen was initiated using short-acting insulin matched to the carbohydrate content of her meals. Three-day calorie counts reveal that FC consumes approximately 1200 calories and 40 g protein per day. A high-calorie, high-protein oral supplement was ordered to help her meet her calorie goals.

Go to questions 6 to 7.

Follow-Up

FC was discharged to home when her weight reached 91 lb (41 kg). She was advised to continue monitoring her blood glucose levels until her posthospitalization office visit. A follow-up bone-density (DEXA) scan was scheduled.

Go to question 8.

Case Questions

1. What factors are most likely contributing to FC's weight loss?
2. What nutritional problems are patients with CF at risk for developing?
3. Is albumin a valid indicator of FC's nutritional status?
4. What is the significance of an elevated blood glucose level?

5. Are FC's current nutrition and vitamin therapy appropriate?
6. Is FC's current enzyme therapy appropriate?
7. What dietary recommendations would you give FC on discharge?
8. What parameters should be used to monitor changes in FC's nutritional status?

Case Answers

1. **What factors are most likely contributing to FC's weight loss?**

    A negative calorie balance accounts for FC's weight loss. Anorexia is compounded by ongoing malabsorption and by increased energy needs due to fever and infections. FC's poor appetite may be due to her current lung infection and to her antibiotic therapy. Decreased appetite in CF patients may also be due to esophagitis, cholelithiasis, salt depletion, and vitamin and mineral deficiencies leading to altered taste (dysgeusia). Psychosocial factors also commonly contribute to anorexia. FC's bulky, foul-smelling stools suggest fat malabsorption. In addition, FC has protein losses due to maldigestion caused by pancreatic enzyme insufficiency. Finally, FC has elevated serum glucose levels. Hyperglycemia is frequently seen with CF exacerbations and can contribute to weight loss.

2. **What nutritional problems are patients with CF at risk for developing?**

    The importance of uncompromised nutritional status in the long-term survival and well-being of patients with CF is well documented. Pancreatic insufficiency occurs in approximately 85% of patients. Analysis of pancreatic secretions reveals a marked decrease in the amounts of water, electrolytes, and enzymes (lipase, protease, and amylase). This results in inadequate digestion of food, producing malabsorption and undernutrition with growth retardation and weight loss. Protein-energy undernutrition impairs immune responses, increases the risk for pulmonary infections, and leads to wasting. Declining respiratory muscle strength may adversely affect survival. Protein deficiency can lead to hypoalbuminemia, which may result in edema.

    Patients with CF are at risk for development of multiple nutrient deficiencies with their associated clinical manifestations. Vitamin K deficiency, which results in coagulopathy, is the most commonly encountered nutrient deficiency. Vitamin E deficiency can lead to hemolytic anemia in infants and to neuropathy, ophthalmoplegia, ataxia, and diminished vibration sense and proprioception in older children and adults. Vitamin D deficiency causes rickets in young children and osteomalacia in adults. Vitamin A deficiency leads to night blindness, conjunctival xerosis, and epithelial keratinization.

    Deficiencies of water-soluble vitamins do not occur as frequently as deficiencies of fat-soluble vitamins. Vitamin B_{12} deficiency produces macrocytic anemia and neuropathy. Pancreatic insufficiency, which occurs when CF patients are not receiving (or are not complying with) enzyme therapy, impairs the digestion of the glycoproteins known as *R binders*, which are necessary for the transfer of vitamin B_{12} to intrinsic factor (IF). Although uncommon even in CF patients, salt depletion leads to lethargy, weakness, dehydration, and metabolic alkalosis. Essential fatty acid deficiency results in desquamation, thrombocytopenia, and poor wound healing.

Osteopenia is also commonly seen in CF patients, which may be due to malabsorption, decreased calcium intake, delayed puberty, reduced physical activity, and medications (e.g., corticosteroids) and to high circulating levels of inflammatory cytokines related to lung infections. FC's DEXA scan revealed very low bone density. According to her 24-hour diet recall, FC's calcium intake was only 800 mg elemental calcium. Her estimated calcium needs were 2000 mg elemental calcium per day; therefore, she was started on an oral calcium supplement to provide 400 mg three times a day. Her serum 25-hydroxy vitamin D level was normal.

3. **Is albumin a valid indicator of FC's nutritional status?**

   The serum albumin indicates visceral protein status. Hypoalbuminemia reflects poor protein intake or increased protein losses, or both, and suggests acute visceral protein depletion. Protein deficiency may develop in as little as 2 weeks. Most commonly, patients with CF are undernourished at the time of diagnosis and throughout their lives, but their albumin levels are normal until the end stages of their disease because the body preserves its visceral protein status in chronically ill patients. Therefore, the clinical diagnosis of undernutrition should be based on physical examination findings, such as temporal and interosseus muscle wasting, and information gathered in the medical and diet history. Similarly, anthropometric results, such as BMI, percent weight change, and diminished TSF and MAMC, reflect fat and muscle wasting due to chronically inadequate protein and energy intake.

4. **What is the significance of an elevated blood glucose level?**

   Hyperglycemia is frequently seen during CF exacerbations and can lead to increased morbidity and mortality in this population. Studies have shown that weight loss and declining pulmonary function can occur several years before the diagnosis of CF-related diabetes (CFRD). Glucose intolerance and CFRD often develop around 18 to 21 years of age in patients with CF. According to the Consensus Conference Report on CFRD, CFRD can be diagnosed by the following criteria: fasting glucose levels of greater than 126 mg/dL on two or more occasions, fasting glucose level greater than 126 mg/dL and a random glucose level of greater than 200 mg/dL, or elevated random glucose levels greater than 200 mg/dL on two or more occasions with symptoms. It is important to treat hyperglycemia aggressively and to monitor fasting glucose levels closely for resolution of glucose intolerance as acute infections resolve.

5. **Are FC's current nutrition and vitamin therapy appropriate?**

    Nutrition Therapy A high-calorie, high-protein, high-fat (30% to 40% of total calories) balanced diet is indicated for patients with CF because of their significant increased work of breathing and potential for malabsorption and maldigestion. Despite her hyperglycemia, calories should not be restricted. Extra salt is needed to replace the large amounts of sodium lost in perspiration. Six small meals per day generally are better tolerated than fewer, larger meals by patients with high caloric requirements. According to the Cystic Fibrosis Consensus Report, a patient whose weight is less than 85% of ideal body weight should receive enteral supplementation via a nasogastric tube (NG) tube or enterostomy. With the addition of oral high-calorie supplements, FC was able to meet her caloric needs.

    Vitamin Therapy Even with appropriate pancreatic enzyme therapy, fat malabsorption and associated fat-soluble vitamin deficiencies may still persist in CF patients. A daily multivitamin supplement enriched in fat-soluble vitamins that are in a water-miscible form to improve absorption is therefore indicated. Typically, CF patients are instructed to consume two times the recommended dietary allowance (RDA) for vitamins and minerals to prevent the associated deficiencies. The revised RDA for vitamin E is 15 mg (22 IU) per day. CF patients are encouraged to supplement their diets with 200 to 400 IU vitamin E per day to ensure adequate absorption of this vitamin. Vitamin K is produced by gut micro-organisms. Antibiotic therapy significantly decreases gut bacteria and, as a result, diminishes vitamin K production. Therefore, vitamin K supplements should be given to all patients receiving chronic antibiotic therapy.

Go to Treatment description at beginning of case.

6. **Is FC's current enzyme therapy appropriate?**

    Malabsorption should be suspected in any patient with CF who reports an increased incidence of foul-smelling, floating stools. Such patients require higher enzyme dosages to help them digest and absorb fat. Currently, FC is taking four capsules per meal and two capsules per snack of Pancrease MT 10 (10,000 units of lipase per capsule). Instead of increasing the number of MT 10s, changing the prescription to MT 16s (16,000 units of lipase per capsule) and altering the dosage to six capsules per meal and three capsules per snack will increase the total units of lipase that the patient receives and minimize the number of capsules the patient must ingest with each meal and snack. The usual recommended dosage is 500 to 2500 units of lipase per kilogram per meal.

7. **What dietary recommendations would you give FC on discharge?**

    Because patients with CF have such high caloric and protein needs (up to 2 times the RDA to prevent undernutrition), it is very important *not* to limit calories to control hyperglycemia. Instead, insulin therapy should be adjusted to optimize glucose control by matching the carbohydrate content of meals and snacks. If patients consume concentrated sweets, these should accompany a meal to reduce the glycemic response. Recent data have suggested that up to 75% of adults with CF have glucose intolerance. Approximately 14% of patients over 18 years of age require insulin therapy to manage hyperglycemia.

On discharge, FC should be instructed to increase her caloric intake with small, frequent nutrient-dense meals and Scandishakes (high-calorie powder supplement to mix with milk) to promote weight gain. Her insulin regimen may need to be adjusted based on her blood glucose levels, which she should continue to monitor at least once a day. Her blood glucose log will be brought to her office visit to assess improvement in glycemic control with the resolution of her acute infection.

Go to Follow-Up description at beginning of case.

8. **What parameters should be used to monitor changes in FC's nutritional status?**

Weight Change Weight should be monitored daily during an inpatient admission and then rechecked at each outpatient appointment. Due to her worsening symptoms and poor appetite, FC's weight was 88 lb (40 kg) when she was admitted to the hospital. Her BMI of 16 kg/m^2 suggested that she was undernourished. She lost an additional 4 lb (1.8 kg), reflecting an 8% weight change from her usual body weight, which is indicative of significant weight loss. Arm anthropometrics (TSF and MAMC) are also useful in screening and following a patient's body fatness and lean body mass. Patients with CF are often hypermetabolic because of their increased work of breathing, inflammatory responses, and infections.

Dietary Intake/Appetite FC's energy requirements are 1800 to 2400 calories per day for weight gain using the Harris-Benedict equation and an activity factor of 1.5 for moderate disease. Her daily intake in the hospital was approximately 1200 calories, a 600-calorie-per-day deficit, which can lead to continued weight loss. Calorie intake should be increased to prevent further weight loss and promote weight gain. FC's intake should be assessed periodically to ensure that her calorie intake is adequate.

Laboratory Data Relevant laboratory data to be monitored are prothrombin time (to assess adequate vitamin K stores), fat-soluble vitamin levels (vitamins A, D, and E levels should be checked annually), and iron stores. Albumin and prealbumin levels can be affected by acute infection and therefore may not reliably detect a change in nutritional status.

See Chapter Review Questions, pages A-30 to A-32.

11

Renal Disease

Jean Stover and Gail Morrison

> **Objectives***
>
> • Describe the specific medical nutrition therapy for acute and chronic renal failure, nephrotic syndrome, and nephrolithiasis.
> • Describe the goals of medical nutrition therapy for patients on hemodialysis and peritoneal dialysis.
> • Identify the impact of various forms of renal replacement therapy and renal transplant on a patient's nutritional status.
> • Explain the importance of regulating the intake of protein, calories, sodium, potassium, phosphorus, fluid, vitamins, and other minerals in patients with renal disease.

Acute Renal Failure

Acute renal failure (ARF) is characterized by a sudden decline in the glomerular filtration rate (GFR) of the kidney due to insults such as infection, exogenous nephrotoxins, trauma, dehydration, and shock resulting in ischemia. Patients with ARF are at high risk for undernutrition because of underlying illnesses, recent surgical procedures, or trauma, all of which place the patient in a catabolic state. In ARF precipitated by major trauma, critical illness, or sepsis, patients frequently undergo metabolic changes that accelerate degradation of protein and amino acids and result in the loss of lean body mass. The dramatic effects of this catabolic state include poor wound healing and increased infection and mortality.

* SOURCE: Objectives for chapter and cases adapted from the *NIH Nutrition Curriculum Guide for Training Physicians* (*http://www.nhlbi.nih.gov/funding/training/naa*).

Medical Nutrition Therapy for Acute Renal Failure

Decisions on implementing aggressive medical nutrition therapy depend on the patient's nutritional status and catabolic rate, the phase of ARF, the amount of urine output, and clinical indications such as uremia or volume overload requiring dialysis or continuous renal replacement therapy (CRRT). Thus, medical nutrition therapy for the patient with ARF must be highly individualized.

Goals are to minimize uremia and maintain the chemical composition of the body as close to normal as possible; preserve body protein stores until renal function returns; maintain fluid, electrolyte, and acid-base homeostasis; and prevent nutritional deficiencies.

Protein

Restricting protein intake to 0.6 to 0.8 g/kg per day is indicated for the patient with ARF whose GFR falls to less than 10 mL per minute and who is not catabolic or on any form of dialysis or CRRT. All forms of dialysis and CRRT contribute to protein losses. The protein intake of patients who are receiving hemodialysis should be liberalized to 1.2 g/kg per day, and patients receiving peritoneal dialysis are encouraged to ingest 1.2 to 1.3 g/kg protein each day. Severely catabolic patients with ARF may have even higher protein needs and require CRRT or aggressive dialytic therapy to allow for sufficient protein intake.

Calories

Caloric requirements for patients with ARF vary depending on the degree of hypermetabolism that is present. Usual recommendations are 35 kcal/kg per day; however, the most accurate determination of caloric requirements is by indirect calorimetry. Patients who have adequate gastrointestinal (GI) tract function but cannot tolerate food by mouth because of altered mental status, anorexia, nausea, or poor compliance should receive nourishment by enteral tube feeding (see Chapter 12). Those with a dysfunctional GI tract require parenteral nutrition (see Chapter 13). Peripheral insulin resistance may cause hyperglycemia in catabolic patients with ARF; therefore, blood glucose levels should be closely monitored. Also, there may be alterations in lipid metabolism in patients with ARF.

Vitamins and Minerals

Vitamin and mineral requirements for patients with ARF vary depending on their nutritional status and whether they are receiving dialysis or CRRT. Serum electrolytes must be closely monitored in all patients with ARF. Initially, serum potassium and phosphate are likely to be elevated and serum sodium lowered in nondialyzed patients who are oliguric (urine output <400 mL per day). Patients with acute intrinsic renal failure (usually defined as acute tubular necrosis and the major cause of ARF) may experience salt and water overload during the oliguric phase and salt and water depletion during the diuretic or recovery phase of the disease, when urine output can exceed 2 to 3 liters per day. In the recovery phase, sodium, potassium, and fluid may need to be replaced to offset urinary losses. Oliguric or anuric patients receiving hemodialysis usually require a sodium restriction of 2 to 3 g per day and a potassium restriction of 2 to 3 g per day. Those undergoing peritoneal dialysis, frequent hemodialysis (>3 times per week), and some forms of CRRT generally have more liberal sodium and potassium allowances. Patients with ARF who are undergoing any form of dialysis or CRRT should receive supplemental water-soluble vitamins above the recommended dietary allowances (RDA) and dietary reference intakes (DRI).

Fluid

Daily fluid intake for oliguric patients should equal urine output plus approximately 500 mL to replace insensible losses; fluid needs increase if the patient has a fever. Most anuric patients can tolerate approximately 1000 mL a day with hemodialysis three times per week. These restrictions may be liberalized in patients who receive continuous or daily peritoneal dialysis or hemodialysis more frequently than three times per week.

Continuous Renal Replacement Therapy

Continuous arteriovenous hemofiltration (CAVH) uses catheters that are placed into a large artery and vein (often the femoral artery and vein). The arterial blood flows through a small filtering device with a large porous membrane where plasma is filtered of water, minerals, and uremic toxins, and albumin and blood products return to the vascular space through the vein. This form of therapy removes large volumes of essentially albumin-free plasmanate, leaving water and electrolytes in a concentration equal to normal serum levels. Parenteral nutrition can be combined with CAVH to provide intravenous nutrition while controlling salt and water balance and removing small amounts of metabolic waste products that accumulate in renal failure.

Continuous arteriovenous hemodiafiltration (CAVHD) combines hemodialysis and hemofiltration simultaneously and removes larger amounts of solutes as well as large volumes of fluid. CAVH and CAVHD use systemic arterial blood flows; other forms of CRRT, including continuous venovenous hemofiltration (CVVH) and continuous venovenous hemodiafiltration (CVVHD), use a pumping machine that may result in less erratic blood flows and ultrafiltration rates.

Chronic Renal Failure (Predialysis)

Medical nutrition therapy goals for patients with chronic renal failure (CRF), before dialysis or renal transplantation, are to retard the progression of CRF while providing adequate calories to maintain or achieve ideal body weight and to prevent or alleviate the symptoms of uremia and restore biochemical, calcium/ phosphorus, vitamin, and iron balance.

Medical Nutrition Therapy for Chronic Renal Failure

Protein

In CRF, as the GFR and excretion of nitrogenous wastes decline, it is necessary to control the level of protein intake while continuing to maintain a positive nitrogen balance. Protein restriction can minimize the symptoms of uremic toxicity by reducing the production of nitrogenous wastes in the blood. A growing body of evidence also suggests that protein restriction early in the course of CRF due to glomerular damage may slow the progression of the disease and delay the need to initiate dialysis therapy. The generally accepted level of protein restriction for patients with GFR less than 25 mL per minute is 0.6 g/kg per day (using an adjusted body weight if the patient is obese).

A more liberal protein intake of 0.8 g/kg per day may be recommended for patients who are in earlier stages of CRF, who will not accept a lower protein diet, or who cannot meet their energy needs with a more restrictive diet. Approximately 50% of high biologic value protein is also generally encouraged to ensure that essential amino acid requirements are met. The biologic value of a dietary protein is determined by its constituent amino acids, with the highest value given to proteins such as eggs, meats, and other animal proteins that contain all essential amino acids. It has also been shown that carefully planned vegetable-based low-protein diets can be used, either alone or alternated with conventional meat-based low-protein diets, to meet the goals of protein restriction for individuals with CRF who are not yet on dialysis. Nutritional status must be monitored closely in patients prescribed protein-restricted diets, especially when they are ingesting 0.6 g/kg per day.

When patients exhibit proteinuria, as in diabetic nephropathy, the daily urinary protein losses can be added to the daily allowance. Additional increased protein needs due to catabolism from the use of glucocorticoid (steroid) therapy or recent surgery may contraindicate limiting dietary protein.

Calories

The recommendations for adequate energy intake for individuals with chronic renal insufficiency who are not yet on dialysis are generally 35 kcal/kg per day to maintain body weight and allow for effective protein utilization. It has been recommended that 30 kcal/kg per day be used for those greater than 60 years of age due to a more sedentary lifestyle. Calories from complex and simple carbohydrates must be included in the diet to provide adequate energy to prevent weight loss. Adding regular carbonated beverages, hard candy, fruit ices, fruit drinks, sugar, honey, and jelly to the diet can be suggested if the use of these specialty products is not feasible.

Lipids

Additional fat, in the form of monounsaturated and polyunsaturated fats, may also be recommended to provide adequate calories for patients with CRF. Since dyslipidemia is found in 20% to 70% of patients with CRF, lipid levels should be monitored and an effort made to keep total cholesterol, low-density lipoprotein (LDL), high-density lipoprotein (HDL), and triglyceride levels within normal limits (see Chapter 7). Pharmacologic therapy may need to be considered to manage lipid levels.

Sodium

As renal failure progresses to a GFR of approximately 10% of normal, renal sodium excretion subsequently falls. Sodium intake may have to be limited to

Table 11-1   Foods with high sodium content.

Bacon	Processed cheeses	Canned soups*
Canned/smoked	Tomato juice*	Vegetable juice*
Cold cuts	Packaged gravy	Worcestershire sauce
Corned beef	Barbecue sauces	Frozen dinners (unless of a "healthy" variety)
Dried beef	Meat tenderizers	Delicatessen salads and meats
Frankfurters	Chili sauce	Olives
Ham	Sauerkraut	Pizza
Salt pork	Chinese food	Bouillon cubes*
Sausages	Pickles	Dried soup mixes
Scrapple	Relish	Salted crackers*
Tongue, smoked meats or fish	Soy sauce	Packaged or prepared casserole dishes
	Tomato sauce	

Canned seafood

Potato chips,* pretzels,* salted popcorn,* salted nuts*

Generally, any labeled food with a sodium content >400 mg per serving is considered high in sodium.

*These items can be purchased "salt-free" or "low sodium" in most grocery stores.

prevent sodium retention, generalized edema, hypertension, and/or congestive heart failure, especially in the advanced stages of renal failure when excretion diminishes. Sodium balance can usually be maintained by limiting sodium intake to 2 to 3 g per day, but occasionally a sodium restriction of 1 g per day is needed. The typical American diet contains between 4 and 8 g sodium per day.

Measuring urinary sodium, via a 24-hour urine collection, may be helpful in determining how much sodium is being excreted. Urinary sodium is reported in milliequivalents (mEq), making it necessary to convert from milligrams to milliequivalents to determine how many milliequivalents of sodium are associated with any given diet. To convert milligrams of sodium to milliequivalents, divide the number of milligrams by the molecular weight of sodium (23 mg Na = 1 mEq Na). For example, assuming that a low-sodium diet is limited to 2000 mg per day, it contains 87 mEq sodium (Table 11-1).

Potassium

The kidney usually handles potassium efficiently until the GFR is significantly reduced (<10 mL per minute). Thus, a dietary potassium restriction may only be necessary during the latter stages of CRF. Exceptions include renal diseases such as diabetic nephropathy and tubulointerstitial nephritis, in which aldosterone deficiency develops and potassium excretion declines (typically seen at a GFR of 50 mL per minute). Use of an angiotensin-converting enzyme (ACE) inhibitor to control blood pressure in some individuals may also require a mild to moderate potassium restriction, even with good urine output. ACE inhibitors suppress the renin-angiotensin system, resulting in decreased aldosterone levels and subsequent elevations in serum potassium levels. Angiotensin receptor antagonists used to control hypertension can also cause hyperkalemia, although the likelihood is probably lower than with ACE inhibitors. When serum potassium levels are consistently greater than 5.0 mEq/L, a potassium-restricted diet of 2 to 3 g per day (51 to 77 mEq per day) should be initiated (Table 11-2).

Calcium and Phosphorus

Renal osteodystrophy refers to the complex lesions of bone, including osteitis fibrosa and osteomalacia, that are present in the majority of patients with CRF. Restriction of dietary phosphorus has been shown to prevent the development of secondary hyperparathyroidism, which is seen frequently in patients with CRF. Phosphorus levels are known to become abnormal in patients with a GFR in the range of 20 to 50 mL per minute. At this level of renal function, glomerular filtration is inadequate to excrete a normal dietary phosphorus load, and a phosphorus restriction of 800 to 1000 mg per day is recommended (Table 11-3). With a protein-restricted diet, this is usually feasible, as animal protein-based foods are also high in phosphorus content. If dairy products are avoided in a vegetable-based low-protein diet using soy products, this level of phosphorus restriction is also feasible.

Generally, calcium carbonate or calcium acetate should also be prescribed with meals as "phosphate binders" to interfere with the absorption of phosphate in the small intestine and to keep the serum phosphate levels within normal range. Currently, sevelamer hydrochloride (Renagel), a nonabsorbed phosphate-binding polymer without calcium or aluminum, can be recommended (Table 11-4). If this medication is used for any length of time before dialysis is initiated, serum bicarbonate levels should be monitored carefully, as it contains chloride and does not provide a "buffering effect."

A combination of sevelamer hydrochloride and calcium acetate is sometimes used to provide phosphate binding without adding significant calcium. Serum calcium levels may not decrease until the GFR is less than 30 mL per minute, thus initially eliminating any need for specific calcium supplementation until later stages of CRF. Since foods rich in calcium (primarily dairy products) are also high in phosphorus content and must be restricted, calcium carbonate and calcium acetate can be used between meals to increase serum calcium levels, if necessary, once serum phosphate levels are normal.

Water Balance and Fluid Restriction

Fluid intake for individuals with CRF should be balanced by their ability to eliminate fluid. As long as the urine output essentially equals the daily fluid intake, fluid balance is maintained. If edema becomes apparent, prescribing loop diuretics often increases sodium and water excretion sufficiently to maintain balance. In the latter stages of CRF, a fluid limit equal to the volume of urine output plus 500 mL per day for insensible fluid losses may be necessary to prevent edema and hyponatremia.

Vitamins and Iron

Protein and mineral restrictions to manage CRF usually result in a diet deficient in vitamins. Supplementation with folic acid (1 mg per day), pyridoxine (5 mg per day), the DRI for other B-complex vitamins, and ascorbic acid

Table 11-2   Foods with high and low to medium potassium content.

HIGH-POTASSIUM VEGETABLES	HIGH-POTASSIUM FRUITS AND JUICES
Artichokes	Apricots
Beans (navy, lentil, kidney, pinto)	Avocados
Broccoli	Bananas
Brussels sprouts	Cantaloupes
Carrots, raw	Dates
French fries	Figs
Greens	Honeydew melons
Lima beans	Mangos
Parsnips	Nectarines
Potato, baked	Oranges, orange juice
Pumpkin	Papayas
Spinach	Prunes
Sweet potato	Raisins
Tomato	Rhubarb
Winter squash (butternut, acorn)	Watermelon
Tomato juice	Apricot nectar
Vegetable juices	Prune juice

OTHER HIGH-POTASSIUM FOODS	
Milk ($>$4–8 oz/d)	Salt substitutes (containing KCl)
Chocolate	Molasses
Nuts	Potato chips
Bran cereal	

LOW- TO MEDIUM-POTASSIUM VEGETABLES	LOW- TO MEDIUM-POTASSIUM FRUITS AND JUICES
Asparagus	Apples, apple juice
Beets	Applesauce
Cabbage	Blueberries
Carrots, cooked	Cherries
Cauliflower	Cranberries, cranberry juice
Celery	Fruit cocktail
Corn	Grapefruits, grapefruit juice (only 4 oz/d)
Cucumber	Grapes, grape juice
Eggplant	Lemons
Green beans	Limes
Green peppers	Peaches, fresh (small)
Kale	Pears, fresh (small), pear nectar
Lettuce	Pineapples, pineapple juice (only 4 oz/d)
Okra	Plums
Onions	Raspberries (1 cup)
Peas	Strawberries (1 cup)
Potato (only when presoaked)	Tangerines
Radishes	
Wax beans	
Zucchini	

Table 11-3   Foods with high phosphorus content.

FOODS	PORTION SIZE	PHOSPHORUS CONTENT (mg)
Dairy		
Cheese, all types	1 oz	110–220
Half-and-half	1/2 cup	110
Custard	1/2 cup	155
Frozen custard	1/2 cup	100
Ice cream	1/2 cup	70–115
Frozen yogurt	1/2 cup	100
Milk, all kinds	1/2 cup	~120
Pudding, instant	1/2 cup	280
Pudding, homemade	2 cups	115
Protein foods		
Eggs	1 large	103
Liver, beef (pan fried)	3.5 oz	460
Peanut butter	2 Tbsp.	100–120
Salmon	3 oz	70–80
Sardines	1	210–240
Tuna	3 oz	140–265
Vegetables		
Baked beans and pork and beans	1/2 cup	140
Dried beans	1/2 cup	130
Chickpeas	1/2 cup	110–140
Lentils, boiled	1/2 cup	180
Soybeans, boiled	1/2 cup	200
Bread and cereals		
Barley	1/2 cup	200
Raisin bran	3/4 cup	150
Cornbread (from mix)	2 1/2" × 1 3/8"	209
Whole-grain breads	1 slice	60
Miscellaneous		
Chocolate	1 oz	65
Nuts, mixed, dry	1 oz	120
Peanuts, dry	1 oz	100
Beverages		
Beer	12 oz	45–150
Colas	12 oz	60

SOURCE: Data from: Pennington J. Food Values of Portions Commonly Used, 17th Edition. Philadelphia: Lippincott, 1998.

Table 11-4   Selected phosphate-binding medications.

MEDICATION	DOSE	CA^{2+} (mg) (ELEMENTAL)	AL (mg)	MANUFACTURER
Calcium carbonate				
Calcium carbonate	1 tablet	500	0	Roxanne
Calci-Chew	1 tablet	500	0	R & D Labs
Calci-Mix	1 capsule	500	0	R & D Labs
Caltrate 600	1 tablet	600	0	Lederle Labs
Oscal 500	1 tablet	500	0	SmithKline Beecham
Nephro-Calci	1 tablet	600	0	R & D Labs
Children's Mylanta	5 mL	160	0	J & J–Merck
Tums–Regular	1 tablet	200	0	SmithKline Beecham
Extra-strength	1 tablet	300	0	SmithKline Beecham
Ultra	1 tablet	400	0	SmithKline Beecham
500	1 tablet	500	0	SmithKline Beecham
Calcium acetate				
PhosLo	1 tablet	169	0	Braintree Labs
Aluminum hydroxide				
Amphogel	5 mL	0	111	Wyeth-Ayerst Labs
Alucap/Alutab	1 capsule/tablet	0	175	3M Pharmaceuticals
Nonabsorbed polymer				
Renagel	1 caplet/tablet	0	0	Genzyme

(60 to 100 mg per day) is often necessary. Because of the kidney's inadequate conversion of vitamin D from 25-hydroxycholecalciferol [25(OH)D$_3$] to its active form, 1,25-dihydroxycholecalciferol [1,25(OH$_2$)D$_3$], supplementation of this active form is often required and highly individualized. Vitamin A, on the other hand, may accumulate as CRF progresses and should not be supplemented. Vitamin preparations designed specifically for individuals with renal failure are available to meet these needs.

In most individuals with CRF, anemia develops, primarily because of the kidney's decreased production of the hormone erythropoietin. This hormone stimulates the bone marrow to produce red blood cells. Many individuals with CRF begin treatment with the human recombinant form of erythropoietin (epoetin alfa) before dialysis is initiated. To promote red blood cell production, iron supplementation is often necessary for patients receiving erythropoietin therapy, which varies depending on iron status.

Dialysis

The goals of medical nutrition therapy for patients on maintenance hemodialysis (HD) and maintenance peritoneal dialysis (PD), including continuous ambulatory peritoneal dialysis (CAPD) and continuous cycling peritoneal dialysis (CCPD), are to maintain:

- Protein equilibrium to prevent a negative nitrogen balance while avoiding excessive weight gain
- Serum potassium and sodium concentrations within an acceptable range and maintaining total body sodium as close to normal as possible
- Fluid homeostasis by preventing fluid overload or volume depletion
- Serum calcium, phosphorus, and parathyroid hormone (PTH) levels within an acceptable range to prevent renal osteodystrophy and metastatic calcification
- Adequate levels of vitamins and other minerals

Medical Nutrition Therapy for Dialysis

Protein

Protein intake for patients undergoing maintenance dialysis must at least equal minimum dietary protein requirements but not worsen the uremic syndrome by causing retention of urea, electrolytes, and various minerals. The loss of amino acids, the catabolic stress of dialysis, and the level of protein intake in the pre-dialysis period may all contribute to poor protein status in the chronic dialysis patient. A protein allowance of 1.2 g/kg per day for HD patients and 1.2 to 1.3 g/kg per day for PD patients often minimizes the accumulation of excessive nitrogenous wastes, maintains a positive nitrogen balance, and replaces the amino acids lost during dialysis. During episodes of peritonitis, patients receiving peritoneal dialysis have increased dietary protein needs as a result of greater losses of protein across an inflamed peritoneum. Many patients on both HD and PD periodically require supplemental commercial or homemade nutritional drinks, bars, or protein powders to achieve adequate protein intake.

Calories

The caloric intake for patients undergoing maintenance dialysis should be adequate to maintain or achieve ideal body weight. Unless the diet provides sufficient calories from carbohydrate and fat, endogenous protein is used for energy production, and the patient develops a negative nitrogen balance and loses significant muscle mass. With PD, calories gained from glucose absorbed from the dialysate must be considered when determining total caloric needs to prevent excess weight gain and obesity. Patients on both HD and PD, however, may also require nutritional supplements to meet caloric as well as protein intake goals.

Lipids

As mentioned previously, lipid abnormalities are frequently prevalent in patients with kidney disease. Commonly, patients undergoing HD present with normal or high total cholesterol, low-density lipoprotein (LDL), and triglyceride levels, and normal or low high-density lipoprotein (HDL) levels. Patients on PD frequently have high total cholesterol, LDL, and triglyceride levels and low HDL levels. Medical nutrition therapy is aimed at normalizing cholesterol and triglyceride levels without adversely affecting protein and overall caloric intakes in dialysis patients. Pharmacologic therapy for dyslipidemia is often initiated to avoid further restrictions to an already complex diet regime.

Sodium and Fluid

Daily sodium recommendations are determined by a patient's blood pressure, weight, and level of kidney function. Excessive ingestion of sodium may promote excessive fluid intake and precipitate edema. The sodium and fluid allowances for patients on maintenance dialysis depend largely on their interdialytic weight gains. For patients on HD, sodium intake is generally restricted to 2 to 3 g per day, with a fluid allowance of 1000 mL per day plus the amount of urine output, if any. This will allow an acceptable fluid weight gain of approximately 1 lb per day. Sodium and water may be removed more easily with PD because it is performed daily or continuously. A more liberal sodium and water intake is therefore possible for PD patients (see Table 11-1).

Potassium

Potassium intake must be individualized to maintain normal serum potassium levels. Patients on maintenance HD usually can maintain serum potassium levels between 3.5 and 5.5 mEq/L with diets containing 2 to 3 g per day (50 to 75 mEq per day). When serum potassium levels are persistently high, despite dietary counseling, the dialysate potassium content may be lowered or a sodium exchange resin added to the medication regime. When serum potassium levels are consistently low (hypokalemia), the dietary intake can be liberalized or dialysate potassium content increased, or both. This is especially important for patients receiving digoxin therapy, as hypokalemia can cause arrhythmias. Patients on maintenance PD usually maintain a normal serum potassium level without restricting potassium intake. If serum potassium levels fall below normal, dietary potassium is increased, and if unsuccessful, potassium supplements may be required.

Calcium and Phosphorus

As renal function diminishes, phosphorus excretion decreases. With a GFR of less than 25 mL per minute, filtration is inadequate to excrete a normal dietary phosphorus load (1000 to 1800 mg). Dialysis therapy does remove phosphorus, but not efficiently enough to allow an unrestricted diet. The goal of medical nutrition therapy is to achieve and maintain a serum phosphate level of approximately 3.5 to 5.5 mg/dL, and a calcium × phosphorus product less than 55. Phosphorus is widely distributed in foods but is found primarily in muscle tissue (meats, poultry, and fish) and dairy products (see Table 11-3). Therefore, reducing dietary phosphorus intake often involves a concomitant reduction in total protein intake. For patients on maintenance HD and PD, in order to allow adequate protein intake, the usual phosphorus restriction is 1000 to 1200 mg per day.

Controlling serum phosphorus by diet alone is usually not possible if the patient is consuming recommended protein levels (1.2 to 1.3 g/kg per day). As a consequence, most dialysis patients are prescribed phosphate binders, such as calcium carbonate, calcium acetate, or the nonabsorbed phosphate-binding polymer, sevelamer hydrochloride, as mentioned for predialysis patients. All of these medications are prescribed with meals and snacks to promote phosphate binding in the gut, which decreases phosphorus absorption. Normal serum calcium levels are maintained by using the above-mentioned calcium medications as well as by adjusting the calcium content of the dialysate solutions or using calcitriol (the active form of vitamin D) therapy, or both. Sevelamer hydrochloride may be a better choice of phosphate-binding medication than calcium-containing binders in efforts to avoid excessive calcium intake and the potential for increased risk of soft tissue and cardiac/vascular calcifications. When serum calcium levels are greater than 10.5 to 11.0 mg/dL, dialysate calcium content can be adjusted downward and calcitriol avoided. Newer vitamin D analogs are also now available that may help suppress the parathyroid glands without producing hypercalcemia and hyperphosphatemia as readily as calcitriol.

Vitamins and Iron

Patients on both PD and HD generally receive supplementation of folic acid (1 mg per day), pyridoxine (10 mg per day), the RDA or DRI for other B-complex vitamins, and ascorbic acid (60 to 100 mg per day) because of probable existing dietary deficiencies of these vitamins and losses occurring during dialysis. Recently, there has been speculation that even higher doses of folic acid may be beneficial for patients with CRF, as this vitamin can reduce serum homocysteine levels, which are two to three times normal in this population. It has not yet been established whether reducing homocysteine levels in predialysis and dialysis patients will improve cardiovascular morbidity and mortality, as this is currently under investigation.

As mentioned above and in the predialysis phase of CRF, dialysis patients also may require supplements containing the active form of vitamin D, administered either orally or parenterally. This therapy is highly individualized. Intermittent "pulse" doses of oral calcitriol (Rocaltrol) or doxercalciferol (Hecterol) are generally used for PD patients to suppress high levels of PTH. Intravenous calcitriol (Calcijex), paricalcitol (Zemplar), or doxercalciferol is used for HD patients and administered intravenously during the treatment.

Iron supplementation for patients receiving either PD or HD is usually necessary if they are undergoing erythropoietin therapy for anemia. Periodic, weekly, or biweekly doses of intravenous preparations of iron dextran, iron gluconate, or iron sucrose are often given to HD patients to sustain a serum transferrin saturation greater than 20% and ferritin greater than 100 ng/mL. Oral iron, because it is poorly absorbed and not always tolerated, is frequently given only to those with intravenous iron allergies. PD patients often benefit from coming to the dialysis facility periodically for intravenous iron when iron stores are decreased. When transferrin saturation is greater than 50% or ferritin levels are greater than 800 ng/mL, or both, iron therapy is discontinued until repeat levels are obtained.

Renal Transplantation

The goal of medical nutrition therapy for patients who have undergone renal transplant surgery is to provide optimal nutrition without exacerbating the metabolic side effects of immunosuppressive drugs and other medical therapy.

During acute tubular necrosis (ATN) or organ rejection, or both, nutrient modifications may be necessary to prevent hyperkalemia and to control hypertension and circulating blood volume.

Medical Nutrition Therapy for Renal Transplant

Protein

Protein catabolism may occur in the postoperative period secondary to the stress of surgery and high doses of steroids and other immunosuppressive medications. The recommended protein intake for these patients is 1.3 to 1.5 g/kg per day in efforts to reach net nitrogen balance. This level may be difficult to attain initially after surgery but is a realistic goal considering the patient may have already been protein depleted before this surgery. A long-term protein intake of approximately 1 g/kg per day is recommended with successful transplantation. It has been suggested that regular exercise may also help overcome some of the muscle wasting due to the catabolism of steroids.

Calories

Adequate calories are necessary in the postoperative period to use the protein ingested to promote wound healing and to withstand rejection, infection, and other complications. The recommended caloric intake for these patients is 30 to 35 kcal/kg per day, based on dry weight or usual body weight (UBW). Because increased appetite is a common side effect of steroid therapy, the long-range goal is weight maintenance with controlled caloric intake once a reasonable weight is achieved. It has been shown that early intensive nutritional counseling and follow-up are successful in preventing unwanted weight gain in the first year after transplant. Also, regular exercise should be encouraged to aid in weight maintenance.

Carbohydrate

Hyperglycemia also may occur as a consequence of high-dose steroids and other immunosuppressive drugs such as cyclosporine and tacrolimus. The patient may then require a diet controlled in carbohydrate content and sometimes oral hypoglycemic agents or insulin therapy. Need for such medications may subside with time, but a calorie-controlled diet should still be encouraged to prevent unwanted weight gain.

Fat

Dyslipidemia frequently occurs after renal transplantation, primarily due to immunosuppressive therapy as well as obesity. Consequently, total dietary fat may need to be limited, with emphasis on decreasing saturated fat and substituting monounsaturated and polyunsaturated fats in the long-term, chronic posttransplant period. Pharmacologic therapy has also been shown to correct dyslipidemia in this population but should be used cautiously in conjunction with immunosuppressive medications.

Sodium, Fluid, and Potassium

If steroid therapy results in sodium and fluid retention, a reduced sodium intake is encouraged (see Table 11-1). In the absence of edema and hypertension, a more liberal sodium intake is acceptable. Fluid generally is not restricted unless ATN or rejection of the transplanted kidney is present. A higher incidence of hyperkalemia with the use of cyclosporine may indicate periodic potassium restriction, even in patients with a good functioning kidney. Rejection or ATN may also require potassium restriction (see Table 11-2).

Calcium and Phosphate

Generally, neither dietary phosphate restriction nor phosphate-binding medication is needed when the transplanted kidney is functioning well. In fact, hypophosphatemia due to increased phosphate excretion and bone uptake sometimes develops in the acute posttransplant period and may require a high-phosphorus diet or phosphate supplementation, or both (see Table 11-3). Calcium supplementation may be required in the chronic posttransplant period because steroid therapy interferes with calcium absorption.

Vitamins and Iron

Renal vitamin preparations may be continued temporarily for the posttransplant patient, especially if dietary restrictions are needed to treat ATN or rejection. Iron therapy may also continue if epoetin alfa administration is necessary to treat anemia.

Nephrotic Syndrome

Nephrotic syndrome, a kidney disorder with many etiologies, is characterized by large quantities of protein (>3.0 g per day) in the urine. In all cases, this proteinuria is a consequence of damage to the glomerular basement membrane, resulting in its increased permeability to protein. Patients often exhibit poor appetite, muscle wasting, and undernutrition (primarily protein deficiency) secondary to these large protein losses. Nephrotic syndrome is also characterized by edema, when it is associated with a decrease in serum albumin, resulting in decreased plasma oncotic pressure. Dyslipidemia, with elevations either in serum cholesterol or triglycerides, or both, also occurs in nephrotic syndrome and correlates with the degree of proteinuria. Medical nutrition therapy for patients with nephrotic syndrome should aim to reduce proteinuria, prevent negative nitrogen balance, control dyslipidemia, and minimize edema.

Medical Nutrition Therapy for Nephrotic Syndrome

Protein

A high-protein diet may exacerbate albumin excretion through the damaged glomerular membrane. A moderate protein restriction is recommended early in the diagnosis of nephrotic syndrome to reduce the amino acid load to the glomerulus, subsequently diminishing the quantity of albumin crossing the damaged glomerular membrane. The currently recommended protein intake for patients on a moderate restriction is 0.8 to 1.0 g/kg per day. This amount may need to be adjusted based on nutritional status, clinical condition, and degree of proteinuria. Vegetarian diets using soy protein rather than meat-based protein may also be beneficial for patients with nephrotic syndrome.

Calories

Adequate calories from nonprotein sources are needed to use protein and promote weight maintenance or weight gain in patients with nephrotic syndrome. Small frequent meals may be better tolerated if ascites is present; caloric needs for weight maintenance are estimated to be 35 kcal/kg per day. Because these patients are often edematous, dry weight should be used for this calculation.

Fat

Dyslipidemia due to increased hepatic protein synthesis and reduced lipoprotein clearance from the blood by lipoprotein lipase is common in patients with nephrotic syndrome. Elevated very-low-density lipoprotein (VLDL), LDL, cholesterol, and triglyceride levels, along with normal or decreased HDL levels, may warrant a dietary fat restriction to less than 30% of total calories, with an equal balance among saturated, monounsaturated, and polyunsaturated fats. Dietary cholesterol should be limited to less than 200 mg per day. Pharmacologic therapy may be necessary if diet has no effect and the nephrotic syndrome is prolonged.

Sodium and Fluid

Controlling edema through sodium restriction and appropriate use of diuretics is essential in the management of nephrotic syndrome. Because edema is commonly associated with nephrotic syndrome, restricting sodium intake to less than 2 g per day may be necessary. The exact level of restriction must be individualized based on the degree of edema (see Table 11-1). Fluid restriction is not generally recommended.

Potassium

Abnormal potassium levels may occur in patients with nephrotic syndrome, depending on the diuretic prescribed to control their edema or if ACE inhibitors are used to control the proteinuria. Monitoring serum potassium levels is essential to determine whether alterations require a low- or high-potassium diet (see Table 11-2).

Calcium

Hypocalcemia frequently occurs in individuals with nephrotic syndrome if they are hypoalbuminemic. Serum calcium measurements include both free calcium and calcium bound to serum albumin. When attempting to determine if a calcium deficiency is present, it is therefore essential to use the following equation to correct the patient's serum calcium level to reflect the degree of hypoalbuminemia:

$$[(\text{Normal albumin} - \text{serum albumin}) (\text{correction factor})] + \text{serum calcium}$$
$$\text{Correction factor} = 0.8$$
$$\text{Normal albumin} = 4.0 \text{ mg/dL}$$

A concurrent vitamin D deficiency may lead to inadequate calcium absorption from the GI tract in a number of these patients. As a result, if the serum calcium level, corrected for the degree of hypoalbuminemia, still falls below normal levels, a calcium deficiency is likely. Vitamin D supplementation may be recommended for these individuals.

Nephrolithiasis

The goals of medical nutrition therapy for patients with nephrolithiasis (kidney stones) are to eliminate the diet-related risk factors for stone formation and prevent the growth of existing stones. The influence of fluid and specific nutrients such as calcium, oxalate, protein, refined carbohydrates, and sodium on the risk factors for calcium stone formation are discussed in the following section.

Medical Nutrition Therapy for Nephrolithiasis

Fluid

First and most importantly, a high fluid intake is the essential component of diet therapy for patients with nephrolithiasis. An increase in urine volume to 2 liters per day or more is needed to maintain a dilute urine and reduce the concentration of stone-forming substances. Producing this volume of urine requires a fluid intake of approximately 2.5 to 3 liters per day. It has been suggested that moderate alcohol intake may reduce the risk of stone formation, whereas apple and grapefruit juice increase the risk. Also, coffee and tea may reduce stone formation, presumably because of the diuretic effect of caffeine.

Calcium

Hypercalciuria (usually idiopathic) is one of the common urinary abnormalities seen in persons who form calcium stones. Although much attention is directed toward the effect of dietary calcium on urinary calcium excretion, in reality most cases of calcium urolithiasis are not attributed to high dietary calcium intake. In fact, a very-low-calcium diet has been shown to increase the absorption and subsequent excretion of oxalate, which promotes formation of calcium oxalate stones in susceptible individuals. Therefore, maintaining a moderate calcium intake in the range of 600 to 800 mg per day should prevent hyperoxaluria and long-term negative calcium balance.

Oxalate

Changes in oxalate excretion are more important than calcium excretion in altering the probability of developing calcium oxalate stones. Oxalate has a greater relative effect than calcium on urine supersaturation of calcium oxalate. Normally, the quantity of oxalic acid excreted in urine does not exceed 10 to 40 mg per day. Only 10% of this amount comes from the diet (Table 11-5); the remainder is a product of endogenous metabolism.

Table 11-5   High-oxalate foods.

Beans	Fruitcake
String, wax	Eggplant
Legume types	Gooseberries
(including baked beans canned in tomato sauce)	Grits (white corn)
Beets	Instant coffee (>8 oz/d)
Blackberries	Leeks
Carob powder	Nuts, nut butters
Celery	Okra
Chocolate/cocoa and other chocolate drink mixes	Peel: lemon, lime, orange
Concord grapes	Raspberries (black)
Dark leafy greens	Red currants
Spinach	Rhubarb
Swiss chard	Soy products (tofu)
Beet greens	Strawberries
Endive, escarole	Summer squash
Parsley	Sweet potatoes
Draft beer	Tea
	Wheat germ

SOURCE: Reprinted with permission from Kasidas GP, Rose GA. Oxalate content of some common foods: determination by enzymatic method. J Human Nutr 1980;34:255.

GI disorders that cause malabsorption are the most common cause of enteric hyperoxaluria. Oxalate absorption tends to be excessive when malabsorbed fat forms soaps and binds calcium in the gut. Free oxalate is then easily absorbed in the intraluminal intestine. Small increases in urinary oxalate concentration greatly increase the potential for crystal formation. Control of dietary oxalate therefore may benefit those susceptible to oxalate stones, because large fluctuations in urinary oxalate are attributable to variations in diet. Oxalate in the urine can be decreased by reducing oxalate in the diet while maintaining enough calcium to achieve a proper balance between these two elements. Thus, eliminating calcium-containing foods is not advisable for patients with calcium oxalate stones. Vitamin C supplements should be discouraged since ascorbic acid breaks down to oxalic acid and is excreted in the kidney.

Protein

A high intake of animal protein, with its acid load (1 mEq hydrogen per 1 g protein intake), increases urinary calcium excretion. In addition, the binding effect of sulfate in dietary protein decreases renal tubular calcium reabsorption. Limiting intake of foods such as meat, fish, poultry, and eggs to achieve a total protein intake of 60 to 70 g per day is recommended in patients with nephrolithiasis.

Sodium

A high sodium intake increases calcium excretion by expanding extracellular fluid volume, increasing the GFR, and decreasing renal tubular calcium reabsorption.

These alterations result in an increased quantity of calcium-containing crystals in the urine. A moderate reduction of high-sodium foods is recommended (2 to 4 g per day; see Table 11-1).

Carbohydrate

Refined carbohydrates are also known to be calciuric, but those that are high in fiber are anticalciuric. Thus, a diet lower in simple sugars and products made from refined flour, but higher in complex carbohydrates made from whole grains, as well as fresh fruits and vegetables, is recommended.

Herbal and Dietary Supplement Use in Renal Disease

In recent years, alternative medicine has become very popular. Patients with renal insufficiency before dialysis, while undergoing dialysis, or after renal transplantation must be very cautious when considering the use of herbal remedies and dietary supplements. These products are not regulated by the Food and Drug Administration (FDA), and, despite the fact that some of them are already known to be unsafe because they are carcinogenic, hepatotoxic, or nephrotoxic, patients may not be getting what they think they are taking. Laboratory analyses have been reported of products that lack their stated ingredients or are contaminated with pesticides, poisonous plants, heavy metals, or conventional drugs. Also, for patients with renal disease, herbal supplements may be especially dangerous due to the unpredictable pharmokinetics of these products.

The potential exists for drug-supplement interactions due to the large number of medications required for most dialysis and transplant patients. One example is St. John's wort, which has led to acute heart and kidney transplant rejection by causing a profound drop in cyclosporine levels (see Chapter 3, Case 1). Also, some herbs and dietary supplements may impair residual renal function or cause unpredictable effects on blood pressure, such as those that occur with yohimbine. Many "herbal diuretics" are promoted in lay publications to "promote urine flow" and "maintain healthy" kidney function. These products include asparagus root, white sandalwood, licorice root, horseradish, juniper berry, lovage root, and watercress. Because they increase urine volume but not sodium excretion, they are not appropriate for treating edema and are contraindicated in patients with hypertension. They are also irritants to renal epithelial cells and are not to be used for patients with renal disease. It is important to ask about the use of herbs and dietary supplements when taking a medication or diet history from all patients, especially those with renal disease.

For a list of references for this chapter, please visit the University of Pennsylvania School of Medicine's Nutrition Education and Prevention Program web site: *http://www.med.upenn.edu/nutrimed/articles.html*

Table 11-6 **Suggested daily nutrient requirements in renal disease.**

	CALORIES	PROTEIN	SODIUM	POTASSIUM	CALCIUM/ PHOSPHATE	VITAMINS/ OTHER MINERALS	FLUID
Acute renal failure	~35 kcal/kg/d Monitor glucose due to potential for hyperglycemia with catabolism	0.6 g/kg IBW/d for nonhyper-catabolic, nondialyzed patient 1.2 g/kg IBW-HD 1.2–1.3 g/kg IBW-PD >1.5 g/kg IBW— very catabolic	2–3 g/d—oliguric with or without 3x/wk HD ≥3g/d—with more frequent HD/daily PD or CRRT Liberalize and possibly replete during diuretic recovery phase	2.0–3.0 g per day—oliguric with or without 3x/wk HD ≥3g/d with more frequent HD, daily PD or CRRT Liberalize and possibly replete during diuretic recovery phase	Supplement calcium and restrict phosphorus as needed to keep serum calcium 8.5–10.0 mg/dL and phosphorus 3.0–5.0 mg/dL	Supplement B-complex + C vitamins if malnourished or being dialyzed ("renal" vitamin) May use standard MVI with TPN	Oliguric—500 mL (insensible) + urine output — nondialyzed 3x/wk HD — 1000 mL/dL + urine output Liberalize with more frequent HD/daily PD/CRRT May need to be encouraged with diuresis (continued)

Table 11-6 (continued)

	CALORIES	PROTEIN	SODIUM	POTASSIUM	CALCIUM/ PHOSPHATE	VITAMINS/ OTHER MINERALS	FLUID
Chronic renal failure predialysis	30–35 kcal/IBW/d (maintenance) May need to increase fat/carbohydrate to increase calories May need to modify fat/cholesterol if dyslipidemic	0.6 g/kg IBW or adjusted IBW/d (noncatabolic) 0.8 g/kg/IBW/d (early CRF or malnourished) May add losses to restrictions if proteinuria 50% high biologic value protein	2–3 g/d may want to measure urinary sodium for better estimate of needs <2 g/d needed	2–3 g/d when serum levels consistently >5.0 mEq/L Restrictions usually not necessary until later stages of CRF unless on ACE inhibitors	Calcium supplementation and phosphorus restriction usually needed when GFR ≤25 mL/min 800–1200 mg/d+ phosphate binders	Supplementation B-complex plus vitamin C if malnourished or diet restrictive ("renal" vitamin) Active form vitamin D if PTH increases or calcium decreases May need iron if on rHuEPO	Unrestricted if good fluid balance with or without diuretics 500 mL + urine output may be needed in later stages of CRF
Hemodialysis	Same as predialysis (CRF) Limit cholesterol—modify fat intake if hyperlipidemic and this does not jeopardize total calorie intake	1.2 g/kg IBW/d May be greater with malnutrition	2–3 g/d	Generally 2.0–3.0 g/d	Supplement calcium as needed to keep serum levels at least 8.5–10.0 mg/dL either PO or IV (on HD) as needed 1000–1200 mg/d phosphorus; use binders as in predialysis to keep serum levels 3.0–5.0 mg/dL	"Renal" vitamin as in ARF; active vitamin D (calcitriol or other vitamin D analog) Iron usually needed with rHuEPO unless ferritin >800 ng/mL or transferrin saturation >50%	Same as in ARF

Peritoneal dialysis	30–35 kcal/kg IBW/d 20/25 kcal/kg IBW/d (weight reduction) Consider glucose absorption with PD	1.2–1.3 g/kg IBW/d May be greater with malnutrition and peritonitis Limit cholesterol/modify fat as needed (see HD)	Generally 2–3 g/d but may be liberalized to >3 g/d if no edema or increased BP	May be unrestricted due to daily removal of potassium May even need to encourage or give supplements if <normal values	As in HD	"Renal" vitamin; oral calcitriol or other vitamin D analog as needed Iron often needed with rHuEPO as in HD	May be able to liberalize >1000 mL + urine output if no edema increased BP
Renal transplant	Generally 30–35 kcal/kg IBW/d Control carbohydrates with hyperglycemia Modify cholesterol/fat in long-term posttransplant period if dyslipidemia	1.3–1.5 g/kg IBW/d postop ideal 1.0 g/kg IBW/d long term with well-functioning kidney	2–3 g/d initially (or with rejection) Liberalize when no edema—increased BP when transplant functioning well	Limit at 2–3 g/d if hyperkalemic with cyclosporine Rx or ATN/rejection	Calcium supplements may be needed if ATN/rejection pretransplant Phosphorus restrictions not needed with well-functioning kidney—may need repletion, may need restriction and binders with ATN/rejection	May continue "renal" vitamin if ATN/rejection or malnutrition pretransplant May need iron if rHuEPO needed	Not usually restricted unless ATN/rejection

(continued)

Table 11-6 (continued)

	CALORIES	PROTEIN	SODIUM	POTASSIUM	CALCIUM/ PHOSPHATE	VITAMINS/ OTHER MINERALS	FLUID
Nephrotic syndrome	Generally 35 kcal/kg IBW/d May need to restrict fat (30% total calories) and cholesterol (300 mg) if dyslipidemia	0.8–1.0 g/kg IBW/d	≥2 g/d	May need to encourage or restrict or monitor serum potassium levels	Probably do not need to supplement calcium (see vitamins) or restrict phosphate	Supplement B vitamins if on a diet <60 g protein/d Vitamin D supplementation if continued hypocalcemia after correction for low albumin	Restriction not usually recommended

IBW, ideal body weight; HD, hemodialysis; PD, peritoneal dialysis; CRRT, continuous renal replacement therapy; MVI, multivitamin injection; TPN, total parenteral nutrition; CRF, chronic renal failure; ACE, angiotensin-converting enzyme; PTH, parathyroid hormone; rHuEPO, human recombinant erythropoietin; PO, by mouth; IV, intravenous; ARF, acute renal failure; BP, blood pressure; ATN, acute tubular necrosis.
SOURCE: Jean Stover, RD, and Gail Morrison, MD. Used with permission. University of Pennsylvania, School of Medicine.

Case 1

Chronic Renal Failure
Advancing to Dialysis

Gail Morrison and Jean Stover

Objectives

- Given the medical history, physical examination, and laboratory data, identify factors affecting the nutritional status of a patient with chronic renal failure.
- Describe the appropriate medical nutrition therapy for a patient with chronic renal failure before initiation and during continuous ambulatory PD or HD.

AB, a 22-year-old college student, presented to the emergency room with headaches and shortness of breath. He was admitted to the hospital for evaluation when he was found to have a blood pressure of 200/120 mm Hg and mild congestive heart failure (CHF) by chest X-ray. AB reports that over the past year, his weight has increased approximately 10 lb (4.5 kg), although his diet has remained unchanged. He attributed this weight gain to decreased exercise and a busy class schedule.

Past Medical History

AB has had no recent viral illness, sore throat, or upper respiratory infection. He has never had rheumatologic symptoms and has no family history of renal disease. He had a history of multiple streptococcal infections of the throat as a child, some of which were treated with antibiotics and some that went undiagnosed. He is currently not taking any medications, vitamins, minerals, or herbal supplements and has no known drug or food allergies.

Social History

AB shares a dormitory room with a fellow student who is in good health. AB denies alcohol, tobacco, and intravenous or oral drug use.

AB's 24-Hour Dietary Recall

Breakfast	Coffee	8 oz (240 mL)
	Whole milk	2 Tbsp.

Lunch	Hamburger and bun	4 oz (113 g)
	French fries	Large
	Iced tea	16 oz (480 mL)
Dinner	2 slices of chicken breast	6 oz (170 g)
	Baked potato	1 medium
	Butter	2 tsp.
	Broccoli, spinach	$\frac{1}{2}$ cup each
	Chocolate cake	1 slice
	Cola soda	16 oz (480 mL)
Snack	Salted nuts	Small bag
	Cola soda	16 oz (480 mL)

Total calories: 2493 kcal
Protein: 110 g (18% of calories)
Fat: 98 g (35% of calories)
Carbohydrate: 303 g (48% of calories)
Potassium: 3487 mg
Sodium: 1648 mg

Review of Systems

General: Fatigue, weakness, shortness of breath
GI: Anorexia

Physical Examination

Vital Signs

Temperature: 97°F (36°C)
Heart rate: 96 beats per minute (BPM)
Respiration: 24 BPM
Blood pressure: 200/120 mm Hg
Height: 5'9" (176 cm)
Current weight: 170 lb (77.3 kg)
Usual weight: 155 lb (70.5 kg) 6 months ago (use for estimated "dry" weight calculations)
General: Well-developed man
Lungs: Decreased breath sounds with faint crackles at the right base
Cardiac: Regular rate and rhythm, systolic murmur at the apex, S_3 gallop
Abdomen: Soft, nontender, no hepatomegaly
Extremities: 3+ peripheral edema on both legs, ring tight on finger
Skin: Warm to touch
Neurologic: Intact, mild asterixis

Initial Laboratory Data

Patient's Values	Normal Values
Sodium: 135 mEq/L	133–143 mEq/L
Potassium: 4.4 mEq/L	3.5–5.3 mEq/L
Chloride: 111 mEq/L	98–108 mEq/L
CO_2: 15 mEq/L	24–32 mEq/L
Calcium: 7.5 mg/dL	9–11 mg/dL
Adjusted calcium: 8.1 mg/dL	9–11 mg/dL
Phosphate: 10.2 mg/dL	2.5–4.6 mg/dL
Blood urea nitrogen (BUN): 108 mg/dL	7–18 mg/dL
Creatinine: 14.0 mg/dL	0.6–1.2 mg/dL
Albumin: 3.2 g/dL	3.5–5.8 g/dL
Hemoglobin: 8.3 g/dL	13.5–17.5 g/dL [11–12 g/dL (CRF)]*
Hematocrit: 24.3%	41%–53% [33%–36% (CRF)]*
Transferrin saturation: 18%	>20% (CRF)*
Ferritin: 142 ng/mL	>100 ng/mL (CRF)*
Mean corpuscular volume: 70 fL	80–100 fL
White blood cells (WBC): 8.7×10^9/L	$4.5–11.0 \times 10^9$/L

Urinalysis: 3+ heme by dipstick, 1+ protein by dipstick

Sediment: 15–20 red blood cells (RBC) per high-power field (HPF),
   3–5 WBC/HPF 2–4 RBC casts and broad waxy casts/HPF

Electrocardiogram: Normal sinus rhythm at 100, no ischemic changes

Chest x-ray: Cardiomegaly, CHF

*These are guidelines established for patients with CRF by the National Kidney Foundation Kidney Disease Outcomes Quality Initiatives (NKF K/DOQI) committees.

Dialysis Treatment Plans

AB received a PD catheter during his hospitalization and began training for CAPD 2 weeks later. At the end of the training period, a diet plan was developed. He would now be receiving four 2-liter PD exchanges daily. The following data were available after 1 week of training.

Laboratory Data No. 2 (after 1 week on CAPD)

Patient's Values	Normal Values
Sodium: 136 mEq/L	133–143 mEq/L
Potassium: 4.5 mEq/L	3.5–5.3 mEq/L
Chloride: 102 mEq/L	98–108 mEq/L
CO_2: 18 mEq/L	24–32 mEq/L

Calcium: 8.8 mg/dL   9–11 mg/dL
Adjusted calcium: 9.4 mg/dL   9–11 mg/dL
Phosphate: 6.0 mg/dL   2.5–4.6 mg/dL
BUN: 70 mg/dL   7–18 mg/dL
Creatinine: 9.2 mg/dL   0.6–1.2 mg/dL
Albumin: 3.3 g/dL   3.5–5.8 g/dL
Hemoglobin: 9.8 g/dL   13.5–17.5 g/dL (11–12 g/mL)*
Hematocrit: 27%   41%–53% (33%–36%)*

*These are guidelines established for patients with CRF by the National Kidney Foundation
Kidney Disease Outcomes Quality Initiatives (NKF K/DOQI) committees.

Go to questions 8 to 9.

Follow-Up

AB did fairly well on CAPD for 3 months until he began to have difficulty with
the drainage of PD fluid through his dialysis catheter. He had repeated doses
of a thrombolytic agent infused into the catheter in an attempt to dissolve the
proteinaceous material, with only minimal success. He eventually had a new
catheter inserted that only worked temporarily before the same problem developed. He was subsequently readmitted to the hospital for an HD catheter and
started regular outpatient hemodialysis treatments. At that time his urine output
had declined to less than 200 mL per 24 hours.

Laboratory Data No. 3 (after 1 week on hemodialysis)

Patient Values   **Normal Values**
Sodium: 138 mEq/L   133–145 mEq/L
Potassium: 4.8 mEq/L   3.5–5.3 mEq/L
Chloride: 106 mEq/L   98–108 mEq/L
CO_2: 22 mEq/L   24–32 mEq/L
Calcium: 9.2 mg/dL   9–11 mg/dL
Phosphate: 8.4 mg/dL   2.5–4.6 mg/dL
Albumin: 3.5 g/dL   3.5–5.8 g/dL
Hemoglobin: 9.3 g/dL   13.5–17.5 g/L (11–12 g/dL)*
Hematocrit: 28%   41%–53% (33%–36%)*
Transferrin saturation: 23%   >20%*
Ferritin: 185 ng/dL   >100 ng/dL*

*These are guidelines established for patients with CRF by the National Kidney Foundation
Kidney Disease Outcomes Quality Initiatives (NKF K/DOQI) committees.

Go to question 10.

Case Questions

1. Based on AB's history, physical examination, and laboratory data, what is the most likely diagnosis?
2. What additional laboratory tests or studies help confirm your diagnosis?
3. What medications are indicated to manage his clinical condition at this time?
4. Based on AB's physical examination, should his current body weight be used to estimate his caloric and protein needs?
5. How can AB's caloric and protein requirements be estimated?
6. What dietary recommendations are indicated before dialysis based on his initial laboratory data values, and what fluid and electrolyte management does AB require?
7. Using AB's laboratory values to estimate renal function and his vital signs and chest x-ray results to determine his hemodynamic status, what are the immediate and long-term treatment modalities you would recommend?
8. What modifications in phosphate-binding medication should be made once AB's phosphate level improves?
9. What dietary modifications are indicated once AB begins receiving CAPD?
10. When AB's dialysis modality changes to HD, what dietary modifications are appropriate based on his weight and laboratory data?

    Predialysis weight: 74 kg (163 lb)

    Estimated dry weight: 70.5 kg (155 lb)

Case Answers

Part 1: Diagnosis and Medications

1. **Based on AB's history, physical examination, and laboratory data, what is the most likely diagnosis?**

    AB has a history of recurrent streptococcal infections in childhood, which most likely increased his risk of developing acute poststreptococcal glomerulonephritis. In approximately 5% to 10% of patients with a history of streptococcal infections and acute glomerulonephritis (AGN), chronic glomerulonephritis (CGN) develops 15 to 20 years after the acute infections. CGN results in a markedly decreased GFR, which prevents sodium and water excretion and causes increased sodium and water retention. The result is volume-induced high blood pressure and, with significant sodium and water retention, eventually CHF. This form of end-stage renal disease is irreversible and not amenable to treatment with any form of drug therapy.

2. **What additional laboratory tests or studies help confirm your diagnosis?**

    Urinalysis The urinalysis having blood and protein by dipstick indicates renal glomerular damage. RBC casts are highly suggestive of glomerulonephritis, and broad waxy casts suggest dilated renal tubules associated with CGN.

24-Hour Urine Collection This procedure reveals the quantity of protein and creatinine excreted over 24 hours. If the amount of urinary creatinine can be measured in a 24-hour urine specimen, a creatinine clearance can be calculated.

Protein Excretion 2.2 g per 24 hours, normal value <200 mg per 24 hours

Creatinine Excretion 900 mg per 24 hours, normal value 1.0 to 1.6 g per 24 hours

Creatinine Clearance Estimation of creatinine clearance can be calculated using the Cockroff-Gault formula. This may be necessary if urine values are incomplete or not available. The calculation gives an adequate estimation of creatinine clearance as long as the serum creatinine value is stable over time.

$$\text{Men: } (140 - \text{age})(\text{weight in kg})/(72)(\text{serum creatinine in mg/dL})$$
$$\text{Women: } (140 - \text{age})(\text{weight in kg})/[(72)$$
$$(\text{serum creatinine in mg/dL})] \times 0.85$$

$$\text{AB's estimated creatinine clearance} = (140 - 22)(77.3\,\text{kg})/(72)$$
$$(14.0\,\text{mg/dL}) = 9121.4/1008 = 9.05\,\text{mL/min}$$
$$(\text{normal creatinine clearance for a male} = 97 - 137\,\text{mL/min})$$

Renal Ultrasound Renal ultrasound revealed small kidneys bilaterally, which indicate irreversible renal disease (9 and 10 cm, right and left, respectively). Only a renal biopsy could actually confirm the diagnosis of CGN, but it is not performed once small kidneys are identified since no treatment can reverse the kidney damage. AB's significantly increased serum phosphate and decreased serum calcium suggest that the GFR is less than 30 mL per minute, indicating significant renal dysfunction. Tests to eliminate other possible causes of CGN include the following.

Complement Levels CH_5O, C_3, and C_4 are within normal limits (makes the diagnosis of membranoproliferative disease, subacute bacterial endocarditis, and acute poststreptococcal glomerulonephritis highly unlikely).

24-Hour Protein Collection Eliminates the diagnosis of nephrotic syndrome. AB's history and physical examination eliminate other causes of CGN such as Alport's syndrome.

3. **What medications are indicated to manage his clinical condition at this time?**

AB should be discharged on the following medications.

Diuretic (generally a loop diuretic) Diuretics control sodium and water balance (as long as AB has urine output).

Phosphate Binder One should consider the use of a phosphate-binding polymer without calcium and aluminum (sevelamer hydrochloride) since AB's serum phosphate level is so high. However, due to the risk of worsening the metabolic acidosis (low CO_2 level) with sevelamer hydrochloride, which contains chloride and no "buffer," calcium acetate could be used instead, or in combination with sevelamer hydrochloride.

Antihypertensive Medication This should be used as necessary to achieve blood pressure less than 140/90 mm Hg. AB's hypertensive medication dosage will decrease as excess sodium and water are removed.

Renal Multivitamin This is a supplement to correct dietary deficiencies seen in patients with CRF.

Epoetin Alfa This should be used for anemia.

Iron Gluconate This should be used intravenously (IV) if feasible, or an oral iron preparation should be used to boost transferrin saturation and support epoetin alfa in RBC production.

Part 2: Nutrition Assessment

4. Based on AB's physical examination, should his current body weight be used to estimate his caloric and protein needs?

   This patient's total body water is elevated, as evidenced by 3+ peripheral edema of the legs and CHF; his current weight therefore does not reflect his "dry" weight. To estimate dry weight, one should first ascertain the patient's usual weight. AB's usual body weight 6 months ago was 155 lb (70.5 kg), and this is the value that should be used to estimate his protein and caloric requirements.

5. How can AB's caloric and protein requirements be estimated?

   The normal estimated total daily caloric requirement is 35 kcal/kg. In AB's case, this amounts to

   $$(35\,kcal)\,(70.5\,kg) = 2468\,kcal/day$$

   Daily protein recommendations for ARF or CRF (not catabolic) without dialysis are 0.6 g/kg. If proteinuria is present, the urinary protein losses can be added to the daily protein allowance. The 24-hour urine collection indicated a protein loss of 2.2 g in AB's case. His daily protein intake therefore should be

   $$(0.6\,g)\,(70.5\,kg) = 42\,g/day + 2.2\,g = 44.2\,g/day$$

6. What dietary recommendations are indicated before dialysis based on his initial laboratory data, and what fluid and electrolyte management does AB require?

   Protein AB's current meal plan, before any treatment intervention, contained 2493 kcal and 110 g protein. To achieve a protein restriction of 45 g per day, the following modifications are recommended:

   • Limit milk in coffee to 1 to 2 oz (30 to 60 mL) per cup.
   • Substitute a plain hamburger on a bun, or an equivalent, such as 2 oz (57 g) of roast beef, turkey, chicken, or rinsed water-packed tuna on two slices of bread, for a cheeseburger at lunchtime.

- Limit the amount of chicken at dinner to 2 oz (57 g).

- Omit all cheese and nuts because they are high in protein, phosphorus, and sodium, and substitute unsalted pretzels or chips as a nighttime snack.

- Replace calories lost from lowering the protein content of the diet by adding sugar to coffee/tea and polyunsaturated fats to potato and vegetables.

Electrolytes AB's total body water and sodium are elevated, as evidenced by 3+ peripheral edema and mild CHF on his chest x-ray. Therefore, a low-sodium diet (2 to 3 g per day) is indicated at this time (which AB is already following). AB's potassium level is within the normal range; thus, no potassium restriction is indicated at this time.

His initial serum calcium and phosphate levels of 7.5 and 10.2 mg/dL, respectively, are a result of decreased GI calcium absorption and phosphate retention. Lowering serum phosphate levels by dietary restriction and phosphate-binding medication will improve serum calcium initially without calcium supplementation between meals.

Because foods high in calcium are also high in phosphate content, supplementing the diet with calcium-rich foods is not feasible at present. Restricting the daily allowance of dietary phosphate to 800 to 1000 mg is indicated (see Table 11-3). The aluminum and calcium-free phosphate-binding polymer was added in small doses in combination with calcium acetate to AB's medication regimen. The goal was to reduce serum phosphate levels to less than or equal to 5.5 mg/dL and to normalize serum calcium levels.

Fluid Given that AB's 24-hour urine output was 700 mL in the hospital, a total fluid intake of 1200 mL per day or 40 oz (700 mL + 500 mL for insensible fluid losses) should be recommended. To stay within the fluid restriction of 1200 mL per day, morning coffee should be limited to 8 oz (240 mL), the lunch beverage to 12 oz (360 mL), the dinner beverage to 8 oz (240 mL), and the snack beverage to 8 oz (240 mL). Allowing for an additional 4 oz (120 mL) of juice with medications is acceptable.

7. **Using AB's laboratory values to estimate renal function and his vital signs and chest x-ray results to determine his hemodynamic status, what are the immediate and long-term treatment modalities you would recommend?**

From these data, AB has a creatinine of 14 mg/dL, blood pressure of 200/120 mm Hg, and CHF. Therefore, AB underwent a single acute hemodialysis treatment, which effectively removes sodium and water as well as the buildup of uremic products secondary to CGN. He chooses CAPD instead of HD for his long-term treatment. CAPD allows him to perform dialysis exchanges himself in his dormitory room and have more freedom during the day rather than receiving HD treatments in an outpatient dialysis unit. A catheter (used to instill PD solution into the peritoneal cavity) was placed during AB's hospitalization. CAPD usually is started 2 weeks after a PD catheter is inserted to allow for adequate wound healing.

8. **What modifications in phosphate-binding medication should be made once AB's phosphate level improves?**

    At this time, since AB's corrected calcium level is reasonable, no change would be made in phosphate-binding medications unless the sevelamer hydrochloride (if being used) was not tolerated or feasible for AB due to cost. A change to all calcium acetate would then be acceptable.

9. **What dietary modifications are indicated once AB begins receiving CAPD?**

    The protein allowance should increase because AB's laboratory values at the start of CAPD exhibit a mildly depleted albumin level at 3.3 g/dL (normal 3.5 to 5.8 g/dL), and CAPD will remove significant amounts of protein. Since AB has been compliant with his previously prescribed low-protein diet, he will now be able to increase his protein intake. A protein intake of 1.2 to 1.3 g/kg per day (based on UBW or dry weight) is 85 to 92 g per day. To reach that goal, the meat, fish, or poultry portions at lunch and dinner need to be increased to 4 oz (113 g), and AB should be encouraged to eat a sandwich with at least 2 oz (57 g) of meat as his nightly snack.

    AB remains at least 11 lb (5 kg) over his previous usual body weight of 155 lb (70 kg). Current weight is 166 lb (76 kg): [170 lb (77 kg) minus the 4 lb (1.8 kg) of PD fluid indwelling]. The same sodium (2 to 3 g per day) and fluid restrictions (1200 mL per day) are indicated until a regular schedule of PD exchanges can be performed. A potassium restriction is still unnecessary because AB's serum potassium level is normal and may drop as a result of continuous removal of potassium with daily PD.

    Phosphorus should still be restricted to maintain phosphate levels between 3.5 and 5.5 mg/dL, but the restriction can be liberalized somewhat to allow a greater protein intake (animal protein sources are the foods highest in phosphate). By continuing to limit milk to no more than 4 oz per day, and limiting cheese and cola sodas to two times per week, AB can achieve the new daily phosphate allowance of 1000 to 1200 mg per day. An extra one or two sevelamer hydrochloride tablets can be prescribed with the night sandwich as well.

10. **When AB's dialysis modality changes to hemodialysis, what dietary modifications are appropriate based on weight and laboratory data?**

    Predialysis weight: 74 kg (163 lb)

    Estimated dry weight: 70.5 kg (155 lb)

    AB has the potential to gain fluid weight between HD treatments, because he receives them only three times per week (his predialysis weight is 3.5 kg greater than his dry weight). In addition, AB's urine output is diminished further because of his renal dysfunction. Thus, his fluid intake should be decreased to 1 L per day, and he should be encouraged to maintain a sodium restriction of 2 to 3 g per day. The recommended daily protein allowance is now 1.2 g/kg for a total of 85 g, which is the lower end of the previous recommendations. Because HD is intermittent, and AB reports that his urine output is minimal, he should be advised to limit his potassium intake to approximately 70 mEq per day. AB can accomplish this goal by eliminating fruits and vegetables that are high in potassium, such as bananas, orange juice, potatoes, and dark-green leafy vegetables. (See Appendix for list of high- and low-potassium foods.) Phosphorus restrictions for HD are similar to those for PD because no significant change is recommended in the protein content of AB's diet. However, because his phosphate level is now rising again, AB is advised to avoid dairy products completely except for 4 oz (120 mL) of milk per day.

See Chapter Review Questions, pages A-32 to A-34.

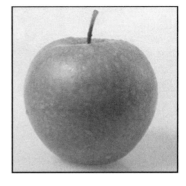

PART IV

Fundamentals of Nutrition Support

12

Enteral Nutrition Support

Judith Fish and Douglas L. Seidner

Objectives*

- Describe the indications and contraindications for enteral nutrition.
- Identify the appropriate enteral formula to meet individual patients' requirements.
- Identify the most appropriate route for tube feeding based on a patient's clinical condition.
- Determine the most appropriate administration method based on feeding route and the patient's clinical condition.
- Select appropriate monitoring tools and methods to identify, treat, and prevent complications of tube feeding.

Tube feeding, or enteral nutrition, is a method of providing nutrition support to patients who are unable to ingest adequate nutrients by mouth. A functional gastrointestinal (GI) tract is necessary to successfully support a patient on tube feeding. This usually means that a patient must have at least 100 cm of small bowel and the condition of the bowel must be adequate for absorption of nutrients. Short-term tube feeding is often used in acute-care settings in patients who are incapable of oral intake due to changes in mental status, poor appetite, or other therapies that prevent eating, such as mechanical ventilation. Guidelines established by the American Society of Parenteral and Enteral Nutrition (ASPEN) recommend initiating nutrition support when patients are expected to (or have) not received adequate oral intake for 7 to 14 days. However, patients who are malnourished or stressed may require earlier initiation of nutrition support. Most institutions provide nutrition screening for patients so that nutrition support is initiated when appropriate.

* SOURCE: Objectives for chapter and cases adapted from the *NIH Nutrition Curriculum Guide for Training Physicians* (*http://www.nhlbi.nih.gov/funding/training/naa*).

Indications and Advantages of Tube Feeding

Patients with a functional GI tract can be fed with a feeding tube. The presence of adequate GI functionality may not be apparent after initial evaluation. In these situations, a cautious trial of tube feeding may be warranted and failure would be a good indication for initiating parenteral nutrition. Tube feeding should not be initiated if a patient has diffuse peritonitis, intestinal obstruction, intractable vomiting or diarrhea, paralytic ileus, or GI ischemia or if the patient is refusing nutrition support. Advances in enteral nutrition have made enteral nutrition possible in conditions such as acute pancreatitis and high-output enterocutaneous fistulas.

Tube feeding offers many potential advantages over parenteral nutrition, including lower rates of infectious and metabolic complications, decreased hospital length of stay, and reduced cost. Research in animals suggests that critical illness leads to a translocation of bacteria and endotoxin from the lumen of the intestine across the mucosal barrier and that this leads to activation of inflammatory pathways and subsequent multisystem organ failure. It has been proposed that the benefits of enteral feeding are, in part, due to a preservation of gut integrity. Studies in patients with burns, head injury, and trauma have shown decreased rates of infection in those receiving enteral nutrition compared to those given parenteral nutrition. Although insufficient numbers of randomized controlled trials are available to make definitive conclusions on the superiority of outcomes of enteral feeding compared to parenteral feeding across all disease states, tube feeding is generally thought to have the least risk for major complications with decreased cost and is therefore the nutrition support therapy of choice when feasible and safe.

Selecting Tube-Feeding Formulas

Tube-feeding formulas can be grouped according to their composition and caloric density. A multitude of formulas are available for enteral nutrition. Since a variety of companies manufacture these products, many formulas are similar between companies. For this reason, many institutions have a formulary that offers a selection of formulas to meet many patients' needs without having excessive inventory. Modular components are also available to add to tube-feeding formulas to modify calorie and protein content to better meet many patients' needs. Some formulas may not fit into one category, and therefore it is best to understand the composition and advantages of each formula (Table 12-1).

Appropriate formulas can easily be selected after defining a patient's nutrient requirements and understanding the composition of available formulas. Nutrient composition and density are important factors to consider when selecting tube-feeding formulas. Other factors that may influence formula decisions include gut function and disease state.

Properties of Tube-Feeding Formulas

Tube-feeding formulas come in a variety of caloric densities (0.8 to 2.0 kcal/mL). Most patients with standard fluid requirements will tolerate a 1.0 to 1.2 kcal/mL

Table 12-1   Classification of tube-feeding formulas.

FORMULA TYPE	CHARACTERISTICS
Polymeric fat	Whole protein, polysaccharide and mixture of sources
Nutrient dense	Polymeric with reduced water (60%–70%)
High nitrogen	Over 15% of calories as protein
Chemically defined	Oligopeptides and free amino acids (elemental) in place of whole proteins, low fat, and/or higher concentration of MCT
Immunomodulating	Added glutamine, arginine, RNA, or marine oils
Hepatic disease	Increased branch chain amino acids and reduced aromatic amino acids
Renal disease	Reduced protein, water, electrolyes, and minerals; may contain few nonessential amino acids
Glucose intolerance	High fat, low carbohydrate, fiber
Pulmonary disease	High fat, low carbohydrate, n-3 fatty acids, and antioxidants

MCT, medium-chain triglycerides; RNA, ribonucleic acid.

formula. Formulas with a caloric density greater than this are well suited for fluid-restricted patients. These formulas provide less water and tend to have a higher viscosity and osmolality. If patients are placed on nutrient-dense formulas to decrease infusion time or volume of tube feeding and additional water is not provided, they are likely to become dehydrated. The amount of water provided by the tube feeding can easily be calculated from the product literature. Most products contain 60% to 80% water. Additional water to meet fluid requirements can be administered as water flushes through the tube during the day or, when applicable, intravenous fluids.

At one time it was thought that tube-feeding formulas with high osmolalities were poorly tolerated. However, tube-feeding formulas generally have osmolalities that are easily tolerated when administered correctly and therefore there is no reason to dilute a formula. Medications with osmolalities over 2000 mOsm may contribute to diarrhea, but tube-feeding formulas of 700 mOsm or less, which account for the majority of tube-feeding formulas, should not contribute to increased stool output.

Nutritional Content of Tube-Feeding Formulas

The type and quantity of carbohydrate, protein, and fat can vary among tube-feeding formulas and should be well understood so that an appropriate formula can be selected for a patient in a given clinical situation. The amount of protein contained in a tube-feeding formula can range from 8% to 25% of total calories. Nitrogen in tube-feeding formulas is supplied as whole protein or partially hydrolyzed protein (peptides) or fully hydrolyzed protein (crystalline amino acids). The products containing hydrolyzed proteins tend to be more expensive. Hydrolyzed proteins are used for patients who are unable to fully digest and absorb protein, such as with Crohn's disease. Formulas containing hydrolyzed proteins should be limited to use for patients who cannot tolerate standard polymeric formula or where a clear-cut advantage for a given indication has been shown (see Table 12-1). Crystalline amino acids are also found in formulas that are designed to have a specific amino acid composition.

Products designed for hepatic encephalopathy have a very specific branch chain–aromatic amino acid ratio. These formulas should only be used for patients with advanced liver disease and hepatic encephalopathy that fail to respond to conventional therapy. Some formulas designed for patients with renal failure restrict fluids, potassium, phosphorus, and magnesium to meet the dietary restrictions of this population. These products should only be used in renal disease when dialysis is inadequate. These products are not nutritionally complete for patients without the appropriate indications and are significantly more expensive. Individual amino acids have recently been added to some formulas with whole protein. For example, glutamine has been supplemented in formulas to promote immune function and improve bowel integrity. Arginine has also been supplemented in some formulas to promote wound healing and immune function. Again, these special products are more expensive, and therefore it is best to use them in well-defined situations.

Carbohydrate and Fat

Carbohydrate and fat are the primary calorie sources in tube-feeding formulas. Most patients will tolerate a standard formula that is 40% to 50% carbohydrate and 25% to 35% fat. Formulas designed for specific disease states may have proportions of carbohydrate and fat content that fall outside this range. Carbohydrate sources come from large molecules such as glucose oligosaccharides, maltodextrin, and hydrolyzed cornstarch. Smaller molecules such as mono- and disaccharides are also available. These molecules require a smaller amount of pancreatic enzymes and intestinal mucosa disaccharidases for adequate digestion. Most commercially made tube-feeding formulas are lactose and gluten free. Some supplements designed for oral intake and infant formulas may contain lactose. Specialty formulas designed to improve glucose control in diabetic patients contain a lower concentration of carbohydrate and are supplemented with fiber. These formulas are useful in those patients who cannot be controlled with a standard polymeric formula and an oral hypoglycemic medication or insulin. These products should not be routinely used for all diabetic patients, as they tend to be higher in fat and are more expensive.

The fat component in tube-feeding formulas has recently been the focus of much research. Previously, most tube-feeding formulas contained one fat source composed primarily of omega-6 fatty acids. Typical sources included corn oil and soybean oil. Recent research has shown the importance of other fatty acids such as omega-3 and medium-chain triglycerides (MCT) in maintaining immune function and maximizing absorption and metabolism efficiency. Now, most tube-feeding formulas contain a mixture of fat sources, such as canola oil, sunflower oil, MCT, and marine oils in addition to corn and soy oils. Many of the formulas designed for patients with malabsorption are low in fat or are supplemented with MCT to minimize symptoms of malabsorption. Formulas should contain a minimum of 4% of calories as long-chain fatty acids to provide a sufficient quantity of essential fatty acids and fat-soluble vitamins.

Formulas designed for respiratory insufficiency contain 40% to 50% of total calories as fat to minimize the production of carbon dioxide through carbohydrate metabolism. These formulas are also nutrient dense for fluid restriction in patients with pulmonary edema. The use of these formulas is usually limited to patients who continue to have respiratory difficulty in spite of standard treatments. Recently, some pulmonary enteral formulas have been supplemented with n-3 fatty acids and antioxidants to downregulate the inflammatory response in patients with acute respiratory distress syndrome (ARDS).

Fiber

Formulas are also available that contain fiber (4 to 20 g/L). Fiber offers many benefits, which include an increase in stool bulk and a source of energy for colonocytes, which may help to normalize bowel function. Fiber has been promoted for the management of diabetics with poor blood sugar control. The benefits of fiber are most useful for patients who require long-term tube feeding. Fiber increases the viscosity of formulas and can contribute to the clogging of feeding tubes. It is best to administer fiber-containing formulas through a tube that is large enough to avoid tube clogging.

Vitamins, Minerals, and Trace Elements

Vitamins, minerals, and trace elements are all included in standard tube-feeding formulas. Most formulas meet the US recommended dietary allowances for these nutrients in 1.0 to 1.5 liters of formula. A vitamin and mineral supplement is appropriate for patients receiving less than the necessary volume in order to meet the requirements.

Selecting the Feeding Route

Several factors are considered when selecting a route for tube feeding. First, it is important to consider the duration of tube-feeding use. Patients who require only 4 to 6 weeks of therapy are managed with a nasogastric or nasoenteric tube, which can be placed with little risk to the patient. These tubes can be easily removed when tube feeding is no longer needed. Patients who require long-term tube feeding often prefer a tube that is less visible and more comfortable. Surgical gastrostomy and jejunostomy tubes are frequently placed in patients who require long-term tube feeding. Because these procedures are performed in the operating room, they are frequently done at the time that the patient is scheduled for another surgical procedure. For patients who are not scheduled for a surgical procedure, a percutaneous endoscopically placed gastrostomy (PEG) or PEG with jejunostomy tube (PEG/J) can be placed without general anesthesia. The surgical and endoscopic methods of tube placement carry some risks, which include bleeding, wound infection, and bowel obstruction. However, these risks are minimized when an experienced physician is performing the procedure and the patient's clinical and nutritional status is not severely compromised.

A feeding tube placed with the tip of the tube in the stomach offers many advantages over a tube placed in the small bowel. Feeding into the stomach is more physiologic and allows feeding to be administered without a feeding pump. Gastric feeding tubes are common in patients who receive home tube feeding. Small bowel feeding tubes, which are ideally placed past the ligament of Treitz, are frequently used for patients with tracheal aspiration, reflux esophagitis, gastroparesis, gastric outlet obstruction, previous gastric surgery, and early postoperative feeding. Tubes have been designed to meet this need and can be placed temporarily via a nasoenteric route or long term through the abdominal wall. Although controversial, many clinicians believe that small bowel tube feeding may decrease the risk of aspiration. Temporary small bowel feeding tubes are generally more difficult to place than nasogastric feeding tubes.

Feeding tubes can be manually advanced into the small bowel at the bedside. Several reports using these techniques have shown good success; however, this requires protocols and adequately trained staff. Radiologic and endoscopic techniques are also used for small bowel tube placement. Nasoenteric feeding tubes can also be directly placed in the operating room if a patient is undergoing abdominal surgery. Confirmation of nasogastric and nasoenteric tube position can be made using a plain film of the abdomen. Radiographic confirmation is recommended when tubes are placed or repositioned.

Administering Tube Feeding

Tube-feeding schedules should be designed around the patient's clinical condition, physical activity, and feeding access. Feeding tubes placed in the stomach allow a large volume (200 to 500 mL) of formula to be administered over 20 to 40 minutes. The small bowel cannot tolerate large volumes given over a short period of time. For this reason, small bowel tube feeding must be administered with a pump over a continuous time period (8 to 24 hours). Most patients who are critically ill receive tube feeding continuously over 24 hours. Patients who are more mobile are good candidates for tube feeding that is cycled nocturnally. This also allows patients who are transitioning to oral intake to avoid suppressing their appetite during the day. Patients with gastric feeding tubes who are physically active may prefer to administer their tube feeding over a short period of time three to five times a day, similar to eating meals. This method, referred to as *intermittent gravity feeding*, offers flexibility and minimal equipment and is popular with patients receiving home tube feeding.

In order to allow for GI adaptation to tube feeding, the feeding volume is increased in a step-wise fashion to a goal rate by the second or third day, depending on tolerance. Continuous tube feeding is generally initiated at 30 mL per hour and increased by 30 mL per hour every 6 to 8 hours to the eventual goal rate as tolerated. Intermittent feedings, via gastric feeding tubes, are usually initiated at 150 to 200 mL over 20 to 40 minutes. The feeding is then advanced by 50 to 100 mL with every feeding to the eventual goal volume as tolerated. Mild bloating and loose bowel movements are common when tube feeding is initiated. If the patient shows any signs of severe intolerance to the feeding, such as diarrhea, elevated gastric residuals, or vomiting, the administration should not be further advanced and may be discontinued, sometimes temporarily, while appropriate clinical evaluation is done.

Monitoring and Complications

Outcome measures, such as length of hospital stay, morbidity, mortality, and costs, are important to track to determine the efficacy of enteral nutrition support. Other measures are used to monitor nutrition support to optimize therapy and minimize complications. Clinical monitoring of patients receiving tube feeding should include metabolic, GI, and mechanical assessment. Feedings received should be compared to prescribed calorie and protein goals. Adjustments in prescriptions should be made with changes in clinical status and activity. If a patient is not responding to the therapy, indirect calorimetry can be used to better define energy needs. Need for nutrition support should also be routinely re-evaluated. Acutely ill patients require daily to weekly monitoring of serum electrolytes, blood urea nitrogen (BUN), creatinine, and glucose. Stable outpatients may only need laboratory tests performed every month.

Because of the risk for refeeding syndrome, it is important to begin tube feeding cautiously and to monitor serum potassium, magnesium, phosphorus, and calcium closely in patients with severe undernutrition. Hyperglycemia may develop in patients with preexisting diabetes or significant stress. These patients can be managed with enteral hypoglycemic agents or insulin and frequent blood glucose monitoring. Excessive carbon dioxide production caused by overfeeding can cause difficulty in ventilatory support and weaning. Calories and carbohydrate provided from tube feeding and other sources such as intravenous fluids should be routinely monitored and adjusted to avoid the complications of overfeeding.

Assessing GI tolerance should include noting any reports of abdominal pain, nausea, vomiting, abdominal distention, or change in stool patterns. Precautions should be undertaken to prevent aspiration. This includes elevating the head of the bed to 30 degrees or greater while the feeding is administered, monitoring for high gastric residual volumes, and placement of postpyloric feeding tubes in high-risk patients and adequate airway management (Table 12-2). Blue dye has been added to tube-feeding formulas to help monitor aspiration of tube feeding. This practice is now being discouraged due to several case reports of mortality caused by blue dye number 1. In order to monitor hydration, it is helpful to routinely evaluate input/output and daily weight. A rapid change in weight may suggest an alteration in hydration and should prompt further investigation.

It is important to monitor the oral intake of patients who are transitioning to an oral diet and to adjust tube-feeding volume accordingly so as to avoid suppressing their appetite and overfeeding. The most common complication of tube feeding in the hospital setting is diarrhea, which is rarely caused by the tube-feeding formula. Likely causes of diarrhea are medications, *Clostridium difficile* colitis, underlying or unrecognized GI disorders, and sometimes the rate of tube-feeding delivery. Medications that may cause diarrhea include antibiotics and elixirs that contain sorbitol (Table 12-3). If diarrhea develops while the patient is receiving tube feeding, it is important to evaluate all the potential causes and treat them appropriately; administering antidiarrheals before checking stool for *C. difficile* toxin and, when appropriate, bacterial cultures can be risky and may lead to toxic megacolon. Constipation is a more common symptom in patients receiving long-term tube feeding, patients receiving high doses of pain

Table 12-2   Aspiration precautions.

Elevate the head of the bed to at least 30 to 45 degrees

Monitor for aspiration contents in the lungs

   Direct observation

   Glucose testing

   pH testing

Monitor gastric residuals (>200 mL warrants holding tube feeding and considering promotility agents)

Consider use of dual-lumen tubes (small bowel feeding with continuous gastric decompression)

Monitor feeding tube placement

   Radiography

   Auscultation of insufflated air

   Observation of fluid pulled from the feeding tube

   Check pH of fluid aspirated from the tube

Monitor and maintain adequate airway cuff pressure

Table 12-3   Examples of medications associated with diarrhea.

Sorbitol-containing medications

Propranolol solution

Acetaminophen elixir

Cimetidine solution

Ranitidine syrup

Bactrim (trimethoprim and sulfamethoxazole) suspension

Furosemide solution

Antibiotics

Neomycin

Clindamycin

Ciprofloxacin

Amoxicillin

Others

Potassium oral solutions

Oral phosphate supplements

Magnesium-based antacids

Promotility agents

medications, and those who are immobile. Fiber-containing formulas and adequate water are most useful in preventing constipation in this population.

Dehydration can occur when patients do not receive adequate fluid via tube feeding, intravenous fluid, and water flushes through the tube. This can occur in patients receiving diuretic therapy and those individuals with unusual losses from drains, stool output, or emesis. Routine monitoring of weight, blood pressure, heart rate, laboratory measures, and clinical status help to identify this problem before it becomes critical.

Clogged and displaced feeding tubes are frequent problems for patients receiving tube feedings. Patients may pull out nasal feeding tubes either intentionally

Table 12-4 Administering medication through a feeding tube.

- Use liquid form of medication whenever possible.
- Consult pharmacy on availability of liquid medication and if tablets are crushable.
- If crushing a medication, crush finely and disperse in warm water if clinically appropriate.
- Flush the feeding tube before and after each medication.
- Consult pharmacy on the timing of medications in relationship to the feeding to avoid drug nutrient reactions.
- Consult pharmacy before administering drugs through a small bowel feeding tube. Some medications require the acidic stomach pH for proper action.
- Medications should not be mixed with enteral formulas.
- Do not crush enteric coated, sustained-released, or timed-released tablets or capsules.
- Do not mix medications together.

or inadvertently. It is important to secure feeding tubes in place and avoid excess tubing that can be tangled with other objects. Percutaneously placed tubes can be displaced as well. If this occurs, a temporary tube must be placed in the ostomy immediately because the site can close quickly. Feeding tubes can become clogged when water flushes are inadequate or medications are administered in the feeding tube inappropriately. It is recommended that feeding tubes be flushed daily and at any time the feeding is stopped or a medication is administered. Medications should be in a liquid form whenever possible, and the tube should be flushed with water after each separate medication administration (Table 12-4). Although there are many theories about how to unclog feeding tubes, warm water or pancreatic enzymes with sodium bicarbonate are the only two methods proven to be effective. It is best to avoid colas and cranberry juice due to their likelihood of leaving a residue that can cause further clogging of the tube.

Conclusion

Tube feeding offers a method of nutrition support to patients who are unable to consume adequate nutrition but have a functional GI tract. Tube feeding has many advantages over parenteral nutrition, and therefore it should be used whenever feasible and clinically safe. A wide selection of formulas, tubes, and administration methods are available. Detailed assessment of the patient's clinical condition, nutrient requirements, and activity will direct selection of feeding route, formula, and administration method. Monitoring metabolic, mechanical, and GI tolerance to tube feeding will guide adjustments in tube-feeding therapy. Following these principles, tube feeding can support patients successfully for as long as the therapy is indicated.

For a list of references for this chapter, please visit the University of Pennsylvania School of Medicine's Nutrition Education and Prevention Program web site: *http://www.med.upenn.edu/nutrimed/articles.html*

Enteral Feeding and Esophageal Cancer

Lisa D. Unger and M. Patricia Fuhrman

Objectives

- Assess the nutritional status of patients with esophageal cancer.
- Assess the nutrition-related metabolic abnormalities that can affect patients with cancer.
- Identify appropriate dietary recommendations for patients with odynophagia due to radiation therapy.
- Understand clinical and metabolic monitoring of patients receiving enteral nutrition support.
- Recognize the benefits of enteral nutrition support in a patient receiving radiation therapy to the head and neck.

CD is a 50-year-old male inpatient at a university hospital. He has recently been diagnosed with esophageal cancer and reports a 25-lb weight loss over the past 6 months due to dysphagia (difficulty swallowing) and loss of appetite. CD is status post esophagectomy and jejunostomy tube placement. Chemotherapy and radiation therapy are planned. During this hospitalization, a swallowing study was performed to rule out a postoperative leak and to assess whether it was safe for CD to resume eating and drinking. After he passed the swallowing test, a liquid diet was initiated, and he was eventually advanced to a regular diet.

Past Medical History

CD has no significant past medical history.

Medications

CD takes no medications.

Social/Diet History

CD lives alone. He denies intravenous drug use and drinks one beer in the evening. CD smoked two packs of cigarettes per day for 30 years (60 pack year history).

He quit 2 years ago. CD's dysphagia worsened over the past 6 weeks, and his appetite became very poor. He reports limiting his intake to juices, broth, and tea over the past month.

Review of Systems

General: Fatigue, weight loss
GI: Poor appetite, dysphagia
Neurologic: No sensory loss
Musculoskeletal: No muscle or joint pain

Physical Examination

Vital Signs

Temperature: 99.0°F (37.2°C)
Heart rate: 80 beats per minute (BPM)
Respiratory rate: 14 BPM
Blood pressure: 120/80 mm Hg
Height: 5'11" (180 cm)
Current weight: 130 lb (59 kg)
Usual body weight: 155 lb (70 kg)
Body mass index (BMI): 18 kg/m^2
Percent weight change: 16% over 6 months [(155–130)/155] × 100

General: Cachectic man in no acute distress
Head/neck: Bilateral temporal wasting
Cardiac: Regular rate and rhythm; no rubs, gallops, or murmurs
Chest: Status post esophagectomy with wound site clean, dry, and intact
Abdomen: Soft, nontender, nondistended; bowel sounds present; jejunostomy tube site clean and dry
Extremities: No edema; general decrease in muscle mass
Neurologic: Alert and oriented to person, place, and time; intact

Laboratory Data

Patient's Values	Normal Values
Albumin: 3.1 g/dL	3.5–5.8 g/dL
Hemoglobin: 13.5 g/dL	13.5–17.5 g/dL
Hematocrit: 40%	40%–52%
BUN: 13 mg/dL	10–20 mg/dL

Creatinine: 0.8 mg/dL   0.8–1.3 mg/dL
Potassium: 3.6 mmol/L   3.5–5.3 mmol/L
Sodium: 136 mmol/L   133–143 mmol/L

Go to questions 1 to 2.

Follow-Up Description

CD was discharged from the hospital able to eat an adequate oral diet. His jejunostomy tube was not removed because in 4 weeks he would be receiving chemotherapy and radiation therapy that could adversely affect his oral intake. CD was instructed to flush his jejunostomy tube daily with 60 mL water to keep it patent (open). Four weeks later, CD began receiving chemotherapy and radiation therapy, and after 2 weeks of these treatments, severe odynophagia (painful swallowing) developed. As a result, his oral diet greatly diminished. Based on a 24-hour recall and usual intake over the past week, CD reported consuming 1/2 cup of flavored gelatin and 6 oz applesauce daily, which totals approximately 200 calories per day with no significant amount of protein, vitamins, or minerals.

Go to questions 3 to 8.

Case Questions

1. What factors are helpful in diagnosing undernutrition in this patient?
2. What nutritional and nutrition-related metabolic abnormalities can affect patients with cancer?
3. What are the possible adverse effects of radiation therapy for esophageal cancer patients and how can they affect CD's nutritional status?
4. In general, what dietary recommendations alleviate odynophagia, as experienced by a patient receiving radiation therapy for esophageal cancer?
5. Since severe odynophagia develops secondary to radiation therapy and CD is eating only approximately 200 kcal per day, what alternative feeding options are available for him?
6. How should an enteral formula be selected, and what issues related to fluid balance should be considered?
7. What clinical and laboratory parameters should be monitored for patients who receive tube feeding?
8. CD asks how long enteral nutrition support is planned. What factors determine when CD's jejunostomy tube can be removed?

Case Answers

Part 1: Diagnosis

1. **What factors are helpful in diagnosing undernutrition in this patient?**

   Based on CD's medical history, he has had a decreased appetite and dysphagia for the past 6 months, with worsening dysphagia over the past 6 weeks. This has limited his intake to juices, broth, and tea over the last month. This diet is inadequate in protein, calories, vitamins, and minerals and has contributed to CD's severe weight loss, resulting in a 16% weight change over the past 6 months. In addition, his BMI is only 18 kg/m^2, indicating that he is currently underweight. Additional evidence that supports a diagnosis of undernutrition includes his cachectic appearance and temporal wasting found on physical examination. Laboratory data shows a decreased albumin level of 3.1 g/dL, indicating mild protein depletion. Although hypoalbuminemia is often associated with nutritional inadequacy, its half-life of 21 days and sensitivity to hydration status and inflammatory processes limit its clinical use as an indicator of short-term nutritional status.

2. **What nutritional and nutrition-related metabolic abnormalities can affect patients with cancer?**

   Patients with cancer and those undergoing treatment can experience symptoms that decrease oral intake, such as dysphagia, alterations in taste and smell, and obstruction of the GI tract that can be caused by tumor growth. In addition, the release of cytokines, such as tumor necrosis factor and interleukins, can lead to decreased intake. Psychological factors, such as depression and anxiety, may also contribute to a decreased appetite.

   Of note, there may be an increase in resting energy expenditure in some oncology patients. Furthermore, an alteration in carbohydrate metabolism with an impaired sensitivity to endogenous insulin and an alteration in lipid metabolism may cause patients with progressive disease to metabolize more fat (have an increased rate of lipolysis), thus depleting fat reserves. The catabolism of endogenous protein and accelerated gluconeogenesis can occur because the normal starvation adaptive mechanism of protein-sparing and reduced energy expenditure may not take place in the cancer patient.

   Go to Follow-Up Description on previous page.

Part 2: Nutritional Management

3. **What are the possible adverse effects of radiation therapy for esophageal cancer patients, and how can they affect CD's nutritional status?**

   Radiation therapy for esophageal cancer can have adverse effects, the most prominent being odynophagia, which can cause CD's oral intake to greatly diminish, eventually affecting his nutritional status.

4. In general, what dietary recommendations alleviate odynophagia, as experienced by a patient receiving radiation therapy for esophageal cancer?

    For odynophagia, the patient should avoid foods with extreme temperatures; foods that are spicy, hot, tart, or high in acid; raw fruits and vegetables; and dry, coarse, and highly salty food. It is recommended that the patient drink liquid nutritional supplements to increase protein and calorie intake. Suggest that the patient try soft, blended foods, such as casseroles, mashed potatoes, soups, scrambled eggs, and yogurt.

5. Since severe odynophagia developed secondary to radiation therapy and CD is eating only approximately 200 kcal per day, what alternative feeding options are available for him?

    Because of severe odynophagia resulting from radiation therapy, CD cannot consume adequate calories and protein. Therefore, he will continue to lose weight and become more undernourished if he depends on oral intake alone. Since his radiation therapy is planned for several more weeks and he has a functional GI tract, he is a good candidate for enteral nutrition support using his jejunostomy tube, which is a long-term feeding tube. After determining his nutrient goals, choose an enteral formula that best meets these goals.

6. How should an enteral formula be selected, and what issues related to fluid balance should be considered?

    A variety of enteral formulas are available, each of which provides different concentrations of calories and protein to meet patients' requirements. The enteral formula for CD should be selected based on his estimated calorie and protein needs for weight gain and protein repletion. His oral intake should also be considered.

    Fluid balance is important to consider, particularly when enteral nutrition is the sole source of fluid intake. It is therefore important to monitor fluid status in all patients receiving tube feedings in order to prevent dehydration. If the tube-feeding regimen does not supply enough water to meet patients' fluid requirements, since the amount of water in tube-feeding formulas varies, additional fluid can be provided with water flushes via the feeding tube several times throughout the day.

7. What clinical and laboratory parameters should be monitored for patients who receive tube feeding?

    It is very important to monitor patients for tube feeding tolerance, hydration, and electrolyte and nutritional status. Physical symptoms that should be monitored include incidence of nausea, vomiting, stool frequency, diarrhea, and abdominal pain. Physical examination should include assessing for abdominal distention or tenderness and evidence of edema or dehydration. Weight changes should also be noted. In addition, serum electrolytes (sodium, potassium, chloride, bicarbonate), calcium, magnesium, phosphorous, BUN, creatinine, and glucose should be monitored *daily* when the patient begins receiving enteral nutrition support. Other parameters that can be monitored on a weekly basis include albumin, prealbumin, and transferrin.

It is important to note that in the first few days of initiating the tube feeding, malnourished patients such as CD may exhibit a refeeding syndrome in which extracellular to intracellular electrolyte shifts of potassium, phosphorous, and magnesium may occur, requiring prompt repletion. Once the patient is metabolically stable, the frequency of monitoring can be decreased as appropriate.

8. **CD asks how long enteral nutrition support is planned. What factors determine when CD's jejunostomy tube should be removed?**

   After his radiation therapy is completed, as CD's odynophagia decreases and his oral intake improves, the tube feedings should be decreased accordingly. Upon follow-up 2 weeks after radiation therapy is completed, CD reports less odynophagia and is able to increase his oral intake. He also follows up with a dietitian, who offers suggestions and recipes for high-calorie, high-protein, soft, easy-to-swallow foods. He is therefore instructed to decrease his tube-feeding regimen through the jejunostomy tube since his oral intake has greatly improved. Additional parameters used to assess his progress include his weight and prealbumin level, both of which continue to increase.

   Two weeks later, he is able to substantially increase his oral diet and begins to drink two cans (480 mL) of a nutritional supplement daily for additional calories and protein. An 8-oz can of this supplement (240 mL) provides approximately 14 g protein and 365 total calories and also contributes vitamins and minerals. Since his oral intake was deemed adequate to meet his nutritional needs, his tube feeding regimen is discontinued. He was monitored for 4 weeks off tube feeding. His oral intake remains excellent, and he continues to gain weight. Since no further radiation therapy was planned, the decision was made to remove the tube.

See Chapter Review Questions, pages A-34 to A-37.

13

Parenteral Nutrition Support

Laura Matarese and Ezra Steiger

Objectives*

- Describe the indications and contraindications for parenteral nutrition support.
- Determine the composition of parenteral nutrition formulas and how the macronutrient, micronutrient, and fluid requirements are calculated.
- Describe appropriate methods for monitoring and management of the complications associated with parenteral nutrition support.

Parenteral nutrition (PN) supplies protein in the form of amino acids, carbohydrate as dextrose, fat, vitamins, minerals, and trace elements to patients when the gastrointestinal (GI) tract is not functional, accessible, or safe to use. It can be infused via peripheral or central veins. The exact route of administration will depend on the length of therapy, nutritional requirements, goal of nutrition therapy, availability of intravenous (IV) access, severity of illness, and fluid status.

Indications and Contraindications

Indications

Due to the potential for serious complications and the expense of parenteral nutrition, its use should be limited to those who would most likely benefit from the therapy. Enteral nutrition should always be considered if the GI tract can be used. Parenteral nutrition should be used when the GI tract is not functional or cannot be accessed and in patients who cannot be adequately nourished by

---

* SOURCE: Objectives for chapter and cases adapted from the *NIH Nutrition Curriculum Guide for Training Physicians* (*http://www.nhlbi.nih.gov/funding/training/naa*).

enteral nutrition. The following conditions may warrant the use of parenteral nutrition:

- Perioperative support in severe malnutrition
- Inflammatory bowel disease
- Short bowel syndrome
- Pancreatitis
- Mechanical intestinal obstruction or pseudo-obstruction
- Severe malabsorption
- Hyperemesis gravidarum
- Mesenteric ischemia
- Enteroenteric fistula

Contraindications

Parenteral nutrition is not indicated when the GI tract is functional, when the patient's prognosis is not consistent with aggressive nutrition support, or when the risks outweigh the benefits.

Peripheral Parenteral Nutrition

Peripheral parenteral nutrition (PPN) is usually reserved for patients requiring short-term PN who are not markedly hypermetabolic or fluid restricted and have adequate peripheral venous access. Osmolarity and compatibility are factors that need to be considered in PPN solutions. Infusion of hypertonic solutions through a peripheral vein may result in phlebitis. The amount of dextrose and amino acids in the solution is generally limited due to the contribution they make to its osmolarity. Although fluid volume of the solution can be increased to reduce osmolarity, this may not be practical or safe in many patients. Because IV fat emulsions are isotonic, PPN solutions generally include lipids, dextrose, and amino acids. They usually do not provide adequate calories and protein for hypermetabolic, fluid-restricted patients but can be helpful for several days until GI function returns or central access is obtained. Peripheral IV access can only be used when infusing solutions less than 900 mOsm/L.

Central Parenteral Nutrition

Central PN is usually indicated in patients who require long-term PN or in fluid-restricted patients, or both. The solutions may be dextrose based (dextrose and amino acids) or lipid based and are infused via a central vein. The decision to include lipids daily in the solution or to administer them separately is based on various factors. Lipid-based solutions are indicated in situations in which restricting the carbohydrate load is desirable, such as in patients with persistent hyperglycemia or hypercapnia. Reducing carbohydrate intake may decrease the production of carbon dioxide, which may facilitate weaning from the ventilator (see Chapter 10). Generally, there is no limit on the osmolarity of these solutions because concentrated solutions can be administered into the central vein, where they are rapidly diluted due to the high flow rate of blood returning to the heart. Central PN is generally indicated over PPN when any of the following conditions are present:

- Long-term (>7 days) PN support is anticipated
- Moderately to severely elevated metabolic rate
- Moderate to severe malnutrition
- Fluid restriction
- Poor peripheral access
- Central access availability

Macronutrient Requirements

Energy

Estimated basal energy requirements are based on an individual's age, sex, height, and weight. Energy expenditure can be estimated through predictive equations. This estimated amount should fall within a range of 20 to 35 kcal/kg.

The Harris-Benedict equation can be used to predict basal/resting energy expenditure (REE) in adults.

REE equation for males:

$$66 + [13.7 \times \text{weight (kg)}] + [5.0 \times \text{height (cm)}] - [6.8 \times (\text{age})] = \text{kcal/day}$$

REE equation for females:

$$655 + [9.7 \times \text{weight (kg)}] + [1.85 \times \text{height (cm)}] - [4.7 \times (\text{age})] = \text{kcal/day}$$

The REE is generally multiplied by a factor (1.2 to 1.75) to account for physical activity. The final number derived is an estimate of total energy expenditure (TEE) as described in Chapter 1. Energy expenditure can also be measured by direct and indirect calorimetry. The calories are then supplied in the PN formula in the form of dextrose, lipid, and amino acids.

Glucose

D-Glucose (dextrose monohydrate), used in PN solutions, provides 3.4 kcal/g. Continuous dextrose infusion should be limited to 5 mg/kg per minute, or 1700 dextrose calories per day (500 g) for a 70-kg patient, which is the maximum rate of glucose oxidation. When glucose oxidation rates are exceeded, fat synthesis will occur, a process that may generate excessive carbon dioxide (CO_2). This may contribute to CO_2 retention in patients with respiratory disease. In addition, exceeding glucose oxidation rates may also contribute to hepatic steatosis, or fat deposition in the liver. Also, one should be sure to take into account dextrose in other IVs.

Lipids

IV fat emulsions supply lipids, which are a source of essential fatty acids (EFAs) and a concentrated source of calories. To prevent essential fatty acid deficiency (EFAD) in adults, 1% to 2% of total calories should come from linoleic acid (omega-6) and approximately 0.5% of calories from alpha-linolenic acid (omega-3). Lipids are often provided daily, supplying fewer than 30% of total calories. In addition to providing a source of EFAs and supply of nonprotein calories, the use of IV lipid emulsions may aid in blood glucose control in the hyperglycemic patient.

Impaired immune response has been associated with high intake of linoleic acid. Additionally, rapid infusion of lipids (>110 mg/kg per hour or 185 g per day for a 70-kg patient) may result in reduced lipid clearance and impaired reticuloendothelial function and pulmonary gas exchange. To minimize these negative effects, fat intake should be restricted to fewer than 30% of total calories. Dietary fat provides 9 kcal/g, a 10% IV lipid emulsion provides 1.1 kcal/mL, a 20% IV lipid emulsion provides 2.0 kcal/mL, and a 30% IV lipid emulsion provides 3.0 kcal/mL. Lipid emulsions should not be given in hypertriglyceridemia-induced pancreatitis or when serum triglyceride values are greater than 400 mg/dL.

Protein (Amino Acids)

The primary function of protein in PN solutions is to maintain nitrogen balance and promote maintenance of lean body mass. Parenteral protein is provided in the form of synthetic amino acids and contains a mixture of essential and nonessential amino acids. Each gram of protein supplies four calories. Protein is often administered based on body weight and stress level:

Mild stress: 0.8 to 1.0 g/kg per day

Moderate stress: 1.5 g/kg per day

Severe stress: 2.0 g/kg per day

Adjustments in protein load should be made according to the patient's tolerance and clinical response and through monitoring of serum transport proteins, nitrogen balance results, and renal and liver function.

Fluid and Electrolyte Requirements

Daily fluid requirements can be estimated from the sum of urine output, GI losses, and insensible water losses from the skin and respiratory tract. Weighing the patient daily is the best means of assessing net gain or loss of fluid. Rapid weight gain or loss (>4 lb [1.8 kg] in 1 week) generally represents fluid changes and not tissue synthesis. Vital signs, such as blood pressure and heart rate, and physical examination changes (e.g., edema, ascites, skin turgor) also offer evidence of fluid status. In general, young adults require 30 to 40 mL/kg per day and the elderly require 30 mL/kg per day.

Electrolytes are routinely added to the PN solutions in amounts sufficient to provide for daily needs. Electrolyte requirements will vary depending on the patient's current electrolyte, renal, and fluid status, as well as the patient's underlying disease process. If the patient had been receiving maintenance IV fluids before starting PN, it is helpful to note the electrolyte composition of these fluids and use this as a guide to prescribe the PN formula. Patients receiving PN may have higher intracellular electrolyte requirements than patients receiving standard IV fluids.

Calcium is essential for normal muscle contraction, nerve function, blood coagulation, and bone mineralization. The usual dose is 9 to 22 mEq per day. Sixty percent of serum calcium is bound to protein, primarily albumin. Therefore, in the presence of a low serum albumin level, a low serum calcium level needs to be adjusted for hypoalbuminemia.

Adjusted calcium level = (4.0 − serum albumin) × 0.8 + serum calcium

When in doubt and when the serum albumin is less than 2.8 g/dL, an ionized calcium level should be obtained. Along with calcium, phosphorus is the major component of bone hydroxyapetite and teeth. Phosphorus is the primary intracellular anion and functions in the metabolism of carbohydrate, fat, and protein. The usual dose is 15 to 30 mM per day. Each milliequivalent of potassium phosphate provides 0.68 Mmol phosphate or 21 mg elemental phosphorus. Each milliequivalent of sodium phosphate provides 0.75 Mmol phosphate or 23 mg elemental phosphorus. The combination of calcium and phosphorus in PN formulas has the potential of forming a precipitate. Thus, it is important to follow appropriate and safe guidelines for maximum calcium and phosphorus additives in a PN formula.

Magnesium functions in enzyme reactions such as glycolysis and in all reactions involving adenosine triphosphate (ATP). Magnesium is often depleted in patients with protein-calorie malnutrition and prolonged IV fluid therapy. Magnesium may also appear low in patients with hypoalbuminemia.

Corrected magnesium level = Mg + 0.005 (40 − serum albumin)

Patients may also have excessive losses from prolonged gastric suction, fistulas, and diarrhea. The usual dose of magnesium sulfate is 8 to 24 mEq per day. Magnesium sulfate provides 8.12 mEq/g magnesium.

Potassium is the major cation of intracellular fluid. The normal dose is 60 to 120 mEq per day. Hypokalemia may result from diuretics, amphotericin B, nasogastric suction, or vomiting. Other medications such as cyclosporine may cause hyperkalemia. The PN solution should provide maintenance potassium requirements. Acute deficits of potassium should be corrected outside of the PN with an IV replacement dose.

Sodium is a major extracellular ion and functions in the maintenance of osmotic pressure and in acid-base balance. The usual dose is 100 to 150 mEq per day. Requirements may be increased when there are excess losses from urine, ostomies, or fistulas or decreased in renal or hepatic failure.

Sodium and potassium may be added to PN solutions in the form of chloride or acetate salts. Chloride is a major extracellular anion and functions in the maintenance of osmotic pressure and acid-base balance. Acetate may be added to PN solutions when clinically appropriate since it is converted to bicarbonate in the liver and functions as a systemic alkalinizer. Bicarbonate should never be added to PN solutions since it is not compatible with other additives and may form a precipitate.

Vitamins, Minerals, and Trace Elements

Vitamins, minerals, and trace elements should be added daily to the PN solution in order to prevent deficiencies. These are given as standard multiple-vitamin and trace element preparations. In the event that vitamin, mineral, or trace element deficiencies or unusual losses occur, they can sometimes be supplemented above the amount normally added to the PN solution.

Medications

PN solutions are complex formulations designed to deliver fluid, electrolytes, and nutrients. Most medications should not be added to the PN solution because of potential instability and incompatibility. Heparin and, when necessary, insulin can be added to the PN solution. Only regular human insulin should be added to PN solutions. Other medications, such as histamine H_2-receptor antagonists and octreotide, can be added to the PN solution when needed.

Parenteral Nutrition Prescription

The base solution can be specified by the actual grams of dextrose, fat, amino acids, and calories, or it can be prescribed as final concentrations. Depending on the facility, individual electrolytes and minerals can be specified or a selection can be made from several standard solutions. In most institutions, the PN prescription is ordered for a 24-hour period.

Infusing Parenteral Nutrition

When using a continuous PN regimen, it is important to determine the desired volume to be delivered at the maintenance rate of infusion to fulfill the patient's caloric and protein needs over a 24-hour period. Occasionally, patients who are clinically and metabolically stable and who exhibit no complications with continuous 24-hour total parenteral nutrition (TPN) may benefit from cycled TPN to increase mobility and ease of care. Cycled TPN generally is infused over a 10- to 16-hour period.

Monitoring and Management of Complications

Catheters

Central access can be obtained via subclavian, jugular vein, or peripherally inserted central catheters (PICC) used for delivery of PN solutions. For long-term access, a Hickman or Broviac catheter or implantable port can be used.

Mechanical complications of catheter insertion may include pneumothorax, hydrothorax, and great vessel injury. To minimize morbidity, obtaining a chest x-ray before using a new central line for PN is important to ensure that the line was correctly placed and that no internal injuries occurred during its insertion.

Infectious Complications

Many hospitalized patients receiving PN have multiple causes for elevations in temperature and sepsis, including intra-abdominal infections, wound infections, urinary tract infections, pneumonia, phlebitis, and drug fever. However, a sudden change in the patient's usual temperature may be an indication of possible catheter-related sepsis. Newly uncontrolled blood sugars may also be a sign of infection. The catheter can be seeded by a remote source or can be the primary source of infection. Catheter-related sepsis can be minimized with meticulous catheter insertion techniques and good catheter care maintenance.

Metabolic

Hyperglycemia may be associated with glucosuria, osmotic diuresis, hyperosmolar nonketotic dehydration, and coma. A blood glucose should be performed four times daily until the patient demonstrates adequate blood sugar control. If a stable insulin requirement exists, insulin can be added to the PN solution to bring blood glucose to acceptable levels. In some instances it may be necessary to reduce the dextrose calories and replace with lipid calories to aid in blood glucose control. Hypoglycemia may be seen in patients after abrupt discontinuation of PN infusion with a high dextrose load. To avoid this problem, infusions can be tapered down over a period of 1 to 2 hours to allow for serum insulin adaptation.

Electrolyte imbalances may occur in severely stressed patients both before and after PN infusions are begun. It is best to correct any existing electrolyte abnormalities before PN is initiated. Close monitoring of electrolytes, magnesium, calcium, and phosphorus during the first few days of PN is important. Corrections for electrolyte imbalances must be made promptly with IV replacements to avoid serious complications, such as seizures, arrhythmias, or even death.

Dehydration and fluid overload are potential complications when PN administration is the primary route of fluid infusion. Fluid overload or edema may be seen in patients with renal failure, liver failure, congestive heart failure, and hypoalbuminemia. Excessive PN volume infusion can significantly exacerbate fluid retention states. Under these circumstances, a concentrated PN solution may be used. Fluid status should be evaluated daily to determine if the patient is dehydrated or at risk for fluid overload. Intake, output, and body weight records should be monitored daily. The physical examination should note the presence of edema, rales, ascites, distended neck veins, and other signs of fluid retention.

Preventing Refeeding Syndrome

Refeeding syndrome may occur in prolonged starvation, resulting in severe imbalances of serum phosphorus, potassium, and/or magnesium as well as fluid and glucose. Once nutrition support begins, increased cellular uptake of electrolytes may cause extremely low serum electrolyte levels. This dramatic shift can lead to generalized fatigue, lethargy, muscle weakness, cardiac dysfunction, and potentially death. The refeeding syndrome can be minimized by initially providing the patient with half of his or her energy requirements. Phosphorus, potassium, magnesium, glucose, and fluid status must be monitored closely in these patients when nutrition support is initiated (Chapter 5, Case 2).

Nutrition parameters, such as albumin, transferrin and prealbumin, may be monitored weekly to help assess the efficacy of therapy.

For a list of references for this chapter, please visit the University of Pennsylvania School of Medicine's Nutrition Education and Prevention Program web site: *http://www.med.upenn.edu/nutrimed/articles.html*

Case 1

Colon Cancer and Postoperative Sepsis

José Antonio Ruy-Díaz and David C. Frankenfield

Objectives

• Describe the appropriate parenteral nutrition recommendations for a patient with colon cancer.

• Assess the nutritional status of a critically ill patient.

• Identify clinical and metabolic parameters used to monitor patients receiving parenteral nutrition.

• Recognize the adverse effects of undernutrition and the associated benefits of providing appropriate nutrition support.

• Recognize the benefits of parenteral nutrition in a malnourished, critically ill, surgical patient.

AJ, a 73-year-old man, presents to the emergency room with 72 hours of abdominal pain of increasing severity. He describes his pain as radiating through the entire abdomen. He also reports nausea and vomiting of gastric contents at least five times during the last 3 days. AJ also reports liquid greenish stools on about eight occasions. He mentions that he has been losing weight for the last 6 months without any explanation.

Past Medical History

AJ had a stroke 2 years ago, leaving as a sequela paresis of his right leg. He currently takes warfarin (Coumadin) and digoxin as medications. He denies drug or food allergies. He had an appendectomy 3 years ago.

Social History

AJ is currently retired from his job as an employee for a commercial organization. He was a heavy alcohol consumer, drinking 34 oz (1000 mL) tequila daily until 10 years ago, when, on advice from his physician, he stopped drinking. AJ smoked 20 cigarettes every day until approximately 10 years ago.

Review of Systems

The review of systems was unremarkable except for nausea, abdominal pain, and weight loss.

Physical Examination

Vital Signs

Temperature: 100°F (38°C)
Heart rate: 96 beats per minute (BPM)
Respiration: 23 BPM
Blood pressure: 100/60 mm Hg
Height: 5'6" (170 cm)
Current weight: 99 lb (45 kg)
BMI: 16 kg/m²
Usual weight: 132 lb (60 kg) 1 year ago
Percent weight change: 25% over 6 months (132–99)/132

General: Thin man who appears in severe distress
Skin: Pale, cold, and dry
Head, ears, eyes, nose, throat (HEENT): Anicteric
Cardiac: Regular rate and rhythm, no murmurs or extra sounds
Pulmonary: Hypoventilation in both lung bases, with rales
Abdomen: Marked abdominal tenderness, particularly in the hypogastrium, with guarding and rebound; distended; no bowel sounds
Extremities: No cyanosis or edema; paresis of right leg
Neurologic: Awake, alert, nonfocal
Clinical studies: An abdominal x-ray showed severely distended loops of the small bowel in right upper quadrant and no air in the rectum. An abdominal ultrasound revealed distended loops of small intestine. No evidence of cholelithiasis (gallstones) was found. Bile ducts appeared normal. The liver looked normal.

Laboratory Data

Patient's Values	Normal Values
Sodium: 139 mEq/L	133–145 mEq/L
Potassium: 5.8 mEq/L	3.5–5.3 mEq/L
Chloride: 110 mEq/L	97–107 mEq/L
CO_2: 27 mEq/L	24–32 mEq/L
Blood urea nitrogen (BUN): 41 mEq/L	10–20 mEq/L
Creatinine: 2.5 mg/dL	0.8–1.3 mg/dL

Glucose: 137 mg/dL	70–110 mg/dL
Albumin: 2.8 g/dL	3.5–5.8 g/dL
Calcium: 7.6 mg/dL	9–11 mg/dL
Adjusted calcium: 8.1 mg/dL	9–11 mg/dL
Magnesium: 1.7 mg/dL	1.8–2.9 mg/dL
Phosphorus: 2.7 mg/dL	2.5–4.6 mg/dL
Amylase: 48 units/dL	60–180 units/dL
Bilirubin: 0.57 mg/dL	0.2–1.2 mg/dL
Aspartate aminotransaminase (AST): 36 U/L	0–40 U/L
Alanine aminotransaminase (ALT): 14 U/L	0–36 U/L
Hemoglobin: 7.9 g/dL	13.5–17.5 g/dL
Hematocrit: 29%	41%–53%
White blood cells: 32 tho/μL	4.0–11.0 tho/μL
Prothrombin time: 27 seconds	<15 seconds
Platelet count: 1,315,000/mm^3	150,000–450,000/mm^3

Hospital Course and Therapy

On admission to the hospital, a nasogastric tube was placed and his nausea and vomiting resolved. He was also placed on NPO (nothing to eat or drink) restrictions. His nasogastric tube drained 800 to 1200 mL of feculent fluid the first day. At the same time, he was rehydrated with IV fluids consisting of D$_5$W 1/2 normal saline. However, 24 hours after admission he continued to experience abdominal pain and his nausea and vomiting recurred when the nasogastric tube was clamped.

The surgical team decided to take AJ to the operating room to perform an exploratory laparotomy. The findings of the procedure were an occlusive tumor mass of 3.9 cm located at the sigmoid colon, with necrosis of the entire colon proximal to the tumor. AJ had a total colectomy, with Hartmann's procedure and an ileostomy. The histopathologic examination reported a well-differentiated adenocarcinoma of the colon, Dukes-Ashley B, with free surgical margins and acute necrotizing colitis proximal to obstructing neoplasm. AJ was transferred to the intensive care unit (ICU) after surgery. He required mechanical ventilation for 5 days. After correction of his volume deficit, AJ's serum creatinine dropped to 1.2 mg/dL. He had no evidence of renal failure.

Case Questions

1. List AJ's possible medical problems demonstrated by his overall clinical picture.

2. What are the possible etiologies of AJ's bowel obstruction?

3. What additional evidence from AJ's physical examination could be used to assess his nutritional status before initiating parenteral nutrition?

4. Why is parenteral nutrition the most appropriate form of nutritional intervention at this point in AJ's clinical course?

5. Using the Harris-Benedict equation, calculate AJ's REE; also calculate AJ's protein requirement and maximum carbohydrate and lipid oxidation rates. How much dextrose and lipid should be ordered in the PN?

6. What biochemical laboratory data should be used to monitor AJ while he is on PN?

7. After AJ's postoperative conditions began to resolve and his bowel sounds showed increased activity, his physician decided that he should begin an oral diet. How should AJ's feeding begin and what recommendations are appropriate on discharge?

Case Answers

1. **List AJ's possible medical problems demonstrated by his overall clinical picture.**

   - Bowel obstruction (mechanical?) as evidenced by distended loops of small intestine and no air in the rectum on abdominal x-rays and feculent fluid obtained from the nasogastric tube.
   - Mesenteric thrombosis? (Consider his past medical history of stroke.)
   - Severe electrolyte imbalance demonstrated by hyperkalemia, elevated BUN, and creatinine.
   - Bilateral pneumonia?
   - Weight loss and severe undernutrition.

2. **What are the possible etiologies of AJ's bowel obstruction?**

   In a compilation of the overall causes of intestinal obstruction (both small and large bowel), taken from 13 reported series comprising a total of 12,731 adult patients, hernia accounted for 40% of the causes of the obstruction, adhesions 29%, intussusception 12%, and cancer 10%. However, in elderly patients, the main cause of large intestinal obstruction is colon cancer (70% of the cases), followed by diverticulitis (5%) and volvulus (10%). The symptoms are often insidious, although in most cases acute obstruction is the direct reason for calling a surgical consult. Diarrhea with the passage of blood and mucus may result from ulceration of the bowel. The occurrence of diarrhea may lead patients to assert that their bowel function is regular, whereas the looseness is secondary to the irritation caused by the constipated feces as in AJ's case.

3. **What additional evidence from AJ's physical examination could be used to assess his nutritional status before initiating parenteral nutrition?**

   Evidence of undernutrition includes decreased food intake, significant weight loss, decreased albumin level, and thin appearance. Serum albumin is low, which could indicate undernutrition but could also indicate hemo-dilution or the presence of an inflammatory response. Undernutrition plays an important role in the rate of postoperative complications that interfere with surgical activity, impairing immune response mechanism. Synthesis and regeneration processes are affected, and the ability to fight infection is altered. The gastrointestinal tract must be supported during critical illness to support rapid cellular turnover rate and the metabolic and immunologic adaptation to stress. Disruption in the ecologic equilib-rium of the gastrointestinal tract often occurs during critical illness. This damaged equilibrium may cause bacterial translocation, sepsis, and the systemic inflammatory response syndrome (SIRS). Bacterial translocation occurs from the small intestine to the mesenteric lymph nodes, trigger-ing a whole cascade of deleterious events that could lead to multiorganic dysfunction syndrome (MODS).

4. **Why is parenteral nutrition the most appropriate form of nutritional inter-vention at this point in AJ's clinical course?**

   AJ has malnutrition, inflammatory metabolism, abdominal sepsis, cancer, and impaired intestinal function. Therefore, PN should be initiated to prevent further undernutrition and as a method for nutrition support.

5. **Using the Harris-Benedict equation, calculate AJ's resting energy expenditure (REE); also calculate AJ's protein goal and maximum carbohydrate and lipid oxidation rates.**

$$REE = 66 + 13.7 \text{ (weight in kg)} + 5 \text{ (height in cm)} - 6.8 \text{ (age)}$$
$$= 66 + 13.7 \text{ (45)} + 5 \text{ (170 cm)} - 6.8 \text{ (73)} = 1035 \text{ kcal/day}$$

Total daily calorie needs with activity factor for in-bed patient
$$= REE \times 1.45 = 1500 \text{ kcal/day}$$

$$\text{Protein goals} = \text{current weight} \times 1.3 \text{ g/kg}$$
$$= 45 \text{ kg} \times 1.45 \text{ g/kg} = 65 \text{ g/day}$$

(Protein restriction based on patient's initial renal parameters; when renal function normalizes, protein goal can be increased to 1.5 g/kg per day.)

Maximum glucose oxidation rate is 5 to 7 g/kg per day; this is 225 to 315 g per day. At 3.4 kcal/g hydrated dextrose, the maximum dextrose oxidation rate is 765 to 1070 kcal per day. Maximum lipid oxidation rate is 2.5 g/kg per day, and fat has 9 kcal/g. The caloric equivalent of this lipid load is 1000 kcal. Many nutrition support practitioners advocate an upper limit of 1.0 g lipid per kilogram body weight, which for AJ would be 45 g (405 kcal per day). Some consideration could be given to eliminating or severely limiting IV fat for the first week, in an attempt to avoid stimulating eicosanoid pathways that would promote inflammation and downregulate cellular immunity. Dextrose infusion should be started in the PN (aim to keep serum glucose maintained at <200 mg/dL). With a total calorie goal of 1500 kcal per day, a protein calorie contribution of 280 kcal per day (70 g amino acid × 4.0 kcal/g), and a lipid intake of 1.0 g/kg body weight, dextrose calorie infusion will be 660 kcal per day (4.4 g/kg per day). The initial infusion can be lower than goal to assess the metabolic response to the PN. Insulin may be necessary to control the blood glucose. Insulin can be added directly to the PN bag based on initial use of sliding scale if requirements remain stable.

6. **What biochemical laboratory data should be used to monitor AJ while he is on PN?**

   • Sodium, potassium, chloride, CO_2, BUN, creatinine, calcium, magnesium, phosphorus, and glucose should be measured daily. Daily electrolyte replacement in PN solution is designed to replenish any losses noted in the previous day's laboratory data. When laboratory data become stable and normal, frequency of checking may be able to be reduced.

   • Liver function tests, albumin or prealbumin weekly, transferrin, and triglycerides every few weeks.

   • A 24-hour urine collection can be made weekly for measurement of urine urea nitrogen. With this information, nitrogen balance can be calculated (nitrogen balance = nitrogen intake − nitrogen excretion), and the protein content of the PN can be adjusted as required.

7. **After AJ's abdominal sepsis and septic complications resolved and his bowel sounds showed increased activity, he was advanced to an oral diet. How should AJ's feeding begin and what recommendations are appropriate on discharge?**

   Oral feedings should begin with a clear liquid diet and be gradually advanced as tolerated eventually to regular food. PN should not be discontinued until AJ tolerates 75% of his requirements through the oral diet; however, PN should be weaned accordingly as oral intake increases in order to avoid overfeeding. Tube feeding should be considered if the patient cannot consume adequate nutrition by mouth but has a functional GI tract. Evaluation of the patient's nutritional progress should be included in any follow-up visits to his physician.

See Chapter Review Questions, pages A-37 to A-39.

Appendix

Food Sources of Fiber

FOOD	SERVING SIZE	TOTAL FIBER PER SERVING (g)
Almonds	1 ounce	3.0
Apple (with skin)	1 medium	3.0
Banana	1 small	1.8
Barley (cooked)	$1/_2$ cup	15.5
Black beans (cooked)	$1/_2$ cup	3.6
Bran muffin	1 = 2 oz	3.9
Broccoli (cooked)	$1/_2$ cup	2.0
Brown rice	$1/_2$ cup	1.7
Brussel sprouts (cooked)	$1/_2$ cup	3.4
Carrots (cooked)	$1/_2$ cup	1.5
Green peas (frozen, cooked)	$1/_2$ cup	3.0
High Fiber Cereals	$1/_3$ to $1/_2$ cup	4.0–10.0
Kidney beans	$1/_2$ cup	5.0
Lentils (cooked)	$1/_2$ cup	4.0
Lima beans (cooked)	$1/_2$ cup	6.8
Mango (fresh)	1 medium	2.2
Navy beans (cooked)	$1/_2$ cup	3.3
Oat bran bagel	$1/_2$ large bagel	1.5
Oatmeal (cooked)	$1/_2$ cup	2.0
Orange (fresh)	1 medium	3.1
Okra (cooked)	$1/_2$ cup	4.1
Peanuts (dry-roasted)	1 ounce	2.2
Pear (with skin)	1 medium	4.3
Pinto beans	$1/_2$ cup	3.4
Pistachios (dry-roasted)	1 ounce	3.0
Plum (fresh)	2 medium	2.4
Raspberries (raw)	$1/_2$ cup	2.9
Spinach (cooked)	$1/_2$ cup	2.0
Strawberries	$1^1/_4$ cup	2.0
Wheat bran	2 Tbsp.	1.6
Whole wheat bread	1 slice	2.3

SOURCE: Adapted from Shills M. Modern Nutrition in Health and Disease. 9th ed. Baltimore: Williams & Wilkins, 1999.

Food Sources of Folate

FOOD	SERVING SIZE	FOLATE (μg)
Asparagus (cooked)	0.5 cup	121.2
Banana (raw)	1 medium	22.5
Bran flakes, Kellogg's	0.75 cup	102.3
Bread, white	1 slice	8.5
Cauliflower	0.5 cup	27.2
Corn flakes, Kellogg's	1 cup	98.8
Corn, sweet (boiled)	0.5 cup	25.4
Egg (boiled)	1 large	22.0
Milk, nonfat/skim	1 cup	12.7
Milk, whole (3.3% fat)	1 cup	12.2
Muffin, English	$^1/_2$ unit	10.5
Orange juice prepared from concentrate	1.0 fl oz	13.9
Peas, green (boiled)	0.5 cup	50.6
Potato (baked with skin)	1 medium	22.2
Rice Krispies, Kellogg's	1.25 cup	116.4
Roll, hamburger/hot dog	1 medium	11.6
Tomato, red (raw)	1 medium	18.4

SOURCE: Adapted from Shills M. Modern Nutrition in Health and Disease. 9th ed. Baltimore: Williams & Wilkins, 1999.

Food Sources of Omega-3 Fatty Acid

FOOD	SERVING SIZE	OMEGA-3 (g)
Canola oil	1 Tbsp.	1.4
Flaxseed oil	1 Tbsp.	6.7
Flaxseeds	1 Tbsp.	2.63
Walnut oil	1 Tbsp.	1.3
Walnuts	$^1/_4$ cup	3.4
Wheat germ oil	1 Tbsp.	0.86
Soybeans (cooked)	$^1/_4$ cup	1.05
Sardines	3.5 oz	1.5
Salmon	3.5 oz	1.9
Tuna, albacore	3.5 oz, raw	2.1

SOURCE: Adapted from Pennington JAT. Food Values of Portions Commonly Used. 17th ed. Philadelphia: Lippincott, 1998.

Food Sources of Vitamin E

FOOD	SERVING SIZE	IU
Almonds, dry roasted	1 oz	7.5
Peanuts, dry roasted	1 oz	2.1
Pistachio nuts, dry roasted	1 oz	1.2
Corn oil	1 Tbsp.	2.9
Safflower oil	1 Tbsp.	4.7
Soybean oil	1 Tbsp.	2.5
Wheat germ oil	1 Tbsp.	26.2
Wheat germ, toasted, Kretschmer	$1/4$ cup	9.8
Broccoli, frozen, boiled	$1/2$ cup	1.5
Spinach, frozen, boiled	$1/2$ cup	0.85
Turnip greens, frozen, boiled	$1/2$ cup	2.4
Mayonnaise, made with soybean oil	1 Tbsp.	1.6
Mango	1 medium	2.3
Kiwi	1 medium	0.85
Oatmeal, instant	1 oz packet	0.21
Sunflower seeds, dried	1 oz	21.3

SOURCE: NIH Clinical Center National Institutes of Health Web site *http://www.cc.nih.gov/ccc/ supplements/vitd.html* accessed February 20, 2003, and Jean A.T. Pennington Food Values of Portions Commonly Used. 17th ed. 1998.

Food Sources of Vitamin E as Alpha-Tocopherol (mg)

FOOD	SERVING SIZE	mg
Almonds (dried)	1 oz (24 nuts; 28 g)	6.72
Avocado	1 medium (173 g)	2.32
Corn oil	1 Tbsp. (14 g)	1.90
Fish sandwich with tartar sauce	183 g	1.83
Mango	1 medium (207 g)	2.32
Margarine, Mazola	1 Tbsp. (14 g)	8.00
Olive oil	1 Tbsp. (14 g)	1.67
Pancakes with butter and syrup	232 g	1.39
Peanuts (dried)	1 oz (28 g)	2.56
Pistachios (dried)	1 oz (47 nuts; 28 g)	0.87
Sunflower seeds (dried)	1 oz (28 g)	14.18
Sweet potato	1 medium	5.93
Wheat germ oil	1 Tbsp. (14 g)	20.30

SOURCE: Adapted from Pennington JAT. Food Values of Portions Commonly Used. 17th ed. Philadelphia: Lippincott, 1998.

Food Sources of Vitamin K

FOOD NAME	SERVING SIZE	PHYLOQUINONE PER SERVING (μg)
Blueberry muffin	1	14
Asparagus	$1/2$ cup	72.0
Broccoli	$1/2$ cup	88.0
Brussels sprouts	$1/2$ cup	225.0
Cabbage	$1/2$ cup	73.0
Carrot	1 medium	12.0
Cauliflower	$1/2$ cup	12.0
Celery (raw)	1 medium stalk	17.0
Coleslaw	1 cup	119.0
Collards	$1/2$ cup	374.0
Green peas	$1/2$ cup	19.0
Mixed vegetables	$1/2$ cup	15.0
Okra	$1/2$ cup	32.0
Spinach	$1/2$ cup	324.0
Summer squash	$1/2$ cup, sliced	4.0
Tomato juice, bottled	8 fl oz (237 mL)	5.6
Tomato, red (raw)	1 medium	4.4
Apple, red	1 medium	2.8
Apricots (raw)	4	4.7
Avocado (raw)	$1/5$ medium	4.3
Grapes, red/green, seedless (raw)	$1\,1/2$ cups	12.0
Pear (raw)	1 medium	8.1
Plums (raw)	2 medium	11.0
Strawberries (raw)	8 medium	2.2
Peach (raw)	1 medium	2.4
Beef liver	100 g	3.0
Ground beef	100 g	2.4
Lamb chop	100 g	4.6
Orange (raw)	1 medium	2.4

SOURCE: Adapted from Pennington JAT. Food Values of Portions Commonly Used. 17th ed. Philadelphia: Lippincott, 1998.

Foods Sources of Purine

FOOD	mg/100 g
Anchovies	363
Liver	233
Sardines	295
Asparagus	50–150
Bread and cereals, whole grain	50–150
Cauliflower	50–150
Fish, fresh and saltwater	50–150
Legumes, beans/lentils/peas	50–150
Meat—beef/lamb/pork/veal	50–150
Mushrooms	50–150
Oatmeal	50–150
Peas, green	50–150
Poultry-chicken/duck/turkey	50–150
Shellfish—crabs/lobster/oysters	50–150
Spinach	50–150
Wheat germ and bran	50–150

SOURCE: Adapted from Pennington JAT. Food Values of Portions Commonly Used. 17th ed. Philadelphia: Lippincott, 1998.

Food Sources of Vitamin D

FOOD	SERVING SIZE	IU
Cod liver oil	1 Tbsp	1360
Salmon, cooked	$3\frac{1}{2}$ oz	360
Mackerel, cooked	$3\frac{1}{2}$ oz	345
Sardines, canned in oil	$3\frac{1}{2}$ oz	270
Milk, fortified	8 fl oz	98
Margarine, fortified	1 Tbsp.	60
Liver, beef, cooked	$3\frac{1}{2}$ oz	30
Dry cereal, fortified	$3/4$ cup	40–50
Egg yolk	1 whole	25

SOURCE: NIH Clinical Center National Institutes of Health Web site *http://www.cc.nih.gov/ccc/supplements/vitd.html* accessed February 6, 2003.

Food Sources of Iron

FOOD	AMOUNT	IRON (mg)
Apple juice	1 cup	1.9
Beef (cooked regular hamburger)	4 oz	2.1
Black beans (dry, cooked)	$\frac{1}{2}$ cup	2.5
Chick peas (dry, cooked)	$\frac{1}{2}$ cup	2.45
Chicken breast (cooked)	3 oz	0.9
Chili with meat and beans	1 cup	4.3
Egg	2 medium	1.4
Instant oatmeal	1 packet	6.7
Pork and beans (dry, cooked)	$\frac{1}{2}$ cup	2.5
Prune juice	1 cup	3.0
Raisin bran	$\frac{3}{4}$ cup or 1 oz	3.5
Scallops	6 units	2.0
Shrimp (fried)	3 oz	1.4
Spinach (cooked)	1 cup	6.4
Spinach (raw, chopped)	1 cup	1.5
Steak	3 oz	2.6
Tomato juice	1 cup	3.0
Tortilla	1 unit	2.2
Tuna (in oil)	3 oz	1.6
Turkey (no skin, light and dark)	3 oz	1.4

SOURCE: Adapted from Pennington JAT. Food Values of Portions Commonly Used. 17th ed. Philadelphia: Lippincott, 1998.

Review Questions

Chapter 1: Overview of Nutrition in Clinical Care

1. Which of the following medical conditions are associated with obesity?
   a) Diabetes
   b) Cardiovascular disease
   c) Osteoarthritis
   d) All of the above

2. When assessing a patient's nutritional status, use of a blood test along with the medical history and physical examination is extremely beneficial. Which of the following serum proteins would be most useful in assessing a patient's nutritional status over the previous 3 months?
   a) Serum transferrin
   b) Serum albumin
   c) Serum prealbumin
   d) Retinol-binding protein

3. What is the major reason why an individual will lose weight on Dr. Atkins New Diet Revolution Program?
   a) Carbohydrates stimulate appetite
   b) Ketosis allows for the breakdown of fatty tissue
   c) Protein and fat increase basal metabolic rate
   d) Caloric deficit (fewer total calories are eaten)

4. The following blood tests and vital signs can be used to diagnose a patient with metabolic syndrome. Indicate whether these values would be high (a) or low (b):

   Glucose

   High-density lipoprotein (HDL) cholesterol

   Triglycerides

   Blood pressure

5. TR is an 80-year-old nursing home patient who is being treated for a pressure ulcer on his back. He was recently diagnosed with marasmus. Which of the following clinical signs is associated with marasmus?

a) Excessive loss of fat and muscle stores
b) Weight gain
c) Increased metabolic rate
d) Edema

6. AB and her husband have a 3-year-old child. Due to the fact that they are both obese with a body mass index (BMI) greater than 30 kg/m^2, what is the likelihood or percent chance that their child will become overweight?

a) 20%
b) 50%
c) 80%
d) 100%

7. Which of the following conditions will increase a patient's nutrient requirements?

a) Asthma
b) Infection/fever
c) Heart disease
d) Multiple sclerosis

8. Mr. D comes to see the pediatrician with his 6-month-old daughter, Jennifer. Jennifer weighs 6.8 kg (twenty-fifth percentile), and her length is 67.5 cm (seventy-fifth percentile). Mr. D expresses concern because he thinks Jennifer is small for her age. Are her weight and length measurements appropriate for her age?

a) Yes
b) No
c) Cannot be determined without Jennifer's dietary intake
d) Cannot be determined without Jennifer's head circumference

9. JR is a 33-year-old man who was diagnosed as being human immunodeficiency virus (HIV) positive 1 year ago. JR's weight history is as follows:

Height = 5′11″ (180 cm)
Current weight = 155 lb (70 kg)
Usual weight (1 year ago) = 170 lb (77 kg)

Using the above data, what is JR's percent weight change from his usual weight?

(*Usual weight – current weight*)/Usual wt

a) 10.5%
b) 5.3%
c) 8.8%
d) 12%

10. Nutritional information may be integrated into the medical history, review of systems, and physical examination. Column A lists topics that should be addressed when evaluating a patient. Match each issue with the appropriate part of the medical workup in Column B.

Column A	Column B
Bleeding gums _____	(a) Family history
Blood pressure _____	(b) Past medical history
Clothes tighter or looser _____	(c) Review of systems

Constipation _____
Grandfather died of heart disease _____
Mother has osteoporosis _____
Sedentary woman _____
Smoker _____
Vegetarian woman _____
Vitamin and herbal supplements intake _____
Weakness and fatigue _____
Well nourished _____

(d) Social history
(e) Physical examination

11. Over the past several decades, overweight and obesity in adults and children have increased dramatically in the United States. Which of the following hypotheses could explain why overweight and obesity have increased?
    a)   Changes in the gene pool
    b)   Increase in calorie intake
    c)   Decrease in sedentary behavior
    d)   All of the above

12. Metabolism of 150 g carbohydrate, 20 g fat, and 10 g protein yields approximately how many kilocalories?
    a)   300 kcal
    b)   550 kcal
    c)   820 kcal
    d)   1100 kcal

13. AM is a 54-year-old postmenopausal woman who wants to lose weight. She is 5′6″ (168 cm) and weighs 190 lb (86.4 kg). What is her BMI? (see Figure 1-2)
    a)   BMI = 19 kg/m^2
    b)   BMI = 24 kg/m^2
    c)   BMI = 31 kg/m^2
    d)   BMI = 36 kg/m^2

14. A 7-month-old baby boy is brought in to his pediatrician by his mother because he is suffering from diarrhea and a loss of appetite. He has a history of multiple respiratory infections. His physical examination reveals an undernourished child with follicular hyperkeratosis on his legs and arms and keratomalacia. Based on these physical examination findings, this infant is most likely deficient in which of the following vitamins or minerals?
    a)   Vitamin A
    b)   Iron
    c)   Vitamin D
    d)   Calcium

15. An obese individual's energy requirement is overestimated by the Harris-Benedict equation because a percentage of adipose tissue is metabolically inactive. What percent of adipose tissue is metabolically inactive in obese individuals?
    a)   5%
    b)   10%
    c)   25%
    d)   50%

Chapter 2: Vitamins, Minerals, and Pytochemicals

1. Match the vitamin/mineral in Column A with the correct food source in Column B. Answers in Column B can only be used once.

    Column A   **Column B**
    Vitamin C _____   (a) Carrots
    Iron _____   (b) Cheese
    Vitamin E _____   (c) Grapefruit
    Potassium _____   (d) Red meat
    Beta-carotene _____   (e) Nuts
    Calcium _____   (f) Bananas

2. Match the vitamin deficiency in Column A with the appropriate clinical presentation in Column B. Answers in Column B can only be used once.

    Column A   **Column B**
    Vitamin K _____   (a) Rickets
    Vitamin A _____   (b) Keratomalacia
    Vitamin D _____   (c) Ecchymosis
    Vitamin C _____   (d) Scurvy
    Thiamine _____   (e) Beriberi

3. Match the mineral deficiency in Column A with the appropriate clinical presentation in Column B. Answers in Column B can only be used once.

    Column A   **Column B**
    Calcium _____   (a) Growth retardation
    Iodine _____   (b) Microcytic anemia, pallor
    Zinc _____   (c) Osteoporosis
    Iron _____   (d) Endemic goiter
    Vitamin B_{12} _____   (e) Pernicious anemia

4. WS is a 55-year-old woman who is complaining of intermittent flushing, itching, and heartburn for several months. Megadosing of which of the following vitamins may result in these symptoms?

    a) Niacin
    b) Riboflavin
    c) Vitamin B_{12}
    d) Vitamin E

5. Vitamin C intake enhances the absorption of which of the following minerals?

    a) Fluoride
    b) Iron
    c) Sodium
    d) Calcium

6. CK is a 45-year-old woman who has received long-term oral antibiotic therapy for a severe infection. As a result, she presents with an elevated prothrombin time (PT). Based on this history, what vitamin deficiency is the most likely cause of the elevated PT?

    a) Vitamin B_{12}
    b) Vitamin C
    c) Vitamin K
    d) Vitamin A

7. Free radicals and antioxidants have received attention because of their high reactivity and ability to denature proteins, lipids, and nucleic acids. Which of the following vitamins exhibit antioxidant properties?

    a) Vitamin B_{12}
    b) Vitamin E
    c) Vitamin B_6
    d) Thiamine

8. Malaborption of fat-soluble vitamins may result from which of the following diseases?

    a) Multiple sclerosis
    b) Cardiovascular disease
    c) Marasmus
    d) Cystic fibrosis

9. MT is a 31-year-old woman who was diagnosed with inflammatory bowel disease and reports occasional blood in her stools. She complains of fatigue and feeling cold, and she chews on ice. Which of the following vitamin or mineral deficiencies should be suspected in this patient?

    a) Thiamine
    b) Phosphorus
    c) Iron
    d) Vitamin E

10. Vitamin and mineral toxicities may result from misuse of supplements or dosage errors. Match the following vitamins and minerals in Column A with the symptoms or clinical presentations that are indicative of the nutrient toxicity in Column B. Answers in Column B can only be used once.

Column A	Column B
Fluoride _____	(a) Tooth mottling
Vitamin B_6 _____	(b) Cracked lips, dry rough skin, alopecia of eyebrows
Vitamin D _____	(c) Oxalate urinary calculi
Vitamin C _____	(d) Anorexia and vomiting
Vitamin A _____	(e) Sensory ataxia, impairment of the lower-limb position

11. Dietary reference intakes (DRIs) were established to help individuals prevent chronic disease through good nutrition habits. Recently, the DRIs have been updated for various vitamins and minerals. What is the new DRI level for folate in nonpregnant women?

    a) 200 μg per day
    b) 300 μg per day
    c) 400 μg per day
    d) 500 μg per day

12. Phytochemicals are naturally occurring compounds found primarily in foods of which origin?

    a) Animal
    b) Plant
    c) Seafood
    d) None of the above

13. Recent evidence has shown that individuals who eat diets rich in phytochemicals may have a lower incidence of which of the following conditions:
    a) Cancer
    b) Bone disease
    c) Ear infections
    d) Alopecia

14. Older adults may have difficulty absorbing calcium and iron because of achlorhydria, which normally occurs with aging. Achlorhydria can be defined as
    a) Absence or reduction of hydrochloric acid production in the stomach
    b) Absence or reduction of lactase enzyme in the small intestine
    c) Absence or reduction of lipase enzyme in the small intestine
    d) Absence or reduction of pepsin production in the stomach

15. Which of the following dietary recommendations would be most helpful for patients with iron-deficiency anemia?
    a) Limit the amount of dairy foods to 1 serving per day
    b) Eat yellow and orange fruits every day
    c) Drink at least one glass of tea every day
    d) Eat lean red meat at least once a week

Chapter 3: Herbal Medicine

1. Many popular herbal remedies have been shown to cause toxicity when used in large doses. Which of the following body organs are most likely to be affected by excessive intakes of herbal remedies?
    a) Heart
    b) Kidney
    c) Liver
    d) All of the above

2. CT is a 25-year-old woman who has had a weight problem since childhood. She is presently taking an herbal supplement that her family physician suggests she discontinue because of the reported adverse effects, which include insomnia, hypertension, tachycardia, tremors, and possibly death. Based on this information, which of the following herbal remedies is CT currently taking?
    a) Ginkgo biloba
    b) Ephedra
    c) Ginger
    d) Milk thistle

3. ST is a 53-year-old woman with hypercholesterolemia. She has currently added soy protein to her diet since her last nutrition consult. Soy protein has been shown to reduce hot flashes and to lower both total and low-density lipoprotein (LDL) cholesterol levels. However, there is current debate over the safety of using soy protein. Which of the following adverse effects has been documented with excessive intakes of soy protein in some experiments?
    a) Increased risk of breast cancer
    b) Increased risk of heart disease
    c) Increased risk of gallbladder disease
    d) Increased risk of pancreatitis

4. JH is a 79-year-old man who is diagnosed with Alzheimer's disease and extreme dementia. The herbal remedy he was prescribed caused him cramps, constipation, and skin rashes. Despite the side effects, an improvement in cognitive function was seen as well as a slight improvement in short-term memory. Which of the following herbal remedies was most likely prescribed?

   a) Ginger
   b) Ginkgo biloba
   c) Ginseng
   d) Phytoestrogens

5. Significant drug-herb interactions have been identified in some clinical settings. Match the following drug/herb in Column A with the potential interaction or side effects in Column B. Answers in Column B can only be used once.

Column A	Column B
St. John's wort (SJW)/serotonin reuptake inhibitor _____	(a) Spontaneous bleeding
Ginseng/warfarin _____	(b) Decreased International Normalized Ratio (INR)
Ginkgo biloba/acetylsalicylic acid (ASA) _____	(c) Hypertension
Garlic/warfarin _____	(d) Decreased serum drug levels
Yohimbine/tricyclic antidepressants _____	(e) Increased INR

6. SJW is one of the most commonly used over-the-counter herbal remedies today. Although it has been widely accepted to treat mood disorders such as depression, several side effects and drug complications are still reported. Which of the following problems are commonly seen in patients taking SJW?

   a) Anorgasmia and frequent urination
   b) Reduced effectiveness of warfarin
   c) Reduced levels of digoxin
   d) All of the above

7. RS is a 28-year-old woman who has recently been diagnosed with depression. The only medication she is currently taking is birth control pills (oral contraceptive). She was also prescribed 400 mg SJW and has been taking this for 6 months. Which of the following potential drug-herb interactions might you expect to see in this patient?

   a) Enhanced drug activity
   b) Intermenstrual bleeding
   c) Decreased drug activity
   d) Hypertension

8. JT is a 27-year-old woman who is planning to get pregnant. Which of the following herbs should be avoided to prevent harm to her future fetus?

   a) SJW
   b) Saw palmetto
   c) Black cohosh
   d) All of the above

9. Herbal therapies have been clinically proven to improve the medical health of some patients. Match the herbal therapy in Column A to the indication for use in Column B. Answers in Column B can only be used once.

Column A	Column B
SJW _____	a) Upper respiratory infection
Ginkgo _____	b) Colic and anxiety
Echinacea _____	c) Mild depression
Black cohosh _____	d) Mild dementia
Chamomile _____	e) Menopausal treatment

10. When deciding whether to recommend herbal therapies to patients, safety issues from the Guidelines for the Use of Herbal Remedies in Clinical Practice must be referenced. Which of the following is not in agreement with these guidelines?

    a) "Natural" does not necessarily mean it is safe.
    b) Herbal remedies should not be used if pregnancy is desired or if currently pregnant.
    c) Infants and children can use herbal treatments.
    d) Elderly patients should be closely monitored if using herbal treatments.

11. Elderly individuals should be supervised by a physician while taking herbal remedies because of the physiologic changes that occur with the aging process. Which of the following physiologic changes normally occur with aging?

    a) Decreased total body water
    b) Decreased renal clearance
    c) Decreased hepatic clearance
    d) All of the above

12. MM is a 52-year-old woman diagnosed with uncomplicated essential hypertension. Her blood pressure has been moderately well treated. In a recent visit to your office, she complains of flatulence and lack of appetite. You noted a significant weight loss and a persistent smell of garlic on her breath and body. Which of the following statements is true regarding the use of garlic as a therapeutic agent (or herbal remedy)?

    a) Garlic does not affect blood pressure or blood coagulation.
    b) The beneficial effects of garlic on blood pressure and cholesterol levels are inconsistent.
    c) Garlic is unsafe in large doses.
    d) Garlic can lead to an increase in lipid levels.

13. Which of the following herbs should be avoided by patients on anticoagulant medication?

    a) Milk thistle
    b) Valerian root
    c) Ginkgo
    d) Chamomile

14. Patients who decide to use an herbal remedy in place of conventional pharmacologic agents should be advised about the use of herbal remedies because

    a) Premarket testing and studies on safety and efficacy are not required with herbal remedies.
    b) Herbal remedies have the potential to interact with standard pharmacologic agents.
    c) The therapeutically active constituent may not be available in sufficient quantity to achieve the desired result.
    d) All of the above.

15. Which of the following dietary recommendations should be provided to all patients receiving warfarin therapy for anticoagulation?
    a) Maintain daily consistency in vitamin K intake
    b) Maintain daily consistency in vitamin C intake
    c) Eat a diet low in vitamin A
    d) Eat a diet low in vitamin D

Chapter 4: Nutrition in Pregnancy and Lactation

1. Megavitamin therapy is a common practice for many people; however, many do not recognize the potential for toxicity. Of the following vitamins, which is most likely to cause teratogenic effects (birth defects in the developing embryo) if taken during pregnancy in doses exceeding the recommended dietary allowances (RDA)?
    a) Vitamin C
    b) Vitamin A
    c) Vitamin B_{12}
    d) Folate

2. According to the RDA, how many additional calories from the diet are required on a daily basis during the second and third trimester of pregnancy?
    a) An additional 100 kcal per day and 300 kcal per day are required from the diet during the second and third trimester, respectively.
    b) An additional 300 kcal per day are required during the remainder of the pregnancy.
    c) An additional 500 kcal per day and 700 kcal per day are required from the diet during the second and third trimester, respectively.
    d) No additional calories are required from the diet in either trimester.

3. HL is a 30-year-old woman who is planning her second pregnancy. She has already delivered an infant with a neural tube defect (spina bifida) and inquires about any measures that can be taken to prevent a neural tube defect from reoccurring in this pregnancy. What vitamin supplement has been shown to decrease the likelihood of neural tube defects in pregnant women?
    a) Folic acid
    b) Thiamine
    c) Vitamin B_{12}
    d) All of the above

4. Abnormalities often occur in the eating habits of women during their pregnancy. Pica is an eating practice that is seen occasionally. Which of the following best describes this eating habit?
    a) Laxative or diuretic use
    b) Following the newest food fad
    c) Binge eating and purging
    d) Eating nonfood items, such as chalk, ice, or detergent

5. Iron controls the production of red blood cells in both the mother and her developing fetus. During which trimester of pregnancy is the requirement for iron the highest?
    a) 1st trimester
    b) 2nd trimester

    c)   3rd trimester
    d)   Iron requirements do not change during pregnancy

6. Weight gain is expected during pregnancy but must be controlled for the health of the mother and the fetus. Approximately how much total weight gain is recommended for a woman with a prepregnancy body mass index (BMI) = 28 kg/m^2 (normal 19.8–26) who is having twins?

    a)   <15 lb (<6.8 kg)
    b)   15–25 lb (6.8–10.0 kg)
    c)   28–40 lb (12.7–18.2 kg)
    d)   35–45 lb (15.9–20.4 kg)

7. RS is a 26-year-old woman who comes into the obstetrics/gynecology (OB/GYN) clinic because she missed her period for 2 months. After a pregnancy test you inform her that she is 7 weeks pregnant. If RS's BMI was 17 kg/m^2 (normal 19.8–26), what is the appropriate amount of weight she should gain during the remainder of this pregnancy?

    a)   <15 lb (<6.8 kg)
    b)   15–25 lb (6.8–10.0 kg)
    c)   28–40 lb (12.7–18.2 kg)
    d)   40–50 lb (18.2–22.7 kg)

8. Gestational diabetes mellitus is commonly seen in approximately 4% of pregnant women. In reviewing a patient's history, which of the following is considered a risk factor for gestational diabetes?

    a)   Individual of African-American descent
    b)   Undernutrition
    c)   Maternal age
    d)   First-degree relative with cardiovascular disease

9. Folate supplementation is important for all women during their childbearing years. Folate is required for cell growth and division and is therefore necessary for fetal and placental development. Which of the following statements most accurately defines why folate is prescribed to women before they become pregnant?

    a)   Folate needs to be consumed for several weeks to build up adequate body stores.
    b)   Folate is not contained in prenatal vitamins.
    c)   The neural tube forms in the first 18 days of conception before the prenatal visit.
    d)   Folate has been shown to help women become pregnant.

10. Breast milk production is primarily influenced by which of the following conditions?

    a)   Breast milk production is influenced by breast size.
    b)   Breast milk production is influenced by maternal age.
    c)   Breast milk production is influenced by infant demand for the breast.
    d)   Breast milk production is influenced by the weight of the infant.

11. Which of the following vitamins may be deficient in a infant's diet who is exclusively breastfed?

    a)   Vitamin A
    b)   Vitamin B$_{12}$

c) Vitamin C
d) Vitamin D

12. CD takes her 3-month-old infant to the pediatrician for his monthly visit, and his weight has remained stable over the last month. He has been exclusively breastfed since birth, and the pediatrician asks to see CD's technique and feeding frequency. CD reports that she feeds him at least 12 to 15 times each day, 5 minutes on each breast. Which of the following statements best explains why the infant is not gaining weight?

a) Transitional breast milk is low in protein and minerals
b) Duration of feeding on each breast is inadequate
c) Frequency of feeding inhibits breast milk production
d) None of the above

13. Which of the following are potential causes of mastitis during breast feeding?

a) Feeding on only one breast
b) Infrequent changing of wet breast pads
c) Tight-fitting bra
d) All of the above

14. Breast milk changes in composition and volume during each infant feeding. Which of the following statements regarding breast milk composition is correct?

a) Breast milk provided when the breast is nearly empty is richest in fat content.
b) The fat content of breast milk provides only 10% of the infant's total energy requirements.
c) Breast milk contains large amounts of iron.
d) The primary carbohydrate source in breast milk is sucrose.

15. According to the RDA, how many additional calories from the diet are required on a daily basis during lactation?

a) An additional 100 kcal per day is required from the diet during lactation.
b) An additional 300 kcal per day is required from the diet during lactation.
c) An additional 500 kcal per day is required from the diet during lactation.
d) No additional calories are required from the diet during lactation.

Chapter 5: Infants, Children, and Adolescents

1. If a child is chronically malnourished, in what order would the following growth parameters be affected?

a) Length first, weight, and head circumference last
b) Weight first, length, and head circumference last
c) Head circumference first, weight, and length last
d) All the growth parameters would be affected equally

2. Which of the following statements represent the benefits of breastfeeding for the infant?

a) Breastfeeding reduces the incidence of overfeeding for infants
b) Breastfeeding reduces the incidence of ear infections for infants
c) Breastfeeding reduces the possibility of intolerance to cow's milk in infants
d) All of the above

3. DB brings her 5-year-old daughter to the pediatrician for evaluation of hyper-cholesterolemia (elevated blood cholesterol levels). She asks if all children with high cholesterol levels will grow up to be adults with high cholesterol. What is your response?

   a) Not all hypercholesterolemic children will grow up to be hypercholesterolemic adults.
   b) All hypercholesterolemic children will grow up to be hypercholesterolemic adults.
   c) Only children who have an immediate family member with heart disease will grow up to be hypercholesterolemic adults.
   d) Only those children who do not strictly adhere to a low-fat diet will grow up to be hypercholesterolemic adults.

4. MT is a 15-year-old girl who has been diagnosed with an eating disorder. Which of the following statements are correct regarding the characteristics of anorexia nervosa or bulimia, or both?

   a) Adolescents who binge and purge food demonstrate weight fluctuations.
   b) Adolescents with anorexia nervosa maintain their body weight significantly below one's normal weight for age.
   c) Bulimia is characterized by a feeling that one cannot control what or how much one is eating.
   d) All of the above.

5. Due to financial problems, Mr. D asks about changing Jennifer's formula to regular cow's milk (whole milk) now that she is 6 months old. Which of the following statements would be an appropriate response?

   a) The early introduction of cow's milk before 1 year of age may induce a low-grade loss of blood from the gastrointestinal (GI) tract.
   b) Although cow's milk is relatively low in iron, it can be introduced before 1 year of age because the iron in cow's milk is very bioavailable.
   c) The high renal solute load of cow's milk helps stimulate the development of an infant's kidneys.
   d) Cow's milk is high in vitamins and minerals, which are needed by infants at 6 months of age.

6. KS is a 14-year-old adolescent who runs cross-country and plays basketball. Al-though most of her friends have begun to menstruate, KS still has not had her first period. KS weighs 44.5 kg (twenty-fifth percentile) and is 171 cm tall (ninety-fifth percentile). Two years previously, KS had been at the fiftieth percentile for weight and ninetieth percentile for height. What is the most likely cause of the lack of menstruation in this adolescent?

   a) KS was born prematurely
   b) KS has a low body fat composition secondary to her running schedule
   c) KS's mother did not gain enough weight during pregnancy
   d) Unknown cause of delayed menstruation

7. Sam was born in Bosnia during the war. He is a full-term baby, weighs 2.8 kg, and is 48 cm long (tenth percentile). His parents were killed, and he is transferred to a local orphanage in the area of the fighting and fed a low-calorie diet. When he is 1 year old, a truce is reached and food shipments are delivered to the area (height and weight are fifth percentile, and he is hypotensive and bradycardic). At this time

Sam has a large appetite and is fed all he will eat. Within a few days heart failure develops. What is the most likely cause of the heart failure?

    a) Sam did not drink enough fluid with his food
    b) Sam is severely malnourished and was not refed slowly
    c) Sam ate too much protein
    d) All of the above

8. Mrs. S brings her 15-year-old daughter, Jane, to see the pediatrician. Jane's grandmother has severe osteoporosis and fell and broke her hip last week. Mrs. S wants Jane to drink milk to prevent her from also developing osteoporosis. Is her request warranted? Which of the following statements is correct?

    a) A large intake of dairy products is not recommended for adolescents, as so many adolescents are lactose intolerant.
    b) Dairy products are not recommended, as they are a significant source of saturated fat, which promotes atherosclerosis and diabetes.
    c) Dairy products are not important for adolescents, as bone mineralization ends before puberty begins.
    d) Dairy products are an efficient source of calcium needed for proper bone mineralization in children and adolescents.

9. "At risk of overweight" in children and adolescents is defined as a body mass index (BMI) at what percentile?

    a) BMI greater than the seventy-fifth percentile
    b) BMI between the eighty-fifth and ninety-fifth percentile
    c) BMI greater than the ninety-fifth percentile
    d) BMI is not used in pediatrics to assess obesity

10. Why does the American Academy of Pediatrics recommend delaying the introduction of solid foods until infants are at least 6 months of age?

    a) Solid foods before 6 months of age may stimulate the development of food allergies.
    b) Solid foods before 6 months of age may increase the amount of iron in the infant's diet.
    c) Solid foods before 6 months of age may lead to overeating in childhood.
    d) Solid foods before 6 months of age may interfere with the quantity of breast milk consumed.

11. DF is a 4-month-old baby who presents with allergic rhinitis and dermatitis. According to her mom she started eating solid foods 2 weeks ago, which included rice cereal mixed with formula, eggs, and pureed fruits. DF was diagnosed with an allergic reaction. Which of the foods below would be the likely cause of these symptoms?

    a) Eggs
    b) Cereal
    c) Formula
    d) Pureed fruits

12. Which of the following recommendations should be given to parents in order to avoid the development of dental caries in children?

    a) Fluoride supplementation if the water does not contain fluoride
    b) Begin brushing teeth when they erupt
    c) Limit concentrated sweets and foods that adhere to the teeth
    d) All of the above

13. During a chronic nutritional deprivation, the body compensates by decreasing the basal metabolic rate (BMR) in order to conserve protein and organ function. Which of the following two physical examination findings are indicative of a decreased basal metabolic rate?

   a) Hypotension
   b) Bradycardia
   c) Hypertension
   d) Tachycardia

14. JP is an 11-year-old significantly overweight boy who comes to see his physician for a routine evaluation. Laboratory tests reveal elevated alanine aminotransferase (ALT) and aspartate aminotransferase (AST) levels. According to these results, which of the following diseases would be an appropriate diagnosis for JP?

   a) Jaundice
   b) Malabsorption
   c) Nonalcoholic steatohepatitis (fatty liver)
   d) Encephalopathy

15. JP's physician believes that dietary and exercise changes are needed in order for him to lose weight and improve his condition. Which of the following is most important to assess before suggesting any dietary and lifestyle changes?

   a) The family's willingness to make changes
   b) The homework schedule of the child
   c) The child's sleep schedule
   d) The teacher's interest in the child

Chapter 6: Older Adults

1. Metabolic changes that are associated with aging include which of the following descriptions?

   a) Lean body mass increases, body fat decreases
   b) Lean body mass decreases, body fat increases
   c) Lean body mass increases, body fat increases
   d) Lean body mass decreases, body fat decreases

2. RH is a 75-year-old man who consumes 2 Tbsp. mineral oil daily to relieve his constipation. Excessive use of laxatives, in particular mineral oil, can lead to which of the following?

   a) Hyperkalemia
   b) Increased appetite
   c) Interference with fat-soluble vitamin absorption
   d) Fatigue

3. Calcium requirements increase as people grow older in order to compensate for the decreased production of $1,25(OH)_2D$ by the kidney and for the accelerated bone mineral losses. The recent dietary reference intake (DRI) recommendation for men and women aged 51 years and older for calcium is

   a) 800 mg per day
   b) 1000 mg per day
   c) 1200 mg per day
   d) 2000 mg per day

4. Potential nutrition-related consequences due to aging are reduction of the absorption and bioavailability of vitamins and minerals. Which of the following age-related physiologic changes can cause these nutritional problems?
   a) Reduced gastric acid secretion
   b) Reduced T-cell function
   c) Reduced glomerular filtration rate
   d) Reduced bone density

5. Activities of daily living (ADLs) reflect an individual's most basic capacity for self-care and may be limited in approximately 10% of older adults. Which of the following are considered ADLs?
   a) Preparing meals
   b) Housework
   c) Feeding
   d) Managing money

6. Constipation is very common in older adults due to decreased gastrointestinal (GI) motility, inadequate fiber and fluid intake, and certain medications. Examples of high-fiber foods that can be recommended to treat constipation include which of the following?
   a) White rice
   b) Pasta
   c) Wheat bran cereals
   d) White bread and rolls

7. The *Determine Your Nutritional Health Checklist* is an important screening tool to identify individuals at risk for which of the following conditions?
   a) Macular degeneration
   b) Incontinence
   c) Poor nutritional status
   d) Arthritis

8. Older adults are frequently prescribed multiple medications to be taken on a daily basis. How can medications affect the nutritional status of older adults?
   a) Alter food intake by decreasing appetite, taste, and smell
   b) Decrease absorption and function of nutrients
   c) Cause GI disturbances such as constipation
   d) All of the above

9. Which of the following is a potential benefit of moderate alcohol intake in older adults?
   a) Increased stress
   b) Reduced bone mineral density
   c) Reduced cardiovascular function
   d) Mood enhancement

10. Older adults experience age-related changes in their GI tract such as decreased gastric acid secretion and motility. The absorption of the protein-bound form of which of the following vitamins is most likely to decline in older adults due to these changes?
    a) Vitamin A
    b) Vitamin C

      c)   Vitamin B_{12}
      d)   Vitamin D

11. Below which of the following body mass index (BMI) values is a patient classified as underweight and may be at risk of undernutrition and infection?

      a)   BMI less than 16 kg/m^2
      b)   BMI less than 18.5 kg/m^2
      c)   BMI less than 22 kg/m^2
      d)   BMI less than 25 kg/m^2

12. Which of the following is the most common chronic disease seen in older adults?

      a)   Cardiovascular disease
      b)   Hearing impairment
      c)   Diabetes
      d)   Cataracts

13. Older adults who smoke are at increased risk for which of the following conditions?

      a)   Obesity
      b)   Car accidents
      c)   Oral health problems and dentures
      d)   Cataracts

14. Polypharmacy is very common among older adults. The most common reason for older adults to take medication is

      a)   Constipation
      b)   Urinary incontinence
      c)   Eczema
      d)   Hypertension

15. Hypogeusia is a common complaint seen in older adults on review of systems. Hypogeusia can be defined as

      a)   Inability to swallow
      b)   Food lacks taste
      c)   Poor night vision
      d)   Hearing loss

Chapter 7: Cardiovascular Disease

1. In Column A is a list of nutrients from the National Cholesterol Education Program (NCEP) Therapeutic Lifestyle Changes (TLC) diet recommended as therapy to lower serum cholesterol. Match the nutrients in Column A with the appropriate recommendation in Column B, assuming a 2000-calorie diet. Answers in Column B may be used more than once.

Column A	Column B
Total fat _____	(a) 50%–60% of total calories
Saturated fat _____	(b) Less than 200 mg per day
Cholesterol _____	(c) 25%–35% of total calories
Carbohydrates _____	(d) Less than 7% of total calories
Monounsaturated fat _____	(e) Up to 20% of total calories

2. Which of the following metabolic diseases can cause a secondary hyperlipidemia?

      a)   Diabetes mellitus

b) Obesity
c) Hypothyroidism
d) All of the above

3. Recent evidence suggests that trans-fatty acids raise low-density lipoprotein (LDL) cholesterol levels when compared to unsaturated fatty acids. Which statement is true concerning trans-fatty acids?

a) Trans-fats are found in partially hydrogenated margarines and shortenings
b) Trans-fats add shelf life and flavor to foods
c) Trans-fats may increase an individual's risk of heart disease
d) All of the above

4. Pharmacologic doses of which of the following vitamins are used to treat elevated cholesterol levels?

a) Vitamin E
b) Thiamine
c) Niacin
d) Folate

5. Which dietary factor is most responsible for raising serum cholesterol levels?

a) Unsaturated fat
b) Saturated fat
c) Protein
d) Simple sugar

6. Which of the following foods contains the highest amount of monounsaturated fat?

a) Whole grains
b) Soybeans
c) Dairy products
d) Avocados

7. Omega-3 fatty acids are used as adjunctive therapy in the management of patients with atherosclerotic vascular disease. In which of the following way(s) does omega-3 fatty acid act to reduce cardiovascular risk?

a) To decrease platelet aggregation
b) To increase clotting times
c) To decrease triglyceride levels
d) All of the above

8. RJ is a 24-year-old man who came to see his primary care physician because his cholesterol level was elevated when he was screened at a student health fair. A lipid profile was done, and his LDL cholesterol was found to be 145 mg/dL and high-density lipoprotein (HDL) 30 mg/dL. His social history is significant for tobacco (six pack year history), and he does not follow any special diet. Assuming that he does not have any other medical problems or a family history of heart disease, what is his target LDL level according to the NCEP Adult Treatment Panel (ATP) III guidelines?

a) 100 mg/dL
b) 130 mg/dL
c) 160 mg/dL
d) 190 mg/dL

9. Which of the following diseases may contribute to the development of hypertension?
    a) Hepatic steatosis
    b) Acute pancreatitis
    c) Obesity
    d) None of the above

10. Hyperhomocysteinemia is an independent risk factor for cardiovascular disease. What vitamin or mineral would be effective in preventing or treating hyperhomo-cysteinemia, or both, in patients with hyperlipidemia?
    a) Niacin
    b) Vitamin E
    c) Folic acid
    d) Magnesium

11. Alcohol consumption has been shown to have both positive and negative effects on the heart. Which of the following statements is correct regarding excessive alcohol consumption (>2 drinks per day for men; >1 drink per day for women)?
    a) Excess alcohol is cardioprotective.
    b) Excess alcohol reduces the risk of cardiomyopathy.
    c) Excess alcohol reduces triglyceride levels.
    d) Excess alcohol increases blood pressure.

12. The Joint National Committee on Prevention, Detection, Evaluation, and Treatment of Blood Pressure (JNC VI) recommends limiting sodium intake to 2400 mg per day for patients with hypertension. Which of the following foods would be considered low sodium?
    a) Canned tuna
    b) Turkey salami
    c) Fresh turkey breast
    d) Potato chips

13. The Dietary Approaches to Stop Hypertension (DASH) sodium diet has been clinically shown to reduce blood pressure levels in moderately hypertensive patients. Which of the following medical nutrition therapies are recommended to reduce hypertension?
    a) Reduce dietary sodium intake
    b) Increase dietary potassium and calcium intake
    c) Moderate alcohol intake
    d) All of the above

14. Heart failure affects approximately 5 million adults in the United States. Medical nutrition therapy for patients with heart failure should be aimed at controlling which of the following?
    a) Controlling sodium and fluid retention
    b) Providing adequate energy, vitamins, and minerals
    c) Repleting protein stores
    d) All of the above

15. Listed below are data from four different patients. Which patient has metabolic syndrome according to NCEP Guidelines?
    a) A hypertensive, nonsmoking male with HDL: 28 mg/dL, triglycerides: 120 mg/dL, fasting glucose: 90 mg/dL, and waist circumference: 35 in.

b) A normotensive, smoking female with an HDL: 40 mg/dL, triglyceride: 100 mg/dL, fasting glucose: 95 mg/dL, and waist circumference: 32 in.

c) A normotensive, smoking female with an HDL: 35 mg/dL, triglyceride: 155 mg/dL, fasting glucose: 90 mg/dL, and waist circumference: 36 in.

d) A hypertensive, nonsmoking male with HDL: 50 mg/dL, triglycerides: 160 mg/dL, fasting glucose: 100 mg/dL, and waist circumference: 35 in.

Chapter 8: Gastrointestinal Disease

1. ST is a 27-year-old man admitted to the hospital with severe Crohn's disease and an unintentional weight loss of 20 lb (9 kg) over the past 2 months despite a good appetite. Assuming that ST has steatorrhea, what is the most likely cause of his weight loss?

   a) Obstruction
   b) Malabsorption
   c) Cancer
   d) Acquired immunodeficiency syndrome (AIDS)

2. Which of the following vitamins is involved as a cofactor for the enzyme necessary for the conversion of pyruvate to acetyl coenzyme A (CoA)?

   a) Thiamine
   b) Vitamin C
   c) Vitamin D
   d) Niacin

3. Medical nutrition therapy for patients with peptic ulcer disease includes which of the following?

   a) Reducing alcohol
   b) Reducing tobacco
   c) Reducing caffeine
   d) All of the above

4. RF, a 62-year-old woman hospitalized with gastric cancer, undergoes gastric surgery (subtotal gastrectomy with gastrojejunostomy). Postoperatively, she complains of diarrhea, cramping, flushing after eating, dizziness, diaphoresis, and early satiety. What is the most likely diagnosis?

   a) Gastritis
   b) Gastroparesis
   c) Dumping syndrome
   d) Lactose intolerance

5. RP, a 75-year-old man, presents to the Veterans Administration Medical Center with significant peripheral neuropathy. His past medical history is significant for a total gastrectomy performed when he was in his forties, after which he was never placed on vitamin supplements. He rarely drinks alcohol. RP's neuropathy is most likely secondary to malabsorption of which of the following vitamins?

   a) Folate
   b) Vitamin A
   c) Pyridoxine (vitamin B_6)
   d) Vitamin B_{12}

6. PR, a 50-year-old woman with chronic pancreatitis, is hospitalized for surgical evaluation. Assuming that PR takes pancreatic enzymes and can tolerate food, what diet order should be prescribed at this time? (only 1 answer)
   a) Low-sodium diet
   b) Low-protein diet
   c) Low-fat diet
   d) Low-fiber diet

7. TI is a 65-year-old man with chronic liver disease and ascites. What dietary recommendation is appropriate for this patient?
   a) Low-sodium diet
   b) High-protein diet
   c) Low-fat diet
   d) Low-fiber diet

8. FG, a 31-year-old, moderately obese woman, complains of gastroesophageal reflux that occurs most often when she is sleeping. Which of the following recommendations may help alleviate these symptoms?
   a) Increasing caffeine intake
   b) Sleeping without a pillow at night
   c) Waiting at least 2 hours after eating to lie down
   d) Increasing consumption of fatty foods

9. TY, a 45-year-old alcoholic, presents to the emergency room (ER) with pain in his stomach. Laboratory tests reveal the following results:

Patient's Value	Normal Value
Hemoglobin: 10 mg/dL	14–16 mg/dL
Mean corpuscular volume: 104 μm^3	84–95 μm^3
Red blood cell folate: 80 ng/mL	280–903 ng/mL

   Using the information below, what type of anemia should be suspected in this patient?
   a) Iron-deficiency anemia
   b) Macrocytic anemia
   c) Hemolytic anemia
   d) Sickle cell anemia

10. Based on your answer to the question above, what is the most likely cause of the anemia seen in this patient?
    a) Iron deficiency
    b) Folate deficiency
    c) Vitamin B_{12} deficiency
    d) Vitamin C deficiency

11. Which of the following enzymes is required for the breakdown of food starches to disaccharides?
    a) Lipase
    b) Maltase
    c) Amylase
    d) Pepsin

12. Which of the following foods would be considered a good source of insoluble fiber?
    a) White bread
    b) Mashed potato
    c) Raisin bran
    d) Watermelon

13. Individuals with celiac disease are advised to avoid all foods containing rye, wheat, and barley because they are especially sensitive to which of the following proteins?
    a) Albumin
    b) Gluten
    c) Soy protein
    d) Casein

14. In one-half of 60- to 80-year-olds and nearly 100% of those over 80, which of the following gastrointestinal disorders develop?
    a) Diverticulosis
    b) Diarrhea
    c) Diverticulitis
    d) Colon-rectal cancer

15. Why do individuals with chronic liver disease have an elevated prothrombin time (PT)?
    a) They are vitamin B_{12} deficient.
    b) They are malabsorbing fat.
    c) Their liver's ability to produce clotting factors is diminished.
    d) They have lost weight.

Chapter 9: Endocrine Disease: Diabetes Mellitus

1. TR is a 60-year-old woman with type 2 diabetes mellitus [height = 5′3″ (1.58 cm), weight = 155 lb (70 kg), body mass index (BMI) = 27.5 kg/m²]. TR questions her doctor about the benefits of exercise. Which statement is correct concerning the benefits of exercise for individuals with type 2 diabetes mellitus?
    a) Exercise improves blood glucose levels by decreasing insulin sensitivity.
    b) Exercise improves blood glucose levels by increasing peripheral glucose uptake.
    c) Exercise may increase serum low-density lipoprotein (LDL) levels.
    d) Exercise causes ketone body production.

2. Patients with type 1 diabetes mellitus who drink alcohol are at increased risk of hypoglycemia. Which statement is correct concerning alcohol consumption in individuals with type 1 diabetes mellitus?
    a) Alcohol requires insulin to be metabolized.
    b) Alcohol should be consumed without food to prevent hyperglycemia.
    c) Alcohol is metabolized similarly to carbohydrates.
    d) Alcohol inhibits gluconeogenesis in the liver.

3. Patients with diabetes mellitus are at increased risk for which of the following diseases?
    a) Liver disease
    b) Cancer

      c)   Cardiovascular disease
      d)   Pulmonary disease

4. The United Kingdom Prospective Diabetes Study has demonstrated that diabetes mellitus is a progressive disease. How has medical nutrition therapy for diabetes mellitus changed over recent years based on this concept?

      a)   Medical nutrition therapy is aimed at an "ideal" nutrition prescription for all patients with diabetes mellitus.
      b)   Medical nutrition therapy is aimed at the achievement of blood glucose and lipid goals.
      c)   Medical nutrition therapy is aimed at reducing the source of carbohydrate in the diet, namely simple sugars, rather than the total daily intake.
      d)   All of the above

5. What is the target range for the premeal plasma glucose values for nonpregnant adults with diabetes mellitus?

      a)   90–130 mg/dL
      b)   100–140 mg/dL
      c)   150–180 mg/dL
      d)   180–200 mg/dL

6. Results of the Diabetes Control and Complications Trial (DCCT) concluded that intensive therapy delays the onset and slows the progression of diabetic retinopathy, nephropathy, and neuropathy in patients with diabetes mellitus. Which of the following was a major adverse effect of this intensive therapy (4 insulin shots per day)?

      a)   Weight loss
      b)   Hypertension
      c)   Polyuria
      d)   Hypoglycemia

7. What is considered an optimal hemoglobin (Hgb) A1C (HgbA1C) for patients with diabetes mellitus?

      a)   HgbA1C less than 7%
      b)   HgbA1C less than 8%
      c)   HgbA1C less than 9%
      d)   None of the above

8. SK, a 68-year-old man of Italian descent with a 5-year history of type 2 diabetes, is presently being treated by diet alone. He is 5'7" (170 cm) tall and weighs 180 lb (81.6 kg). His BMI is 28 kg/m^2. Current laboratory data reveal a fasting blood glucose of 183 mg/dL. SK loves olive oil and asks the doctor whether he may use it as much as he wants because it is high in monounsaturated fats. Considering his current status, which of the following responses is the best?

      a)   Olive oil may be consumed in unlimited amounts since it is cardioprotective.
      b)   Olive oil should be limited because it is calorically dense and may lead to weight gain.
      c)   Olive oil should be avoided because SK has diabetes.
      d)   None of the responses is correct.

9. In the absence of insulin, excessive fatty acids are released and ketone bodies are produced by the liver from acetyl coenzyme A (CoA). This occurs in starvation and uncontrolled diabetes mellitus. Which of the following are examples of ketone bodies?
   a) Acetaldehyde
   b) Pyruvic acid
   c) Beta-hydroxybutyric acid
   d) Lactic acid

10. One serving of carbohydrate (80 calories) is equivalent to how many grams of carbohydrate?
    a) 5 g
    b) 10 g
    c) 15 g
    d) 20 g

11. The Diabetes Prevention Program, a national study comparing lifestyle to medication, demonstrated that lifestyle changes can have a significant impact on delaying or preventing the onset of type 2 diabetes. In this study how much weight loss was associated with improvement in glycemic control in patients with type 2 diabetes mellitus?
    a) Less than 3% weight loss
    b) 5% to 7% weight loss
    c) 10% to 15% weight loss
    d) 20% weight loss

12. Individuals who are at increased risk for insulin resistance include which of the following?
    a) Patients with a history of hypercholesterolemia
    b) Patients with a "pear-shaped" body
    c) Patients with a first-degree relative with type 2 diabetes
    d) Patients with a first-degree relative with hypertension

13. Which of the following best describes how patients with type 1 diabetes can prevent the onset of diabetic ketoacidosis (DKA)?
    a) Continue taking insulin injections when sick
    b) Avoid hypoglycemia
    c) Avoid alcohol
    d) Increase dietary fat intake

14. GR is a 26-year-old man with type 1 diabetes mellitus. He is presently on an intensive insulin regimen to achieve tight glycemic control. Over the past 6 months, GR has gained 10 lb and seeks nutrition counseling. Which of the following situations would likely have contributed to GR's recent weight gain?
    a) Increased physical activity
    b) Inadequate insulin therapy
    c) More frequent hypoglycemic episodes
    d) Decreased carbohydrate intake

15. Individuals with poorly controlled type 1 diabetes mellitus, evidenced by blood glucose levels greater than 250 mg/dL and urinary ketones, can have a negative response to exercise. This is because in the presence of insulin deficiency which of the following occurs?

a) Hepatic glucose output is decreased, and peripheral use of glucose is decreased.

b) Hepatic glucose output is increased, and peripheral use of glucose is decreased.

c) Hepatic glucose output is increased, and peripheral use of glucose is increased.

d) Hepatic glucose output is decreased, and peripheral use of glucose is increased.

Chapter 10: Pulmonary Disease

1. Respiratory quotient (RQ) is the ratio of carbon dioxide (CO_2) produced to oxygen consumed. Which of the following macronutrients tends to produce more CO_2 per oxygen consumed?

   a) Fat
   b) Carbohydrate
   c) Protein
   d) All macronutrients produce equivalent amounts of CO_2

2. RL is a 12-year-old girl with cystic fibrosis. She has had multiple infections and is receiving antibiotics. For which of the following vitamin deficiencies is RL at risk due to chronic antibiotic therapy?

   a) Vitamin K
   b) Vitamin A
   c) Vitamin B_{12}
   d) Thiamine

3. Why is osteopenia increasingly prevalent in patients with cystic fibrosis?

   a) High calcium intake
   b) Impaired lung function
   c) Increased physical activity
   d) Chronic steroid therapy

4. BC is a 63-year-old man admitted to the hospital with severe respiratory disease. Over the past 2 months, he has lost 10% of his usual body weight and has become more debilitated. What is the most likely cause of weight loss in this patient?

   a) Increased metabolism due to work of breathing
   b) Malabsorption
   c) Cigarette smoking
   d) Increased CO_2 retention

5. How does poor nutritional status compromise pulmonary function?

   a) Decreases muscle strength
   b) Impairs cellular resistance to infection
   c) Diminishes lung function
   d) All of the above

6. Which of the following are potential side effects of medications used to treat chronic obstructive pulmonary disease (COPD)?

   a) Gastric irritation
   b) Nausea and vomiting

      c) Dysgeusia and dry mouth
      d) All of the above

7. TL, a 9-year-old boy with cystic fibrosis, is brought to his pediatrician reporting weakness and lethargy. His mother reports increased stool output, a recent weight loss of 8 lb, and an abnormal prothrombin time (PT). Based on the chief symptom, the physical examination, and the laboratory information, what is the most likely cause of this patient's weight loss?

      a) Anemia
      b) Heart failure
      c) Malabsorption
      d) Liver disease

8. Medical nutrition therapy for patients with obstructive sleep apnea syndrome (OSAS) should focus on which of the following?

      a) Weight reduction
      b) Protein repletion
      c) Vitamin and mineral deficiencies
      d) Fluid repletion

9. TR undergoes a successful lung transplant and is prescribed cyclosporine when discharged from the hospital. Which of the following side effects of cyclosporine therapy commonly occurs that may require nutritional intervention?

      a) Hypokalemia
      b) Hyperglycemia
      c) Hyperlipidemia
      d) Hypomagnesemia

10. Long-term prednisone treatment is often used after lung transplantation. Which of the following is a common complication of prednisone therapy that may require nutritional intervention?

      a) Hyperglycemia
      b) Anorexia that may lead to weight loss
      c) Hypoglycemia
      d) Hyponatremia

11. What is the primary reason why patients with cystic fibrosis require extra dietary sodium?

      a) To reduce their blood pressure
      b) To replace losses from increased sputum production
      c) To replace losses in perspiration
      d) To prevent osteoporosis

12. GF is a 48-year-old man who underwent a lung transplant 5 months ago. He is 5'7" and weighs 190 lb. He is currently taking prednisone (steroid) and cyclosporine (antirejection medication). What factor(s) may have contributed to the weight gain in this patient?

      a) Increased appetite secondary to steroid use
      b) Increased dietary sodium intake
      c) Increased metabolic rate following surgery
      d) Increased potassium intake

13. AR is an 8-year-old girl recently diagnosed with cystic fibrosis who is brought to her pediatrician complaining of weakness and lethargy. She presents with a recent weight loss of 7 lb. Which of the following dietary recommendations would be appropriate to improve AR's nutritional status?

    a) Extra salt
    b) High calorie, high protein
    c) Addition of vitamin and mineral supplements
    d) All of the above

14. Individuals with COPD have increased work of breathing and may therefore be hypermetabolic. Breathing may cause how much of an increase in their energy expenditure?

    a) Twofold increase
    b) Fivefold increase
    c) Tenfold increase
    d) Twentyfold increase

15. A patient who is receiving mechanical ventilation for more than 7 days, whose gastrointestinal (GI) tract is functioning normally, should be fed in which of the following ways?

    a) Peripheral parenteral nutrition support.
    b) Enteral nutrition support via a nasogastric tube.
    c) Parenteral nutrition via a central line.
    d) It is not necessary to feed patients receiving respiratory support.

Chapter 11: Renal Disease

1. Protein is restricted in the diet for an individual with chronic renal failure (CRF) before dialysis is initiated for which of the following reasons?

    a) To preserve lean body mass
    b) To prevent weight loss
    c) To minimize the symptoms of uremia
    d) All of the above

2. The goal of medical nutrition therapy for patients with nephrolithiasis (kidney stones) is to eliminate the diet-related risk factors for stone formation. Which of the following recommendations is most critical for patients with a history of kidney stones?

    a) Increasing fluid intake
    b) Increasing oxalate intake
    c) Decreasing calcium intake
    d) Decreasing magnesium intake

3. Hyperlipidemia frequently occurs after renal transplantation. Which of the following factors is the most likely cause?

    a) Immunosuppressive therapy
    b) Antihypertensive therapy
    c) Weight gain
    d) All of the above

4. KJ is a 52-year-old man who is admitted to the hospital with chronic renal failure secondary to diabetic nephropathy. He complains of fatigue and weakness, and

his blood pressure is elevated. Laboratory values indicate a serum potassium of 4.0 mEq/L. Which of the following diets is most appropriate for KJ at this time?

    a)   2 to 3 g sodium
    b)   No concentrated sweets
    c)   2 to 3 g potassium
    d)   All of the above

5. KJ may be at risk for development of hyperkalemia before the onset of end-stage renal disease due to which of the following medications or other therapies, or both, that he is taking to control his high blood pressure?

    a)   Dietary salt substitutes
    b)   Angiotensin-converting enzyme inhibitors
    c)   Potassium-sparing diuretics
    d)   All of the above

6. KJ has a 24-hour urinary sodium excretion of 200 mEq. How many milligrams of sodium is KJ consuming? (Molecular weight of sodium = 23 mg.)

    a)   9200 mg
    b)   4600 mg
    c)   2300 mg
    d)   1300 mg

7. GN is a 46-year-old woman receiving hemodialysis (HD). She is 5'3" (160 cm) and weighs 110 lb (50 kg). Considering that GN is receiving HD three times per week, how much protein should she be consuming daily?

    a)   Less than 50 g protein per day
    b)   55–70 g protein per day
    c)   75–90 g protein per day
    d)   More than 90 g protein per day

8. The kidney plays an essential role in the metabolism of which of the following vitamins?

    a)   Vitamin A
    b)   Vitamin B_{12}
    c)   Vitamin B_6
    d)   Vitamin D

9. PF is a 50-year-old woman with nephrotic syndrome. Her lipid levels are significantly elevated. Which of the following mechanisms below explains the elevated lipid levels in patients with nephrotic syndrome?

    a)   Defect in the low-density lipoprotein (LDL) receptor, resulting in increased LDL levels
    b)   Increased lipoprotein clearance from the blood by lipoprotein lipase
    c)   Decreased hepatic protein synthesis
    d)   Decreased lipoprotein clearance from the blood by lipoprotein lipase

10. The anemia of chronic renal failure is characteristically normochromic and normo-cytic. It is due mainly to which of the following mechanisms?

    a)   Decreased erythropoietin production
    b)   Blood loss due to dialysis procedure
    c)   Vitamin B_{12} deficiency
    d)   Folate deficiency

11. CV is a 45-year-old man who has recently undergone a renal transplant. He has been prescribed a steroid and immunosuppressive medication to prevent tissue rejection. Which of the following dietary therapies may be recommended once the renal allograft is functioning (2 best answers)?
    a) Calcium supplementation
    b) Phosphate restriction
    c) Sodium restriction
    d) All of the above

12. Medical nutrition therapy for patients with calcium oxalate stones includes which of the following recommendations?
    a) Low-calcium diet (<500 mg per day)
    b) Low-sodium diet (<1500 mg per day)
    c) Low-oxalate diet
    d) Low-fiber diet

13. Many commercial foods are higher in sodium than consumers would expect. Which of the following foods have a high sodium content (>400 mg per serving)?
    a) Tomato juice
    b) Ham
    c) Soy sauce
    d) All of the above

14. SP is a 50-year-old man with CRF. SP's glomerular filtration rate (GRF) has begun to fall below 50 mL per minute. Phosphorus is not being excreted normally, and its intake must be restricted. Medical nutrition therapy was suggested to improve his condition. Which of the following foods contains the highest amount of phosphorus?
    a) Yogurt
    b) Apples
    c) Bacon
    d) Waffles

15. MR is a 30-year-old man who has been diagnosed with acute poststreptococcal glomerulonephritis. He presents with a blood pressure of 210/124 mm Hg, significant weight loss, and peripheral edema. His laboratory results include calcium, 6.9 mg/dL; phosphate, 8.5 mg/dL; albumin, 3.1 g/dL; and hemoglobin, 8.3 g/dL. Based on the given information, which of the following nutritional recommendations would you suggest?
    a) Increase milk intake to improve calcium intake.
    b) Decrease the amount of sugar and polyunsaturated fat.
    c) Decrease protein intake.
    d) Add more high-phosphate foods.

Chapter 12: Enteral Nutrition Support

1. DE, a 76-year-old woman, is being treated for severe depression and anorexia. A nasogastric tube is placed for nutrition support. One reason the nasogastric tube was chosen over other routes of intestinal access in this patient is that
    a) Long-term tube feeding is expected.
    b) Risk of aspiration is high.

c) The stomach is emptying normally.
d) Short bowel syndrome was present.

2. In which of the following conditions is enteral nutrition contraindicated for a patient with chronic inflammatory bowel disease?
   a) Presence of a high-output, enterocutaneous fistula
   b) Severe anorexia
   c) Small bowel that is less than 100% functional
   d) Absent gag reflex

3. ES, a 76-year-old woman, recently had a mild stroke that left her unable to swallow without aspirating. She is currently malnourished, with a body mass index (BMI) of 16 kg/m². What type of access should be placed for feeding?
   a) Nasogastric tube
   b) Peripherally inserted catheter (PIC) line for peripheral parenteral nutrition (PPN)
   c) Nasojejunal tube
   d) Subclavian catheter for total parenteral nutrition (TPN)

4. JL, a 35-year-old man with acquired immunodeficiency syndrome (AIDS), is hospitalized for pulmonary disease. Because his appetite has declined drastically, a nasogastric tube is placed to provide nutrition support. Which formula is most appropriate for this patient?
   a) Calorically dense
   b) Fiber containing
   c) Half strength
   d) Low fat

5. A 68-year-old woman was admitted to the hospital with dehydration and weight loss due to severe depression. She refuses to eat and has a very low oral intake for the past 8 days. What type of nutrition support should be considered?
   a) Peripheral parenteral nutrition
   b) Tube feeding via a surgically placed jejunostomy
   c) TPN
   d) Tube feeding via nasogastric tube

6. Some tube-feeding formulas are classified by the disease that they are designed to treat. Match the formula types in Column A with the specific characteristic it has in Column B. Answers in Column B can only be used once.

Column A	Column B
Glucose intolerance _____	(a) Reduced protein, water, electrolytes, and minerals
Hepatic disease _____	(b) High fat, fiber, low carbohydrate
Renal disease _____	(c) High fat, n-3 fatty acids, and antioxidants
Pulmonary disease _____	(d) Increased branch chain amino acids and reduced aromatic amino acids
Immunomodulating _____	(e) Added glutamine, arginine, or ribonucleic acid (RNA)

7. A 51-year-old man is 48 hours past partial laryngectomy. He is unable to swallow due to the inflammation around the surgical incision. His past medical history includes tobacco and alcohol abuse. He has a functioning gastrointestinal tract. What type of tube-feeding formula is most appropriate?

    a) Pulmonary
    b) Polymeric
    c) Elemental
    d) Hepatic

8. A 26-year-old man is status post a motor vehicle accident, with fractured ribs and a closed-head injury. Respiratory failure has developed, and he is now ventilator dependent. He is lying flat on a rocking bed. He has active bowel sounds and a nasogastric tube for gastric decompression. What two types of enteral access are initially appropriate?

    a) Surgically placed jejunostomy
    b) Percutaneous endoscopic gastrostomy tube
    c) Postpyloric nasoenteric tube
    d) Percutaneous endoscopic jejunostomy tube

9. A 56-year-old man is status postesophagogastrectomy for esophageal cancer. A jejunostomy feeding tube was placed in the operating room. He has been tolerating a continuous feeding regimen and is now preparing for discharge. What type of feeding schedule is appropriate for this patient?

    a) Intermittent gravity
    b) 24-hour continuous
    c) Daytime cycle
    d) Night cycle

10. A 40-year-old man with multiple sclerosis has been stable on home tube feeding. He is administering the feeding intermittently. Recently, he was started on antibiotics for cellulitis. For the last 3 days, he is complaining of frequent, watery stools. What is the appropriate recommendation at this time?

    a) Stop tube feeding
    b) Switch to a nutrient-dense formula
    c) Evaluate stool cultures
    d) Begin strong antidiarrheal medications

11. An 80-year-old man with dysphagia due to a recent stroke was initiated on a standard polymeric tube-feeding formula. He has a history of coronary artery disease and congestive heart failure. Since initiation of the tube feeding, ankle edema has developed. What changes in the tube feeding should be recommended at this time?

    a) Switch to a continuous administration
    b) Switch to a pulmonary formula
    c) Switch to a nutrient-dense formula
    d) Hold tube feeding

12. Which of the following formula components is most useful for individuals with Crohn's disease?

    a) Water-soluble fiber
    b) Hydrolyzed proteins
    c) Restricted potassium, phosphorus, and magnesium
    d) Arginine

13. CT is a 60-year-old woman who has been diagnosed with esophageal cancer. The patient has had a significant weight loss secondary to her difficulty in swallowing. Which of the following is the best indication for initiating enteral nutrition support?
    a) She claims to have a strong appetite but just cannot swallow well.
    b) She has a BMI of 22 kg/m².
    c) She has a well-nourished appearance.
    d) She has an albumin level of 3.7 g/dL.

14. EC is a 59-year-old man who has been recently diagnosed with esophageal cancer and more recently with odynophagia. He is referred to a nutritionist in an attempt to improve his nutritional status. Which of the following suggestions is the most appropriate?
    a) All foods are acceptable for this patient
    b) Increase carbohydrates daily
    c) Drink liquid nutritional supplements to increase protein and calorie intake
    d) Increase fruit and vegetable intake

15. Assuming that the gut works, which of the following statements best explains the benefit of using enteral compared to parenteral nutrition support?
    a) Enteral nutrition better maintains bowel integrity compared to parenteral nutrition.
    b) Enteral nutrition is less expensive in product, administration, and monitoring compared to parenteral nutrition.
    c) Critically ill patients receiving enteral nutrition have a decreased length of stay in the hospital compared to patients receiving parenteral nutrition.
    d) All of the above.

Chapter 13: Parenteral Nutrition Support

1. Central parenteral nutrition is indicated for patients who require long-term nutrition support for greater than which number of days?
    a) 2 days
    b) 4 days
    c) 7 days
    d) 10 days

2. Patients with persistent hyperglycemia or hypercapnia may require which of the following specialized solutions?
    a) Reduced carbohydrate, increased lipids
    b) Reduced protein, increased carbohydrate
    c) Reduced lipids, increased protein
    d) Reduced fiber, increased lipids

3. Peripheral parenteral nutrition (PPN) is used for patients who require short-term nutrition support. Which of the following factors is necessary for patients to receive PPN?
    a) Adequate bowel function
    b) Adequate peripheral venous access
    c) Adequate dietary intake
    d) Adequate cardiac function

4. MB, a 52-year-old woman, underwent an uncomplicated cholecystectomy 24 hours ago. Her abdominal examination reveals distention, and no bowel sounds are audible. This patient was well nourished before admission. What type of nutrition support should she receive?

    a) PPN
    b) Nasogastric feedings
    c) Total parenteral nutrition (TPN)
    d) No nutrition support but re-evaluate on a daily basis

5. TPN may be indicated in which of the following conditions?

    a) Colon cancer
    b) Hyperemesis gravidarum
    c) Congestive heart failure
    d) Multiple sclerosis

6. Which of the following is the maximum rate of continuous glucose (dextrose) infusion for parenteral nutrition solutions?

    a) 1 mg/kg per minute
    b) 3 mg/kg per minute
    c) 5 mg/kg per minute
    d) 10 mg/kg per minute

7. Which of the following electrolytes or minerals cannot be added to TPN solutions due to instability?

    a) Calcium
    b) Magnesium
    c) Bicarbonate
    d) Potassium

8. Treatment of hyponatremia may include which of the following?

    a) Increased sodium concentration in TPN
    b) Fluid restriction
    c) Non-TPN intravenous replacement of losses
    d) All of the above

9. Infusion of hypertonic solutions through a peripheral vein may result in which of the following?

    a) Edema
    b) Phlebitis
    c) Aspiration
    d) Varicose veins

10. Which of the following are potential complications of TPN?

    a) Infection/sepsis
    b) Rhabdomyolysis
    c) Alopecia
    d) Gynecomastia

11. Linoleic acid and alpha-linolenic acid are added to parenteral nutrition solutions to prevent which of the following conditions?

    a) Keratomalacia
    b) Essential fatty acid deficiency

      c)   Hypotension

      d)   Bradycardia

12.   Patients who are at risk of fluid overload, such as those with renal disease, liver failure, or congestive heart failure, may need which of the following types of solutions?

      a)   Excess carbohydrate solution

      b)   Excess sodium and potassium solution

      c)   Concentrated solution

      d)   Reduced amino acid solution

13.   Which of the following statements explains why is it important to monitor calcium and phosphorus additives in a parenteral nutrition formula?

      a)   Calcium and phosphorus may not be absorbed.

      b)   Calcium and phosphorus may form a precipitate.

      c)   Too much calcium could delay wound healing.

      d)   Too much phosphorus could lead to refeeding syndrome.

14.   Which of the following mechanical complications may occur in patients receiving parenteral nutrition via a central vein?

      a)   Pneumothorax

      b)   Congestive heart failure

      c)   Tachycardia

      d)   Aspiration

15.   When estimating a patient's daily fluid requirements, which of the following is usually included in the calculation?

      a)   Urine output

      b)   Gastrointestinal (GI) losses

      c)   Insensible losses from skin and the GI tract

      d)   All of the above

Review Answers

Chapter 1: Overview of Nutrition in Clinical Care

1. d
2. b
3. d
4. a, b, a, a
5. a
6. c
7. b
8. a
9. c
10. e, e, c, c, a, a, d, d, d, d, c, e
11. b
12. c
13. c
14. a
15. c

Chapter 2: Vitamins, Minerals, and Phytochemicals

1. c, d, e, f, a, b
2. c, b, a, d, e
3. c, d, a, b, e
4. a
5. b
6. c
7. b
8. d
9. c
10. a, e, d, c, b
11. c
12. b
13. a
14. a
15. d

Chapter 3: Herbal Medicine

1. d
2. b
3. a
4. b
5. d, b, a, e, c
6. d
7. b
8. d
9. c, d, a, e, b
10. c
11. d
12. b
13. c
14. d
15. a

Chapter 4: Nutrition in Pregnancy and Lactation

1. b
2. b
3. a
4. d
5. c
6. d
7. c
8. a
9. c
10. c
11. d
12. b
13. d
14. a
15. c

Chapter 5: Infants, Children, and Adolescents

1. b
2. d
3. a
4. d
5. a
6. b
7. b
8. d
9. b
10. a
11. a
12. d
13. a, d
14. c
15. a

Chapter 6: Older Adults

1. b
2. c
3. c
4. a
5. c
6. c
7. c
8. d
9. d
10. c
11. b
12. a
13. c
14. d
15. b

Chapter 7: Cardiovascular Disease

1. c, d, b, a, e
2. d
3. d
4. c
5. b
6. d
7. d
8. c
9. b
10. c
11. d
12. d
13. c
14. d
15. c

Chapter 8: Gastrointestinal Disease

1. b
2. a
3. d
4. c
5. d
6. c
7. a
8. c
9. b
10. b
11. c
12. c
13. b
14. a
15. c

Chapter 9: Endocrine Disease: Diabetes Mellitus

1. b
2. d
3. c
4. b
5. a

6. d
7. a
8. b
9. c
10. c
11. b
12. c
13. a
14. c
15. b

Chapter 10: Pulmonary Disease

1. b
2. a
3. d
4. a
5. d
6. d
7. c
8. a
9. c
10. a
11. c
12. a
13. d
14. c
15. b

Chapter 11: Renal Disease

1. c
2. a
3. a
4. d
5. d
6. b
7. b
8. d
9. d
10. a
11. a, c

12. c
13. d
14. a
15. c

Chapter 12: Enteral Nutrition Support

1. c
2. a
3. c
4. d
5. d
6. b, d, a, c, e
7. b
8. a
9. d
10. c
11. c
12. b
13. a
14. c
15. d

Chapter 13: Parenteral Nutrition Support

1. c
2. a
3. b
4. d
5. b
6. c
7. c
8. d
9. b
10. a
11. b
12. c
13. b
14. a
15. d

Index

ANSWER SHEET/ENROLLMENT FORM FOR DIETITIANS AND DIETETIC TECHNICIANS

Continuing Professional Education: Level III Self-Study Learning Activity for 35 ADA Credits

MEDICAL NUTRITION & DISEASE, 3rd edition
Edited by Lisa Hark, PhD, RD and Gail Morrison, MD

This self-study learning activity is pre-approved for <u>35 credits</u> by the American Dietetic Association, Commission on Dietetic Registration (www.cdrnet.org). **You may use this book for 35 CPE credits even if you have completed Medical Nutrition & Disease 1st or 2nd edition.**

Follow the instructions below.

1.   Read *Medical Nutrition & Disease*, 3rd edition, and complete the test questions in the back of the book after completing each chapter (pp. A-7 to A-39). Write the correct answers on the dietitian answer sheet (next page).

2.   Grade yourself using the answers in *Medical Nutrition & Disease*, 3rd edition (pp. A-40 to A-42). Successful completion of this independent learning activity requires that you attain at least 80% correct. If you do not attain this score, retest yourself again and indicate the corrected score on the form. Please note, credits are awarded for completion of the entire book only, not for individual chapters.

3.   If you are participating in the ADA Professional Development Portfolio, **you do not need to submit this form to ADA.** Complete the Certificate of Completion and keep a copy.

4.   If you are not a Portfolio participant yet, please complete the information below and the answer sheet on the next page and return this form to:
     American Dietetic Association
     Commission on Dietetic Registration (CDR)
     120 South Riverside Plaza Suite 2000
     Chicago, IL. 60606-6995
     312-899-0040 Ext 5500 • Fax: 312-899-4772

THERE ARE NO ADDITIONAL CHARGES FROM ADA TO PROCESS THIS FORM. MORE THAN ONE DIETITIAN MAY READ THE BOOK AND COPY THIS FORM AND THE ANSWER SHEET. THIS INDEPENDENT LEARNING ACTIVITY IS VALID UNTIL DECEMBER 31, 2007.

YOU MAY USE THIS BOOK FOR CPE CREDITS EVEN IF YOU HAVE COMPLETED MEDICAL NUTRITION & DISEASE 1st or 2nd EDITION.

Name _____ Credentials _____

ADA Registration # _____ Date completed _____

Address _____

City _____ State _____ Zip _____

Phone # _____ Fax # _____

Email _____

Keep a copy of these forms for your records. ADA requires 6 to 8 weeks for processing. Additional questions to Dr. Lisa Hark, please call 215-349-5795 or email to lhark@mail.med.upenn.edu. For more information, contact our web site at http://www.med.upenn.edu/nutrimed.

Continuing Professional Education Certificate of Completion for Dietitians and Dietetic Technicians

Title of Program: Medical Nutrition and Disease, 3rd Edition
Edited by Lisa Hark, PhD, RD and Gail Morrison, MD

Program Provider's Name: Lisa Hark, PhD, RD (lhark@mail.med.upenn.edu)
Approved for 35 CPE Credits from January 1, 2004 to December 31, 2007
Learning Need: Medical Nutrition Therapy   Code: 5000   CPE Level: 3

ATTENDEE COPY

Participant's Name

Registration Number

Date Completed

Continuing Professional Education Certificate of Completion for Dietitians and Dietetic Technicians

Title of Program: Medical Nutrition and Disease, 3rd Edition
Edited by Lisa Hark, PhD, RD and Gail Morrison, MD

Program Provider's Name: Lisa Hark, PhD, RD (lhark@mail.med.upenn.edu)
Approved for 35 CPE Credits from January 1, 2004 to December 31, 2007
Learning Need: Medical Nutrition Therapy   Code: 5000   CPE Level: 3

STATE LICENSURE COPY

Participant's Name

Registration Number

Date Completed

ANSWER SHEET FOR REGISTERED DIETITIANS

Medical Nutrition & Disease: Chapters 1–13 questions located in Appendix pp. A-7 to A-39.
Fill in the correct answers and grade yourself when finished.
Expiration date: December 31, 2007
Complete the other side. No additional self-reporting form is needed.
More than one dietitian may read the book and copy these forms. There are no fees.
Credits are awarded for completion of the entire book only, not for individual chapters.

Chapter 1	Chapter 2	Chapter 3	Chapter 4
1)	1)_, _, _, _, _, _	1)	1)
2)	2)_, _, _, _, _	2)	2)
3)	3)_, _, _, _, _	3)	3)
4)_, _, _, _	4)	4)	4)
5)	5)	5)_, _, _, _, _	5)
6)	6)	6)	6)
7)	7)	7)	7)
8)	8)	8)	8)
9)	9)	9)_, _, _, _, _	9)
10)_, _, _, _, _, _, _, _	10)_, _, _, _, _	10)	10)
11)	11)	11)	11)
12)	12)	12)	12)
13)	13)	13)	13)
14)	14)	14)	14)
15)	15)	15)	15)

Chapter 5	Chapter 6	Chapter 7	Chapter 8
1)	1)	1)_, _, _, _, _	1)
2)	2)	2)	2)
3)	3)	3)	3)
4)	4)	4)	4)
5)	5)	5)	5)
6)	6)	6)	6)
7)	7)	7)	7)
8)	8)	8)	8)
9)	9)	9)	9)
10)	10)	10)	10)
11)	11)	11)	11)
12)	12)	12)	12)
13)_, _	13)	13)	13)
14)	14)	14)	14)
15)	15)	15)	15)

Chapter 9	Chapter 10	Chapter 11
1)	1)	1)
2)	2)	2)
3)	3)	3)
4)	4)	4)
5)	5)	5)
6)	6)	6)
7)	7)	7)
8)	8)	8)
9)	9)	9)
10)	10)	10)
11)	11)	11)_, _
12)	12)	12)
13)	13)	13)
14)	14)	14)
15)	15)	15)

Chapter 12	Chapter 13
1)	1)
2)	2)
3)	3)
4)	4)
5)	5)
6)_, _, _, _, _	6)
7)	7)
8)	8)
9)	9)
10)	10)
11)	11)
12)	12)
13)	13)
14)	14)
15)	15)

Correct_____/195 × 100 = _____%

Completion of this independent learning activity requires that you attain at least 80% correct (156 correct answers out of 195). If not, retest yourself and indicate the corrected score on the form.
Answers to these questions are located in *Medical Nutrition & Disease, 3rd Ed.* on pages A-40 and A-42.
Questions, please call Lisa Hark, PhD, RD at 215-349-5795, lhark@mail.med.upenn.edu